Rhinosinusitis with Nasal Polyposis

Advances in Oto-Rhino-Laryngology

Vol. 79

Series Editor

Patrick J. Bradley Nottingham

Rhinosinusitis with Nasal Polyposis

Volume Editors

Bradford A. Woodworth Birmingham, Ala.
David M. Poetker Milwaukee, Wis.
Douglas D. Reh Baltimore, Md.

38 figures, 30 in color, and 9 tables, 2016

With a foreword by David W. Kennedy, Philadelphia, Pa.

KARGER

Basel · Freiburg · Paris · London · New York · Chennai · New Delhi · Bangkok · Beijing · Shanghai · Tokyo · Kuala Lumpur · Singapore · Sydney

I dedicate this book to my wife and children whose love and support have provided me a constant source of inspiration.
Bradford A. Woodworth, MD

I dedicate this book to my parents for giving me the foundation I needed, to my wife for her constant love and support, and to my trainees for helping me continue to learn.
David M. Poetker, MD

I would like to dedicate this book to my father, David, who taught me the value of hard work, to my mentors for their training and constant guidance, to my residents and fellows who continue to help me discover and grow, and to my wife for her constant support.
Douglas D. Reh, MD

Bradford A. Woodworth, MD
James J. Hicks Professor of Otolaryngology
Department of Otolaryngology – Head and Neck Surgery
University of Alabama at Birmingham
BDB 563, 1720 2nd Avenue South
Birmingham, AL 35294 (USA)

David M. Poetker, MD
Associate Professor
Zablocki VAMC, Department of Surgery
Department of Otolaryngology and
Communication Medical College of Wisconsin
9200 West Wisconsin Avenue
Milwaukee, WI 53226 (USA)

Douglas D. Reh, MD
Associate Professor
Department of Otolaryngology – Head and Neck Surgery
Johns Hopkins Medicine
601 North Caroline Street, 6th Floor
Baltimore, MD 21287 (USA)

Library of Congress Cataloging-in-Publication Data

Names: Woodworth, Bradford A., editor. | Poetker, David M., editor. | Reh, Douglas D., editor.
Title: Rhinosinusitis with nasal polyposis / volume editors, Bradford A. Woodworth, David M. Poetker, Douglas D. Reh.
Other titles: Advances in oto-rhino-laryngology ; v. 79. 0065-3071
Description: Basel ; New York : Karger, [2016] | Series: Advances in oto-rhino-laryngology, ISSN 0065-3071 ; vol. 79 | Includes bibliographical references and indexes.
Identifiers: LCCN 2016021979| ISBN 9783318058536 (hard cover : alk. paper) | ISBN 9783318058543 (electronic version)
Subjects: | MESH: Rhinitis | Sinusitis | Nasal Polyps
Classification: LCC RF361 | NLM WV 335 | DDC 616.2/05--dc23LC record available at https://lccn.loc.gov/2016021979

www.karger.com
Printed in Germany on acid-free and non-aging paper (ISO 9706) by Kraft Druck GmbH, Ettlingen
ISSN 0065–3071
e-ISSN 1662–2847
ISBN 978–3–318–05853–6
e-ISBN 978–3–318–05854–3

Contents

Foreword

We are all aware that chronic rhinosinusitis (CRS) is not a disease but rather a pantheon of disorders that present with symptoms and signs, which fulfill a broad set of diagnostic criteria. In this book, the authors focus on one important, currently acknowledged phenotype with which we all wrestle in day-to-day patient management, namely, nasal polyposis. It is said that if you had only a limited number of nasal polyp patients in an otolaryngology practice, then the practice would continue to be busy as a result of the need for repeated surgeries. We are now beginning to be able to classify the disorders in this phenotype and to improve our understanding of it. It has been recognized for long now that eosinophilic polyposis responds better to steroids than neutrophilic polyps respond. However, as our knowledge of the nasal polyposis phenotype and many subtypes keeps evolving, we continue to learn that different subtypes of nasal polyposis benefit from varied therapeutic approaches and that armed with such knowledge, we can significantly improve patient outcomes. Endoscopic evaluation has enabled us to follow the disease, even when it is asymptomatic or minimally symptomatic, and manage polyposis with a variety of therapeutic options, without the need for frequent revision surgical interventions.

In this book, the authors provide important practical knowledge for treating physicians. This book also serves as an important academic update reference on nasal polyposis. Divided into three sections, the book covers differential diagnosis, new discoveries in etiology and advances in medical and surgical therapy. In the interest of focusing primarily on new knowledge, the authors elected not to include more established theories regarding polyp formation, such as the role of staphylococcal endotoxins, but do include newer areas such as the influence of P-Glycoprotein function, local immunity, vitamin D deficiency and acquired cystic fibrosis transmembrane conductance regulator deficiency, to name but a few. Sections on differential diagnosis, allergic fungal rhinosinusitis, AERD and cystic fibrosis sinusitis are of particular value to the practicing otolaryngologist, as will be the chapters on immunomodulators, topical therapies and advances in surgery. Sections covering the new discoveries in etiology are invaluable to the subspecialist, a resident preparing for the boards and academic otolaryngologists.

Nasal polyposis is at the forefront of a new era in which the many different manifestations of CRS and of nasal polyposis are appropriately classified and differentially managed. I congratulate the authors in compiling this informative volume and look forward to additional editions as our knowledge and our therapeutic options continue to further evolve.

David W. Kennedy
Rhinology Professor
Perelman School of Medicine
University of Pennsylvania
Philadelphia, Pa., USA

Woodworth BA, Poetker DM, Reh DD (eds): Rhinosinusitis with Nasal Polyposis.
Adv Otorhinolaryngol. Basel, Karger, 2016, vol 79, pp 1–12 (DOI: 10.1159/000444957)

Differential Diagnosis of Chronic Rhinosinusitis with Nasal Polyps

Nyall R. London Jr. • Douglas D. Reh
Johns Hopkins Department of Otolaryngology, Head and Neck Surgery, Baltimore, Md., USA

Abstract

Nasal polyps are semi-translucent mucosal outgrowths of the paranasal sinuses which typically arise in the setting of chronic rhinosinusitis (CRS). Nasal polyps are also associated with asthma, aspirin sensitivity, cystic fibrosis and allergic fungal rhinosinusitis (AFS). The majority of nasal polyps are bilateral and characterized by tissue edema and eosinophil infiltration. Patients with nasal polyps often present with complaints including nasal obstruction, congestion, rhinorrhea or altered sense of smell. The differential diagnosis ranges from benign masses such as schneiderian papilloma, antrochoanal polyp, angiofibroma and encephalocele to malignant neoplasms such as squamous cell carcinoma (SCC), esthesioneuroblastoma, nasal lymphoma and rhabdomyosarcoma. These lesions may have a similar appearance as nasal polyps and particular attention to an alternative diagnosis for nasal polyps should be entertained if the mass is unilateral or congenital in nature. Workup for patients with a unilateral mass should include radiographic imaging, possible biopsy and careful follow-up when appropriate. Here, we review the disease etiology of nasal polyps and describe the approach to the patient with nasal polyps with emphasis on differential diagnosis and workup.

Introduction

Nasal polyps are semi-translucent mucosal outgrowths of the paranasal sinuses, which typically arise in the setting of chronic rhinosinusitis (CRS). The majority of nasal polyps are characterized by tissue edema and infiltration with eosinophils [1]. Most are found bilaterally and are typically located near the middle meatus or ethmoid cells. Patients suffering from chronic rhinosinusitis with nasal polyps (CRSwNP) often complain of nasal obstruction, congestion, rhinorrhea or altered sense of smell, most likely due to the obstruction caused by these polyps. Patients with chronic rhinosinusitis without nasal polyps

(CRSsNP) may share these overlapping symptoms but more typically complain of facial pain or headache [2]. At the center of the pathogenesis of CRS is the disruption of sinonasal mucosa homeostasis. The sinonasal mucosa undergoes constant exposure to airborne microbes and inflammatory triggers and dysregulation of the innate immune response may lead to chronic inflammation [3]. It is not completely understood why some patients develop polyps while others do not; however, it is typically regarded as multifactorial and thought to stem from dysregulation of the interface between the sinonasal mucosa and the lymphoid system [4].

Factors that may contribute to polyp generation include cytokine mediators, innate immune dysfunction, infectious agents, a genetic predisposition, environmental exposures and other inflammatory or obstructive diseases. While CRSsNP is characterized by a T-helper type 1 (Th1) response driven by interferon-γ (IFN-γ), CRSwNP is characterized by a T-helper type 2 (Th2) response driven by interleukin-5, eotaxin and eosinophil accumulation [5]. Furthermore, the decreased expression of Toll-like receptor 9 (TLR-9) and interleukin-22 receptor (IL-22R) has been suggested to contribute to CRSwNP potentially through an inappropriate anti-microbial sinonasal response [3]. Increased colonization of polyps with *Staphylococcus aureus (S. aureus)* has been reported and has been suggested to be a common inciting event in polyp formation. IgE directed against exotoxins derived from *S. aureus*, or such exotoxins themselves acting as super-antigens, may upregulate inflammatory mediators or enhance inflammatory cell recruitment to the nasal mucosa sufficient to promote polyp formation [2, 6]. A genetic predisposition favoring polyp formation has also been reported including human leukocyte antigen (HLA) associations as well as the identification of a specific single nucleotide polymorphism in the promoter region of tumor necrosis factor-alpha (TNF-α) resulting in increased expression [6–7]. Other suggested mechanisms include dysfunction in mucociliary clearance as decreased mucociliary clearance has been found in patients with nasal polyposis [8]. A predisposition toward nasal polyposis is also associated with asthma. Indeed, the prevalence of symptoms of CRS in asthmatics has been reported to be near 70% [9]. Aggressive treatment of CRSwNP has been shown to reduce the severity of asthma as indicated by an improvement in the forced expiratory volume at 1 second (FEV_1) and reduction in systemic steroid usage [10]. These findings support the unified airway theory where stimuli in either the lower or upper respiratory tract trigger similar pathologic inflammatory changes throughout the airway [11]. Additional known causes of nasal polyposis include aspirin sensitivity, cystic fibrosis and allergic fungal rhinosinusitis.

Approach to the Patient with Nasal Polyps

Chronic rhinosinusitis is characterized in the recent updated clinical practice guidelines by 2 or more of the following symptoms including nasal obstruction (most common), facial pain, discolored nasal drainage and hyposmia for >12 weeks [12]. This diagnosis is supported by objective findings of sinonasal inflammation. The workup starts with obtaining a history by confirming the presence of and eliciting the severity of the aforementioned symptoms. In order to objectively assess the degree of sinonasal inflammation and the presence of nasal polyps, nasal endoscopy is most effective [13]. Nasal endoscopy allows one to better assess the status of the middle meatus, mucociliary drainage pathways, the nasopharynx and evaluation of nasal polyps as well as the presence of concurrent infection [13]. CT scan is regarded as the initial imaging modality of choice and provides significantly improved radiographic analysis than sinus x-rays. However, CT scan should not be used as an initial assessment but rather to corroborate the physician's

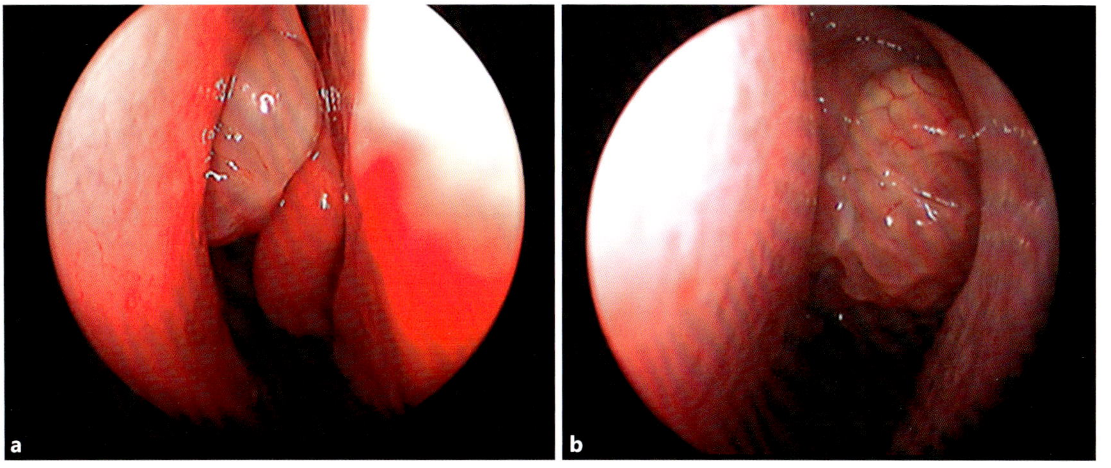

Fig. 1. Differential diagnosis of nasal polyps. **a** Semi-translucent polyp of the middle meatus. **b** Inverted papilloma characterized by a papillomatous appearance on nasal endoscopy. Reprinted with permission from American Journal of Allergy and Rhinology, May/June 2014, vol. 28, No. 3: Maintenance of Certification, p. S28.

findings on history, physical examination and nasal endoscopy [13].

Although polyps are typically found bilaterally and may have a characteristic semi-translucent appearance, one can easily be fooled by a multitude of other possible etiologies with a similar appearance (fig. 1). The differential diagnosis of an intranasal mass includes benign causes such as schneiderian papilloma, antrochoanal polyp, angiofibroma and encephalocele as well as malignant causes such as squamous cell carcinoma (SCC), esthesioneuroblastoma, nasal lymphoma and rhabdomyosarcoma (table 1) [14]. Mistaking a malignant process for a benign nasal polyp could lead to poor outcomes, but in-office biopsy of an unrecognized 'benign' encephalocele or highly vascular mass could lead to equally dangerous bleeding or cerebrospinal fluid leak [15]. Therefore, it is important to maintain a broad differential diagnosis in evaluating a patient with an intranasal mass, particularly if the mass is unilateral, congenital or there are other associated complaints such as rapid growth, epistaxis and cranial nerve deficits. In these cases, one should also obtain an MRI to evaluate the soft tissue extent and

Table 1. Differential diagnosis of nasal polyps

Benign
Nasal polyp
Mucous retention cyst
Antrochoanal polyp
Mucocele
Dacryocystocele
Nasal dermoid
Glioma
Encephalocele
Osteoma
Schneiderian papilloma
Juvenile nasopharyngeal angiofibroma
Hemangiopericytoma
Capillary hemangioma
Cavernous hemangioma
Vascular malformation
Granulomatosis with polyangiitis
Sarcoidosis
Malignant
Squamous cell carcinoma
Adenoid cystic carcinoma
Adenocarcinoma
Esthesioneuroblastoma
Chordoma
Lymphoma
Melanoma
Rhabdomyosarcoma
Fibrous histiocytoma

potential vascularity of any neoplasm. This chapter introduces and describes many of the more common differential diagnoses associated with nasal polyps, which will be discussed in further detail in later chapters.

Benign Intranasal Masses – Cysts

In addition to nasal polyps, there are other benign cysts that can arise from paranasal sinus mucosa. Retention cysts are thought to be due to obstruction of a mucosal duct or seromucinous gland resulting in dilatation of the duct and ultimately cyst formation [16, 17]. Retention cysts are quite common, with a prevalence of up to 35.6% [16]. They are lined with epithelium, most frequently arise in the maxillary sinus, and are often asymptomatic. As such, a retention cyst is often discovered incidentally and appears on CT scan as a dome shaped, homogenous, sharply defined mass, without adjacent bony destruction [17] (fig. 2). Retention cysts are self-limiting and do not require treatment unless a patient becomes symptomatic. It is important to differentiate these from other lesions that require surgical excision such as an inverting papilloma. On endoscopy, a retention cyst typically appears as a clear, thin-walled, cystic mass that will generate a gush of clear or yellow fluid with cyst rupture.

A similar and perhaps related process is the antrochoanal polyp. This lesion is most often unilateral and arises from the mucosa of the maxillary sinus. These lesions usually protrude through an accessory ostium of the maxillary sinus, through the middle meatus, extend into the choanae and may result in nasal obstruction. It has been suggested based on comparing the contents and microarchitecture of the antrochoanal polyp with a maxillary retention cyst that these may be similar entities [16, 18]. When removing these lesions, it is essential to remove the entire lesion at their base in the maxillary sinus to avoid recurrence. As such, a maxillary antrostomy with complete removal of the pedicle is recommended.

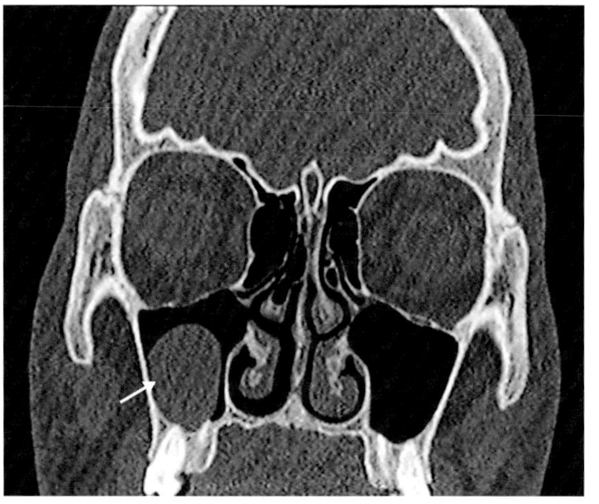

Fig. 2. Mucous retention cyst. Coronal CT scan shows a dome shaped, homogenous, sharply defined mass, without adjacent bony destruction consistent with a mucous retention cyst.

A mucocele is an expansile cyst-like structure of the paranasal sinuses arising from obstruction of the ostium of a sinus and the persistent accumulation of mucous and secretions. Mucoceles are usually located in the frontal or ethmoid sinus [17]. The most common reason for obstruction is sinus surgery or trauma but may include other obstructive causes such as osteoma or other neoplasms. In contrast to a retention cyst, a mucocele causes local remodeling and resorption of surrounding bone without destructive changes that would suggest malignancy [19]. Imaging often demonstrates an expansile process with complete opacification of the sinus (fig. 3). Due to their progressive and degradative nature, these lesions nearly always require surgical intervention.

Dacrocystocele, also known as nasolacrimal duct cyst, is a congenital benign cause of intranasal mass and nasal obstruction, typically presenting in infancy. A dacrocystocele may arise from incomplete canalization of the nasolacrimal system during gestation, resulting in accumulation of fluid and dilatation of the nasolacrimal duct

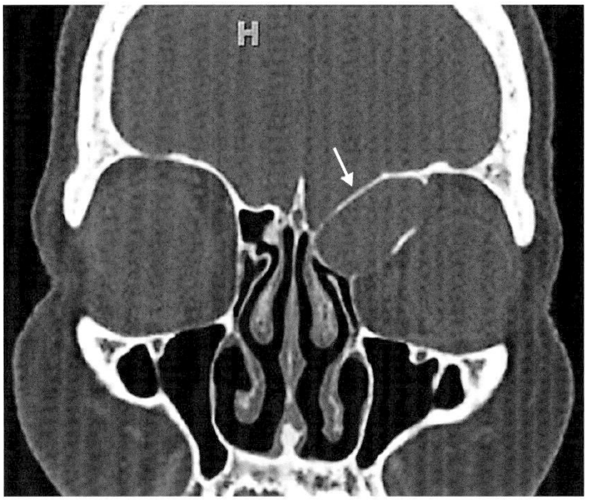

Fig. 3. Differential diagnosis includes mucocele. Coronal CT scan shows complete opacification of the left frontal sinus along with local remodeling and thinning of the surrounding bone consistent with a mucocele.

[20]. Dacrocystoceles are most frequently unilateral with a higher incidence in females. They typically present with epiphora and bluish cystic mass near the medial canthus and may have an intranasal component appearing as a bluish cystic mass on nasal endoscopy. As neonates are obligate nasal breathers, intranasal components of these cysts may cause respiratory compromise therefore necessitating surgical intervention [20].

Benign Intranasal Masses – Congenital Midline and Intracranial Nasal Masses

Congenital midline nasal masses include nasal dermoid, glioma and encephalocele. A nasal dermoid is composed of ectoderm and mesoderm components and forms due to persistent patency of the foramen cecum or through protrusion of dura through the foramen cecum [20]. These masses may have an intranasal component but typically present as a mass along the nasal dorsum. Nasal dermoids are typically addressed surgically because they can become infected, which may lead to meningitis or intracranial infection [20]. Similarly, gliomas are benign congenital midline nasal masses that may arise through the foramen cecum and may possess an intranasal component. In contrast, however, nasal gliomas comprise glial cells and fibrovascular connective tissue [20]. It should be clarified that a nasal glioma is different from an intracranial glioma, which is a hyperplastic process of the brain. A nasal glioma may present as a white non-compressible and non-pulsatile mass that may protrude from the nostril and cause nasal obstruction. A third congenital and potentially midline nasal mass is an encephalocele. An encephalocele develops from a defect in the skull base resulting in the herniation of meninges and brain with a persistent subarachnoid connection [20]. This is in contrast to nasal gliomas, which have lost their intracranial connection. Encephaloceles are often classified based on their etiology (traumatic, iatrogenic, spontaneous) or location of the skull base defect namely frontoethmoid, occipital, cranial vault or basal. On nasal endoscopy, nasal encephaloceles may appear as compressible bluish masses which transilluminate [21]. Failure to distinguish an encephalocele from a nasal polyp prior to biopsy may lead to cerebrospinal fluid leak, meningitis or other poor outcomes. CT is helpful to identify the bony defect where the encephalocele enters the nasal cavity from while MRI delineates the soft tissue and CSF extension from their dural origins. After imaging is performed, encephaloceles are often resected in conjunction with neurosurgery and the skull base defect repaired [22].

Benign Intranasal Masses – Neoplasms

The most common benign sinonasal tumor is the osteoma [23]. These are slow growing, arise from osseous tissue and may cause sinonasal obstruction. The frontal sinus is the most common site of involvement [24]. Osteomas often remain asymptomatic until they reach a certain size or become obstructive. They can become large and may have intracranial or intraorbital involvement. Symptomatically these patients typically present with headache and facial pain. Surgical indications for removal are symptomatic, obstructive and/or expanding osteomas. On CT scan, these appear as radiodense, well-circumscribed lesions that may have adjacent lytic bone destruction [24]. While osteomas are typically covered with normal mucosa and may appear as a mucosal mass on endoscopy, they are rarely mistaken for a nasal polyp and are typically picked up as an incidental finding on a sinus CT.

Papillomas of the sinonasal tract are often referred to as 'Schneiderian' papillomas in reference to the Schneiderian membrane or embryologic derivative from which the sinonasal respiratory epithelium arises [25]. These are subdivided into 3 subgroups based on histologic appearance and include inverted, exophytic and oncocytic [30]. The inverted papilloma is characterized on histology by its endophytic or inverted epithelial nests into the stroma with an intact basement membrane. The etiology of these neoplasms, as well as factors contributing to malignant transformation, is uncertain and debated in the literature. Proposed mechanisms include increased inflammation, cell cycle dysregulation, Human papilloma virus (HPV) infection, and remodeling of cell-cell interactions [25, 31]. For example, increased contralateral nasal inflammation has been demonstrated suggesting an underlying basal increase in inflammation in those with IP. An increase in the inflammatory marker cyclooxygenase-2 (COX-2) has been reported in IP with SCC versus IP alone. Increased proliferation as measured by Ki67 as well as increased markers of apoptosis and apoptosis inhibition have been reported in IP. Furthermore, HPV was detected in 37.8% of cases of IP and expression of epithelial cadherin (E-cadherin) an intercellular junction protein was decreased in IP with SCC versus IP [31].

Inverted papillomas are most commonly situated in a similar location as nasal polyps, predominately the lateral nasal wall, ethmoid and maxillary sinuses [25]. They typically present as a unilateral polyp and may be found in up to 4% of all nasal polyps [14]. These lesions have a characteristic papillomatous appearance on nasal endoscopy (fig. 1). While inverting papillomas are benign, they have a small incidence of malignant conversion, with 9.1% having a focus of SCC [31]. The current management is endoscopic resection with assistance from an external approach if necessary to achieve complete resection [25]. Many staging systems have been developed based largely on the recommended surgical management to be used or the prognosis for the risk of recurrence and include the Krouse, Kamel et al., Han et al. and Cannady et al. staging systems [26–29]. A major problem is recurrence and the best time to achieve full resection is during the first attempt; thus it is important to recognize this process early during surgical resection [32].

Juvenile nasopharyngeal angiofibroma (JNA) is a locally aggressive benign vascular tumor of unknown etiology. These are found exclusively in adolescent males and generally arise in the lateral nasopharynx, in the pterygopalatine fossa from vessels originating from or near the sphenopalatine artery [33]. Nasal endoscopy may demonstrate an erythematous, vascular mass that may protrude into the nasal cavity [33] (fig. 4). Due to the high vascularity of these lesions, an MRI scan is recommended prior to any intervention in suspected individuals. In the case of JNA, MRI may be a better diagnostic method than biopsy and provide the diagnosis without risking catastrophic bleeding. These tumors are locally aggressive and can expand from the sphenopalatine foramen medially into the nasal cavity, laterally into the masticator space or superiorly with intracranial extension (10–20%) [33]. There are multiple staging systems that have been employed to describe JNAs, including Radowski, Onerci and Synderman with the highest stage representing intracranial extension. Traditionally, these tumors have been resected via sub-labial or alternatively a midface de-gloving approach. Technological advanc-

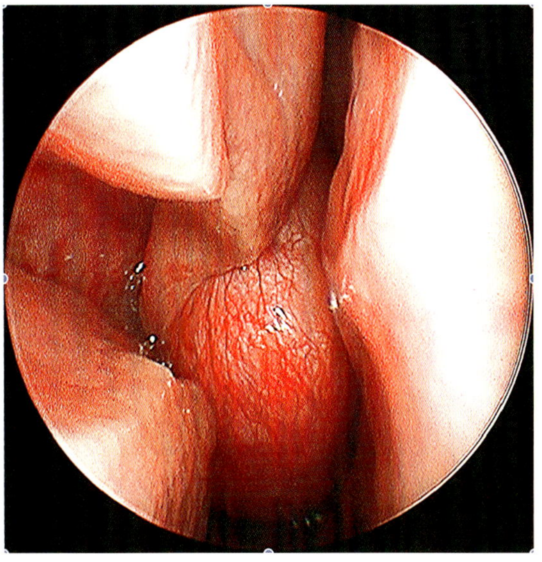

Fig. 4. Redundant Nasal endoscopy shows an erythematous, vascular mass protruding into the nasal cavity from the sphenopalatine foramen consistent with JNA.

es have allowed even advanced cases to be performed endoscopically, and this has become the preferred approach with open approaches used for laterally extending tumors [34, 35]. Due to their vascularity, pre-operative embolization of feeding vessels from the sphenopalatine artery is recommended. A subclass of extranasopharyngeal angiofibroma known as nasal septal angiofibroma appear similar to JNA on histopathology but differ in the location of the mass and the lack of a male sex predilection [36]. These unilateral nasal masses respond well to wide local excision from either an endoscopic or open approach [36].

A hemangiopericytoma is another rare benign vascular tumor. While typically found elsewhere in the body, approximately 25% of these tumors are found in the head and neck [37]. Sinonasal hemangiopericytomas have a rubbery appearance but are variable in color [37]. Usually these tumors are benign but have been known to occasionally possess malignant potential. Hemangiopericytomas are also relatively radiation resistant, thus treatment is surgical. Unfortunately, these tumors have a high degree of recurrence that can occur late.

Benign Intranasal Masses – Other

Benign vascular growths of the sinonasal cavity are rare but include capillary hemangioma, cavernous hemangioma and vascular malformations. Whereas vascular malformations are typically present at birth and do not spontaneously regress, hemangiomas are small or absent at birth, undergo a rapid proliferative phase and may occasionally stabilize or expand later in life [38]. Patients usually present with symptoms including recurrent epistaxis, nasal obstruction or unilateral nasal mass. On examination, the mass typically possesses a bluish or purple coloration [39]. It is important to appropriately diagnose these lesions as benign as they may appear similar to malignant vascular tumors such as angiosarcoma or hemangiopericytoma [38]. Furthermore, biopsy of these lesions may potentially lead to profuse or catastrophic bleeding [39]. In removing these lesions, endoscopic resection with or without pre-operative embolization have been described [38, 39]. If the capillary hemangioma has arisen from the nasal septum, it is important to also resect the perichondrium of the nasal septum to help reduce the risk of recurrence [39].

Systemic autoimmune or inflammatory processes should remain on the differential diagnosis. Churg–Strauss syndrome (CSS) is one example of a vasculitis which can cause severe nasal inflammation, erosion of sinonasal structures and nasal polyposis. A diagnosis of CSS is confirmed when 4 of the 6 following criteria are present: asthma, eosinophilia >10%, paranasal sinus abnormality, pulmonary infiltrates, mononeuritis or polyneuropathy and tissue biopsy demonstrating vasculitis with extravascular eosinophils [40]. Therefore, workup for suspected CSS includes a complete blood count to assess for hype-

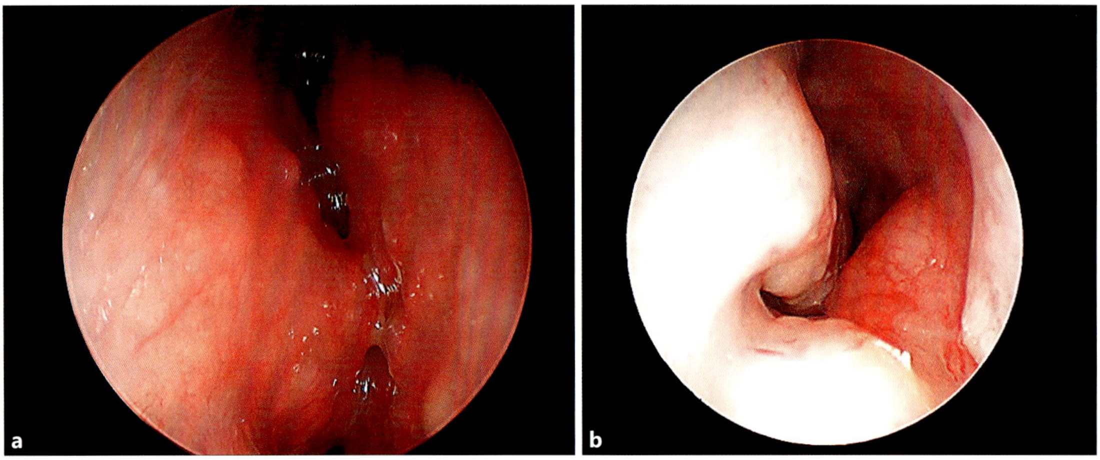

Fig. 5. Endoscopic findings in sinonasal sarcoidosis. **a** Cobblestoning of sinonasal mucosa frequently seen in sarcoid-related inflammatory sinusitis. **b** A nodule that when biopsied showed non-caseating granuloma consistent with sarcoidosis. Reprinted with permission from American Journal of Allergy and Rhinology, May/June 2014, vol. 28, No. 3: Maintenance of Certification, p. S35.

reosinophilia, imaging of the chest to assess for pulmonary infiltrates, and biopsy of suspicious lesions. Treatment of the sinonasal manifestations of CSS can often be managed with sinonasal irrigations and intranasal steroids. In cases of severe nasal polyposis, patients may benefit from surgical intervention [40].

Although they rarely produce nasal polyps, another example of granulomatous disease is granulomatosis with polyangiitis (GPA, formerly Wegener's granulomatosis) which can have various otolaryngologic manifestations including sinonasal, laryngeal and otologic involvement. In extreme cases, granulomatosis with polyangiitis may present with a saddle nose deformity, but more commonly presents as severe inflammation with extensive granulation tissue, crusting and concurrent infection. There can also be erosion of the sinonasal structures including the nasal turbinates or a nasal septal perforation [41]. Diagnosis can be made on the basis of these findings and c-ANCA antibodies are nearly always present in GPA patients [40]. Biopsies may show medium vessel vasculitis but rarely are helpful in making the diagnosis of GPA. Surgery should be avoided in patients with active disease [42]. Treatment for granulomatosis with polyangiitis includes medications such as cyclophosphamide and rituximab rather than surgical intervention [41].

A second example of granulomatous disease is sarcoidosis, which produces otolaryngologic manifestations such as salivary gland dysfunction in a minority of patients [40]. Sinonasal symptoms include chronic crusting, nasal obstruction and epistaxis and may appear on nasal endoscopy as cobblestoning of the mucosa or as a pearly nodule (fig. 5). Diagnostic procedures include tissue biopsy, which may demonstrate non-caseating granulomas and serum angiotensin converting enzyme levels which may be elevated. It is important to rule out infectious etiologies such as tuberculosis. Nasal sarcoidosis is typically treated and well controlled with topical steroids [40].

Malignant Intranasal Masses

Sinonasal carcinomas include SCC, adenoid cystic carcinoma and adenocarcinoma [43]. An association has been reported with industrial or occupational exposures including materials such as formaldehyde, wood dust and asbestos. Similar to carcinoma of the oropharynx, an association has been reported with human papilloma virus (HPV). In contrast to carcinoma of the oropharynx, there appears to be less of a link between smoking and alcohol use. Unfortunately, sinonasal carcinomas typically have a poor prognosis as they present at a late stage due to a lack of symptoms. They have been shown to be radiosensitive and late stage sinonasal carcinoma is typically treated with multiple modalities. With advances in endoscopic techniques, a growing number of tumors can be resected with an endoscopic or a combined open approach while maintaining the important principle of achieving a tumor free margin [44].

Esthesioneuroblastoma, also known as olfactory neuroblastoma, is a rare malignancy of the sinonasal cavity and anterior skull base most likely arising from the basal neural cells of the olfactory mucosa [45]. The presenting symptoms most commonly include epistaxis and nasal obstruction but may also include signs consistent with CRS such as facial pain, headache and anosmia. Additional symptoms such as diplopia, proptosis or neurologic symptoms may be caused by compression or invasion of adjacent structures [45]. Biopsy of esthesioneuroblastoma reveals small blue cells that may be arranged in glandular rings (called Flexner–Wintersteiner rosette) and interdigitating neural processes [45]. Many staging systems have been proposed including Kadish, Biller and Dulguerov (table 2) [46]. Esthesioneuroblastoma can be metastatic and is often treated with a combination of surgical management (endoscopic and/or open approach), radiation therapy and chemotherapy.

A chordoma is a malignant, slow growing tumor with locally aggressive characteristics. These tumors are thought to arise from notochord tissue and almost always are found to have arisen in bone [47]. Most chordomas are found in the sacrum, but may be found in the clivus or posterior skull base

Table 2. Staging systems for esthesioneuroblastoma

Modified Kadish	
A	Confined to nasal cavity
B	Extension to paranasal sinuses
C	Extension beyond paranasal sinuses
D	Metastatic spread
Biller	
T1	Confined to nasal cavity/paranasal sinuses (excluding sphenoid) with or without erosion of anterior fossa bone
T2	Extension into orbit or protrusion into anterior fossa
T3	Brain involvement but resectable with negative margins
T4	Unresectable
Dulguerov	
T1	Confined to nasal cavity and/or paranasal sinuses, sparing most superior ethmoid cells
T2	Confined to nasal cavity and/or paranasal sinuses (including sphenoid) with extension to or erosion of the cribriform plate
T3	Extension to orbit or protruding into anterior fossa
T4	Brain involvement

as well. On nasal endoscopy, these have been known to appear as a blue-grey gelatinous mass with lobulated contours [47]. These are typically treated with surgical excision either through endoscopic, open or combined approach followed by postoperative radiation therapy. In spite of this treatment approach, recurrence rates remain high.

Sinonasal lymphoma is a rare and challenging entity in the differential diagnosis of nasal masses. The appearance of sinonasal lymphoma on endoscopic examination may vary greatly from polypoid to ulcerative to granulomatous [48]. Patients often present with symptoms consistent with a nasal mass but others may have symptoms consistent with CRS such as rhinorrhea. Even when a diagnosis of sinonasal lymphoma is anticipated, pathologic diagnosis can be difficult due to the co-existence of CRS or significant necrosis from adjacent tissue destruction. This can necessitate multiple and deep biopsies in order to obtain adequate tissue [48]. Sinonasal lymphoma is often treated by chemotherapy rather than surgery with radiation therapy reserved for aggressive cases [49].

Sinonasal melanoma should remain on the differential diagnosis and carries a poor prognosis due to delayed patient presentation. Sinonasal melanoma appears often as a friable or polypoid mass with 50% having some type of dark, melanotic color. They may remain asymptomatic in the early stages [50]. This entity typically arises in the nasal septum and turbinates with 2 types described, melanotic and amelanotic [51]. Sinonasal melanoma has the best outcome when managed by surgical resection with negative margins. It can be even more difficult to treat than cutaneous melanoma given its close proximity to vital structures while mucosal melanoma much less frequently expresses the BRAF mutation and therefore sinonasal melanoma often has a poor response to BRAF-targeted therapies [50].

Approach to the Patient with Nasal Polyps – Workup

We have detailed many, but not all, of the sinonasal entities that may mimic nasal polyps. When evaluating a patient with nasal polyps, it is important to obtain a good history, physical examination and nasal endoscopy as this will guide the differential diagnosis. If the mass is found on nasal endoscopy to be unilateral or there are associated cranial neuropathies, one's level of concern should be raised for an alternative diagnosis rather than benign nasal polyp. As with masses of the head and neck, biopsy should be performed to confirm the diagnosis. However, one should consider imaging prior to biopsy as improper biopsy of an encephalocele or vascular anomaly for example could be catastrophic. Typically CT scan is the primary imaging modality as these determine the extent of the mass and delineate any bony breakdown. If a neoplasm or encephalocele is suspected, an MRI can assess the extent of soft tissue involvement and any local extension such as intracranial or intraorbital invasion. Lastly, in workup for patients with CRS recalcitrant to medical management, one should consider potential alternative diagnoses.

Conclusion

Nasal polyps are benign sinonasal outgrowths often associated with CRS. While these may have a characteristic translucent appearance, they can be difficult to distinguish alone from other etiologies on nasal endoscopy. Clinical suspicion should be raised in patients whose polyps are unilateral, unresponsive to medical management, or associated with cranial neuropathies. Imaging should be performed prior to biopsy if intracranial involvement or a vascular lesion is suspected.

References

1 Ryan MW: Chronic rhinosinusitis with nasal polyposis; in Johnson JT, Rosen CA, Bailey BJ (eds): Bailey's Head and Neck Surgery: Otolaryngology, ed 5. Philadelphia: Wolters Kluwer Health / Lippincott Williams & Wilkins, 2014, pp 525–534.

2 Georgy MS, Peters AT: Nasal polyps. Allergy Asthma Proc 2012;33:S22–S23.

3 Lane AP: The role of innate immunity in the pathogenesis of chronic rhinosinusitis. Curr Allergy Asthma Rep 2009;9:205–212.

4 Chaaban MR, Walsh EM, Woodworth BA: Epidemiology and differential diagnosis of nasal polyps. Am J Rhinol Allergy 2013;27:473–478.

5 Huvenne W, van Bruaene N, Zhang N, van Zele T, Patou J, Gevaert P, Claeys S, van Cauwenberge P, Bachert C: Chronic rhinosinusitis with and without nasal polyps: what is the difference? Curr Allergy Asthma Rep 2009;9:213–220.

6 Bernstein JM: The inflammatory process in nasal polyposis: genetics, molecular biology, and electrophysiology; in Onerci TM, Ferguson BJ (eds): Nasal Polyposis, 2010.
7 Rajguru R: Nasal polyposis: current trends. Indian J Otolaryngol Head Neck Surg 2014;66(suppl 1):16–21.
8 Coromina J, Sauret J: Nasal mucociliary clearance in patients with nasal polyposis. ORL J Otorhinolaryngol Relat Spec 1990;52:311–315.
9 Bresciani M, Paradis L, Des Roches A, Vernhet H, Vachier I, Godard P, Bousquet J, Chanez P: Rhinosinusitis in severe asthma. J Allergy Clin Immunol 2001;107:73–80.
10 Batra PS, Kern RC, Tripathi A, Conley DB, Ditto AM, Haines GK 3rd, Yarnold PR, Grammar L: Outcome analysis of endoscopic sinus surgery in patients with nasal polyps and asthma. Laryngoscope 2003;113:1703–1706.
11 Krouse JH: The unified airway. Facial Plast Surg Clin North Am 2012;20:55–60.
12 Rosenfeld RM, Piccirillo JF, Chandrasekhar SS, Brook I, Ashok Kumar K, Kramper M, Orlandi RR, Palmer JN, Patel ZM, Peters A, Walsh SA, Corrigan MD: Clinical practice guideline (update): adult sinusitis. Otolaryngol Head Neck Surg 2015;152(2 suppl):S1–S39.
13 Fokkens WJ, Lund VJ, Mullol J, Bachert C, Alobid I, Baroody F, Cohen N, Cervin A, Douglas R, Gevaert P, Georgalas C, Goossens H, Harvey R, Hellings P, Hopkins C, Jones N, Joos G, Kalogjera L, Kern B, Kowalski M, Price D, Riechelmann H, Schlosser R, Senior B, Thomas M, Toskala E, Voegels R, Wang de Y, Wormald PJ: European position paper on rhinosinusitis and nasal polyps 2012. Rhinol Suppl 2012;3:1–298.
14 Hennessey PT, Reh DD: Chapter 9: benign sinonasal neoplasms. Am J Rhinol Allergy 2013;27(suppl 1):S31–S34.
15 Cingi C, Demirbas D, Ural A: Nasal polyposis: an overview of differential diagnosis and treatment. Recent Pat Inflamm Allergy Drug Discov 2011;5:241–252.
16 Giotakis EI, Weber RK: Cysts of the maxillary sinus: a literature review. Int Forum Allergy Rhinol 2013;3:766–771.
17 Pierse JE, Stern A: Benign cysts and tumors of the paranasal sinuses. Oral Maxillofac Surg Clin North Am 2012;24:249–264.
18 Maldonado M, Martinez A, Alobid I, Mullol J: The antrochoanal polyp. Rhinology 2004;42:178–182.
19 Scangas GA, Gudis DA, Kennedy DW: The natural history and clinical characteristics of paranasal sinus mucoceles: a clinical review. Int Forum Allergy Rhinol 2013;3:712–717.
20 Adil E, Huntley C, Choudhary A, Carr M: Congenital nasal obstruction: clinical and radiologic review. Eur J Pediatr 2012;171:641–650.
21 Tirumandas M, Sharma A, Gbenimacho I, Shoja MM, Tubbs RS, Oakes WJ, Loukas M: Nasal encephaloceles: a review of etiology, pathophysiology, clinical presentations, diagnosis, treatment and complications. Childs Nerv Syst 2013;29:739–744.
22 Woodworth BA, Schlosser RJ, Faust RA, Bolger WE: Evolutions in the management of congenital intranasal skull base defects. Arch Otolaryngol Head Neck Surg 2004;130:1283–1288.
23 Harvey RJ, Sheahan PO, Schlosser RJ: Surgical management of benign sinonasal masses. Otolaryngol Clin North Am 2009;42:353–375.
24 Celenk F, Baysal E, Karata ZA, Durucu C, Mumbuc S, Kanlimaka M: Paranasal sinus osteomas. J Craniofac Surg 2012;23:433–437.
25 Anari S, Carrie S: Sinonasal inverted papilloma: narrative review. J Laryngol Otol 2010;124:705–715.
26 Krouse JH: Development of a staging system for inverted papilloma. Laryngoscope 2000;110:965–968.
27 Han JK, Smith TL, Loehrl T, Toohill RJ, Smith MM: An evolution in the management of sinonasal inverting papilloma. Laryngoscope 2001;111:1395–1400.
28 Kamel R, Khaled A, Kandil T: Inverted papilloma: new classification and guidelines for endoscopic surgery. Am J Rhinol 2005;19:358–364.
29 Cannady SB, Batra PS, Sautter NB, Roh HJ, Citardi MJ: New staging system for sinonasal inverted papilloma in the endoscopic era. Laryngoscope 2007;117:1283–1287.
30 Thompson LD: Schneiderian papilloma of the sinonasal tract. Ear Nose Throat J 2015;94:146–148.
31 Krouse JH: Endoscopic treatment of inverted papilloma: safety and efficacy. Am J Otolaryngol 2001;22:87–99.
32 Woodworth BA, Bhargave GA, Palmer JN, Chiu AG, Cohen NA, Lanza DC, Bolger WE, Kennedy DW: Clinical outcomes of endoscopic and endoscopic-assisted resection of inverted papillomas: a 15-year experience. Am J Rhinol 2007;21:591–600.
33 Zanation AM, Mitchell CA, Rose AS: Endoscopic skull base techniques for juvenile nasopharyngeal angiofibroma. Otolaryngol Clin North Am 2012;45:711–730.
34 Blount A, Riley KO, Woodworth BA: Juvenile nasopharyngeal angiofibroma. Otolaryngol Clin North Am 2011;44:989–1004.
35 Gallia GL, Ramanathan M Jr, Blitz AM, Reh DD: Expanded endonasal endoscopic approach for resection of a juvenile nasopharyngeal angiofibroma with skull base involvement. J Clin Neurosci 2010;17:1423–1427.
36 Garcia-Rodriguez L, Rudman K, Cogbill CH, Loehrl T, Poetker DM: Nasal septal angiofibroma, a subclass of extranasopharyngeal angiofibroma. Am J Otolaryngol 2012;33:473–476.
37 Dahodwala MQ, Husain Q, Kanumuri VV, Choudhry OJ, Liu JK, Eloy JA: Management of sinonasal hemangiopericytomas: a systematic review. Int Forum Allergy Rhinol 2013;3:581–587.
38 Kovalerchik O, Husain Q, Mirani NM, Liu JK, Eloy JA: Endoscopic nonembolized resection of an extensive sinonasal cavernous hemangioma: a case report and literature review. Allergy Rhinol (Providence) 2013;4:e179–e183.
39 Sheppard LM, Mickelson SA: Hemangiomas of the nasal septum and paranasal sinuses. Henry Ford Hosp Med J 1990;38:25–27.
40 Kohanski MA, Reh DD: Chapter 11: granulomatous diseases and chronic sinusitis. Am J Rhinol Allergy 2013;27(suppl 1):S39–S41.
41 Knopf A, Chaker A, Stark T, Hofauer B, Lahmer T, Thurmel K, Bas M: Clinical aspects of granulomatosis with polyangiitis affecting the head and neck. Eur Arch Otorhinolaryngol 2015;272:185–193.

42 Lebovics RS: Sinonasal complications of vasculitic diseases. Cleve Clin J Med 2002;69(suppl 2):SII152–SII154.
43 Haerle SK, Gullane PJ, Witterick IJ, Zweifel C, Gentili F: Sinonasal carcinomas: epidemiology, pathology, and management. Neurosurg Clin N Am 2013;24:39–49.
44 Poetker DM, Toohill RJ, Loehrl TA, Smith TL: Endoscopic management of sinonasal tumors: a preliminary report. Am J Rhinol 2005;19:307–315.
45 Ow TJ, Bell D, Kupferman ME, Demonte F, Hanna EY: Esthesioneuroblastoma. Neurosurg Clin N Am 2013;24:51–65.
46 Roxbury CR, Ishii M, Gallia GL, Reh DD: Endoscopic management of esthesioneuroblastoma. Otolaryngol Clin North Am 2016;49:153–165.
47 Fernandez-Miranda JC, Gardner PA, Snyderman CH, Devaney KO, Mendenhall WM, Suarez C, Rinaldo A, Ferlito A: Clival chordomas: a pathological, surgical, and radiotherapeutic review. Head Neck 2014;36:892–906.
48 Yen TT, Wang RC, Jiang RS, Chen SC, Wu SH, Liang KL: The diagnosis of sinonasal lymphoma: a challenge for rhinologists. Eur Arch Otorhinolaryngol 2012; 269:1463–1469.
49 Peng KA, Kita AE, Suh JD, Bhuta SM, Wang MB: Sinonasal lymphoma: case series and review of the literature. Int Forum Allergy Rhinol 2014;4:670–674.
50 Khan MN, Kanumuri VV, Raikundalia MD, Vazquez A, Govindaraj S, Baredes S, Eloy JA: Sinonasal melanoma: survival and prognostic implications based on site of involvement. Int Forum Allergy Rhinol 2014;4:151–155.
51 Szewczyk-Bieda MJ, White RD, Budak MJ, Ananthakrishnan G, Brunton JN, Sudarshan TA: A whiff of trouble: tumours of the nasal cavity and their mimics. Clin Radiol 2014;69:519–528.

Douglas D. Reh, MD
Department of Otolaryngology – Head and Neck Surgery
Johns Hopkins Medicine
601 North Caroline Street, 6th Floor
Baltimore, MD 21287 (USA)
E-Mail dreh1@jhmi.edu

Woodworth BA, Poetker DM, Reh DD (eds): Rhinosinusitis with Nasal Polyposis.
Adv Otorhinolaryngol. Basel, Karger, 2016, vol 79, pp 13–20 (DOI: 10.1159/000444958)

Allergic Fungal Rhinosinusitis: The Latest in Diagnosis and Management

Patricia A. Loftus · Sarah K. Wise

Department of Otolaryngology, Head and Neck Surgery, Emory University, Atlanta, Ga., USA

Abstract

Allergic fungal rhinosinusitis (AFRS) is the most common form of fungal sinusitis in the United States. Its pathophysiological basis is associated with a predisposed person's type I IgE-mediated allergic response to inhaled mold spores that are ubiquitous in the environment. AFRS is a well-recognized type of chronic, recurrent, and non-invasive hypertrophic sinus disease that affects immunocompetent hosts, most commonly young African American males. There are 5 main criteria used for the diagnosis of AFRS, one being the presence of nasal polyposis. A review of the current literature was performed in order to provide the most up-to-date knowledge regarding the background, diagnosis, management, recent research, and controversies surrounding AFRS. Although much is known about the pathophysiology and etiology of this disease, controversy exists regarding the importance of type I hypersensitivity in AFRS, as humoral immunity and immunoglobulin-independent pathways may also contribute. The potential role of local sinonasal IgE production in the pathophysiology of AFRS is an area of discussion, as is the role of preoperative antifungal medication in improving postoperative patient outcomes. Recent advancements in the diagnosis of AFRS include identification of genes and proteins unique to or over-expressed in AFRS patients. Although AFRS is a well-known and well-described cause of nasal polyposis, controversy still exists regarding this diagnosis. Advances in research may eventually resolve any diagnostic controversies in AFRS.

Introduction

Chronic rhinosinusitis (CRS) is often classified into 2 major groups: CRS *with* nasal polyposis (CRSwNP) and CRS *without* NP (CRSsNP). The CRSwNP group can be further divided into nasal polyposis associated with eosinophilic inflammation and nasal polyposis associated with neutrophilic inflammation. Nasal polyposis in cystic fibrosis patients typically falls into the latter category, while aspirin-exacerbated respiratory disease (AERD) and allergic fungal rhinosinusitis (AFRS) fall into the former category [1]. This chapter will focus on the pathophysiology, diagnosis, management, and latest research regarding AFRS.

Background

AFRS was first described in the early 1980s when Millar et al. [2] observed that the sinus contents from 5 CRS patients had a similar pathological appearance to that of allergic bronchopulmonary aspergillosis (ABPA), an allergic or hypersensitive pulmonary reaction to the fungus *Aspergillus fumigatus*. In 1983, 2 years after Millar et al. [2] had reported their findings, Katzenstein et al. [3] retrospectively reviewed 119 sinus specimens, of which 6% showed septate fungal hyphae, eosinophils, and mucin. Katzenstein et al. [3] called the disease process 'allergic Aspergillus sinusitis' and also likened it to ABPA. When Dematiaceous fungal species such as *Bipolaris, Alternaria, and Curvularia* were found to be the primary organisms involved in this disease process, the term 'allergic fungal sinusitis' was applied [4, 5]. With the general broadening of the term 'chronic sinusitis' to 'chronic rhinosinusitis', signifying involvement of both the nose and sinuses in the pathophysiology, the term most commonly used today is 'allergic fungal rhinosinusitis' [6].

AFRS is the most common form of fungal sinusitis in the United States, with the other forms of fungal sinusitis being acute invasive fungal sinusitis, chronic invasive fungal sinusitis, and fungus ball. AFRS is now a well-recognized type of chronic, recurrent, and *non-invasive* hypertrophic sinus disease that affects immunocompetent hosts [7]. It is generally accepted that AFRS represents a hypersensitive, exuberant, local inflammatory response to extramucosal fungi that are chronically present within the nasal and paranasal sinus cavities, rather than an infectious process [8].

Pathophysiology

The pathophysiological basis of AFRS has commonly been associated with a predisposed person's allergic response to inhaled mold spores that are ubiquitous in the environment [9]. Sinonasal eosinophilia and inflammation perpetuates a cycle of chronic edema, mucociliary dysfunction, stasis of secretions, and super-infection, secondary to improper functioning of the sinonasal mucosa from the inflammatory response to fungus [10].

Symptoms of AFRS progress slowly over time. Patients present with complaints of nasal obstruction, facial pressure, hyposmia or anosmia, and postnasal drip. AFRS patients may also present with proptosis or telecanthus from bony remodeling in the periorbital area. These patients often relay that their symptoms have been refractory to intense medical treatment and prior surgical management [11, 12].

Epidemiology

Studies have shown that, compared to other forms of CRS, AFRS is a disease that affects a younger patient population. Wise et al. [13] compared an AFRS cohort to CRSsNP and non-AFRS CRSwNP cohorts and found that the mean age at presentation of the AFRS group (28 years) was 15 and 20 years younger that the CRSsNP and CRSwNP groups, respectively. This study also demonstrated that AFRS preferentially affects the African American (AA) population and individuals of lower socioeconomic status. Thahim et al. [14] corroborated these findings, illustrating that their AFRS cohort presented at a young age (average of 20.75 years) and were of poor socioeconomic status (80% of the cohort). There was also a male predominance associated with this disease process (2.3:1), which has also been documented in other studies, such as a retrospective review of 93 AFRS patients by Miller et al. [15] that showed a 1.4:1 M:F ratio. This latter study also reported an average patient age of 29 years and found that AAs were the most commonly affected race (59% of cohort). Similarly, Lu-Myers et al. compared 93 AFRS patients to 93 CRS with and without nasal polyposis patients and found that both CRS groups were predominantly white ($p \leq 0.0001$), were older at the time of diagnosis ($p \leq 0.0001$), and had a higher county-based income per capita ($p = 0.004$) as compared to the AFRS group. Unlike the AFRS population, there were no associations found between socioeconomic status and demographics in the CRS population [16].

A study by Ferguson et al. [17] in 2000 demonstrated that the highest percentage of AFRS cases occurred in the southern United States and along the Mississippi basin where the environment is warm and humid, with Memphis, TN, reporting the highest percentage of AFRS cases at 23% over 2 years. According to the literature, worldwide prevalence is highest in Mumbai, India, with one study citing a final diagnosis of AFRS in 8.2% of patients undergoing sinus surgery for nasal polyposis [18].

Diagnosis

The most commonly cited diagnostic criteria for AFRS was published in 1994 by Bent and Kuhn [19]. These criteria include (1) type I IgE-mediated hypersensitivity, (2) nasal polyposis, (3) characteristic computed tomography (CT) findings, (4) eosinophilic mucus, and (5) positive fungal smear. It should be noted that it may take months to years to establish all 5 of these criteria. Although the 1994 Bent–Kuhn criteria are most often used to define AFRS for research studies, some experts debate the importance of fungus and the role of allergy in AFRS. These diagnostic controversies will be further discussed below.

IgE-Mediated Type I Hypersensitivity (Gell and Coombs)

IgE to fungal antigens can be measured in patients' serum and helps to distinguish AFRS from other forms of eosinophilic CRS [11]. As mentioned above, controversy exists over the importance of type I hypersensitivity in AFRS pathophysiology, as humoral immunity and immunoglobulin-independent pathways may contribute. For example, fungal-specific IgG is elevated in AFRS [11, 20], and elevated IgG3 levels specific to *Alternaria alternata* and *Aspergillus fumigatus* were shown to distinguish eosinophilic rhinosinusitis from control groups in a study by Pant et al. [21]. To further add to the diagnostic controversy, not all AFRS patients necessarily have a positive skin test to fungal antigens [22, 23] and/or an elevated total IgE [10]. Therefore, it is hypothesized that immune mechanisms other than fungal allergy play a role in the pathogenesis of AFRS. For example, Clark et al. [24] cultured significantly higher levels of *Staphylococcus aureus* from AFRS patients versus non-AFRS patients (63.2 and 24.1%, respectively), and Bachert et al. [25] demonstrated increased IgE to *Staphylococcus aureus* enterotoxin in certain groups of nasal polyp patients.

The potential role of local sinonasal IgE production should also be considered. A study by Wise et al. [26] in 2008 showed a significant increase in total and fungus-specific IgE staining in AFRS sinus epithelium and subepithelium as compared to controls and to CRSsNP patients. Furthermore, Chang and Fang [27] demonstrated that a group of AFRS patients all had a negative serum IgE response to Aspergillus, but 85.7% of the same patients had maxillary sinus tissue-specific immunoglobulin E (sIgE) to Aspergillus, and Collins et al. [28] illustrated that AFRS patients were significantly more likely to have fungal-specific IgE in sinus mucin (17 of 24, 71%, $p = 0.02$) versus non-AFRS patients.

Nasal Polyposis

Nasal polyposis is classically seen with the initial presentation of AFRS and can certainly be evident with disease recurrence. Postoperative AFRS patients often do not have gross polyposis, provided their disease is under control [29].

Imaging

CT scan shows heterogeneous opacification of the sinuses with central hyperattenuation, which is best seen in soft tissue windows. The bony walls of the paranasal sinuses are often expanded, demonstrating bony erosion and remodeling with a 'pushing border' (fig. 1), especially in the area of the lamina papyracea and skull base. Skull base and orbital erosion are much more common in cases of AFRS as compared to other types of sinusitis. For example, Ghegan et al. [30] reported a 56% incidence of skull base or bony orbital erosion in AFRS patients as compared to an incidence of only 5% in non-AFRS CRS patients. Furthermore, AA males were 15.0 times more likely to have bony erosion with intracranial and intraorbital extension than whites and AA females combined. Similarly, Wise et al. [31] developed an objective method for quantifying radiologic bone erosion in AFRS patients using a 24-point scoring system that included all 8 sinuses and the frontal and sphenoid intersinus septae, and found that males scored higher than females ($p = 0.001$) and AA scored higher than Caucasians ($p = <0.001$) in regards to bone erosion. Lastly, a retrospective study again led by Ghegan et al. [32] considered the impact socioeconomic factors might play in the incidence of bony erosion in AFRS patients and found that there were no significant correlations between bone erosion and socioeconomic factors such as percentage below the poverty level, median household income, population percentage of AAs, or number of physicians per 1,000 residents. However, in a retrospective analysis of 93 AFRS patients in 2014, Miller et al. [15] did find a correlation between bone erosion and residence in counties with lower income per capita ($p = 0.01$) and poorer quality housing ($p = 0.02$). Furthermore, patients with orbital or cranial involvement resided in more rural counties ($p = 0.01$) with less primary care providers per capita ($p = 0.02$).

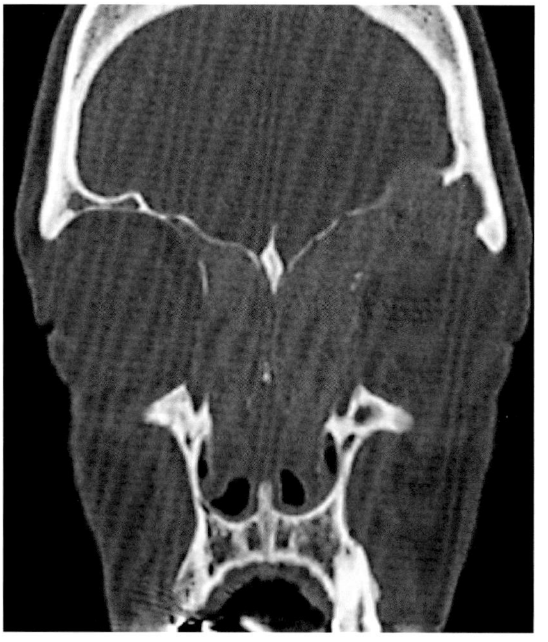

Fig. 1. Radiographic changes in a patient with recurrent AFRS following previous surgery.

On MRI, the sinuses have a peripheral high-intensity signal consistent with inflamed mucosa and a central low signal on both T1 and T2 that corresponds to areas of eosinophilic fungal debris. Fungal debris has lower water content and, therefore, little to no MRI signal [33, 34].

Eosinophilic Mucin

Grossly, the allergic/eosinophilic mucin found in AFRS is thick and tannish-brown colored, described by some as a peanut butter appearance and consistency. Histologically, this mucus consists of degranulating eosinophils in a background of mucin and fungal hyphae. The breakdown product of degranulating eosinophils is termed Charcot–Leyden crystals [11].

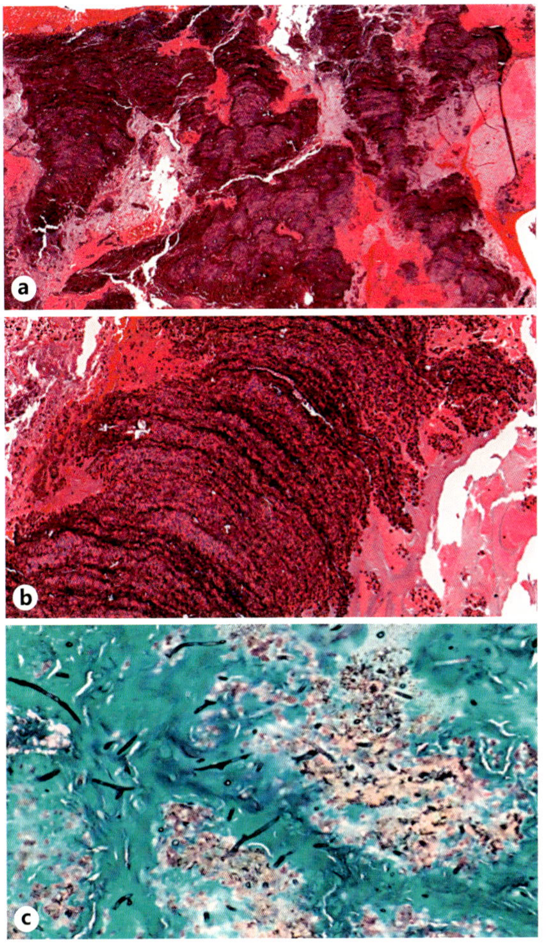

Fig. 2. AFRS allergic mucin on histopathology. (**a**) Low-magnification H&E stain, (**b**) high-magnification H&E stain, (**c**) GMS stain.

Positive Fungal Smear
Nasal polyp tissue and allergic mucin specimens removed during surgery are sent to pathology. Eosinophilic mucin should be evaluated for fungal elements, which requires special fungal stains (fig. 2). Although some experts advocate that a fungal *culture* can be used in place of a fungal smear [22], others do not agree with this [35], citing the fact that most of the population will have positive fungal cultures from their sinuses using modern culture techniques. For example, Ponikau et al. [36] showed that 100% of normal and healthy volunteers were positive for fungi on culture, with an average of 2.3 different organisms per volunteer. Therefore, fungal culture is unlikely to be helpful in the diagnosis of AFRS and a fungal smear should instead be used.

Although other diagnostic criteria have been published for AFRS, the Bent and Kuhn criteria are the most widely accepted and most commonly used. Bent and Kuhn [19] also described 6 associated criteria that can occur in AFRS patients, but need not be present to make the diagnosis: (1) asthma, (2) unilateral predominance, (3) radiographic bone erosion, (4) fungal culture, (5) Charcot–Leyden crystals, and (6) serum eosinophilia.

The European position paper on rhinosinusitis and nasal polyps from 2012 acknowledges that of the above criteria, only type I hypersensitivity and characteristic CT findings are unique to AFRS and distinguish it from other forms of sinus disease. Questions regarding the immunology of AFRS as compared to CRS and the relevance of fungal-specific IgE in this disease process remain unanswered [37].

Genetics and Protein Expression

Both past and current research has focused on the genetic and immunological basis of AFRS. For example, Orlandi et al. [38] performed a DNA microarray analysis on sinus mucosa samples in AFRS and non-diseased patients and found 38 genes or potential genes expressed in the AFRS patient samples that were not expressed in the non-diseased patient samples, while Schubert et al. [39] performed HLA DNA genotyping on a group of AFRS patients and found that 66% of patients with AFS carried at least one HLA-DQB1 *03 allele.

In another study, surface-enhanced laser desorption/ionization time-of-flight mass spectrometry (SELDI-TOF-MS) proteomic profiling of serum samples was able to identify patients with AFRS out of a group of patients with chronic sinusitis, with 84% sensitivity and 90% specificity [40]. Lastly, in 2013, Den Beste et al. [41] compared epithelial cell samples from AFRS patients and non-inflammatory control patients and demonstrated a 41% mean decrease in transepithelial resistance in AFRS cells, a finding that was also associated with decreased expression of 2 tight junction proteins and increased expression of a leaky tight junction protein.

In terms of immunology, Ebert et al. [42] found enhanced production of protease-activated receptors (PARs) in AFRS patients as compared to non-diseased controls. PARs cause an increased production of inflammatory cytokines and potentiate Th2 responses, which are characteristic findings in AFRS. Ayers et al. [43] demonstrated that patients with AFRS and CRSwNP have an increased number of local dendritic cells in sinus mucosa samples as compared to controls without CRS. Similarly, Mulligan et al. [44] reported insufficient vitamin D3 levels in patients with AFRS and CRSwNP, levels that inversely correlated with the number of mature dendritic cells in tissue samples and the amount of bone erosion on CT scan, and concluded that vitamin D3 has a role in the immunopathology of AFRS. Lastly, Laury et al. [45] found significantly increased levels of periostin – which is an extracellular matrix protein associated with eosinophil accumulation – in AFRS sinus tissue samples as compared to CRSsNP and control samples by both immunofluorescence ($p < 0.001$) and PCR ($p = 0.011$).

Although much progress has been made in this field, no testing has been recommended on a routine basis for patients suspected of having AFRS, and research in this area is ongoing.

Management

The standard treatment of AFRS is endoscopic sinus surgery with nasal polypectomy and removal of all eosinophilic mucin and fungal elements. Close follow-up and postoperative medical management is necessary to keep the disease in a dormant state in order to allow normal mucosal function to resume. However, the optimal medical management both preceding and following surgery is controversial.

Considering *preoperative* medical management, Patro et al. [46] recently studied the efficacy of preoperative treatment with itraconazole for AFRS patients by comparing an AFRS cohort treated with 1 month of itraconazole followed by sinus surgery to a control cohort of AFRS patients who did not receive itraconazole prior to surgery. Results showed a statistically significant decrease in SNOT-20 scores and Lund–McKay scores for the itraconazole treatment group, as well as reduction in hyperdensities on CT scan, decreased polyp size, and reduced fungal burden as compared to the control group. The authors concluded that the impressive results of preoperative treatment of AFRS patients with itraconazole deserve further research.

For postoperative management, oral steroids are considered the mainstay of treatment, with studies showing that tapering doses prevent early recurrence and produce both subjective and objective postoperative improvement in AFRS patients [47]. A systematic review of the literature in 2014 by Gan et al. [48] concluded that postoperative systemic and standard topical nasal steroids are recommended in the medical management of AFRS, and that nonstandard topical nasal steroids, oral antifungals, and immunotherapy are options in cases of refractory AFRS. Recommendations for topical antifungals and leukotriene modulators could not be offered from the available current literature. However, a study by Khalil et al. [49] *did* demonstrate that the use of topical fluconazole following sinus surgery significantly reduced recurrence rates of AFRS, while postoperative oral antifungals did not demonstrate this effect. Overall, both oral and topical steroids are considered the mainstay of treatment following endoscopic sinus surgery for AFRS, with consideration of antifungals and immunotherapy in refractory cases.

In regards to immunotherapy using fungal antigens, when combined with surgery and standard of care medical management with corticosteroids, this treatment has been shown to prevent recurrences of AFRS and decrease the need for future corticosteroid treatment [50]. It has also been shown to reduce the reaccumulation of crusts and allergic mucin within the sinuses, as well as decrease the use of topical and systemic steroids [51] and decrease the rate of postoperative AFRS exacerbations and subsequent operations for this disease process [52].

Prognosis

In most cases, visualizing recurrent disease on nasal endoscopy in the office setting precedes return of the patient's clinical symptoms, stressing the need for continued follow-up to promote the best patient outcomes [53]. However, AFRS is known to be a chronic disease that may recur even after intense surgical and medical management and appropriate follow-up. Continued research in this area will hopefully lead to improved treatment options and better patient outcomes, with a focus on improving quality of life for patients with this chronic disease.

References

1 Chaaban MR, Walsh EM, Woodworth BA: Epidemiology and differential diagnosis of nasal polyps. Am J Rhinol Allergy 2013;27:473–478.
2 Millar JW, Johnston A, Lamb D: Allergic Aspergillosis of the maxillary sinuses. Thorax 1981;36:710.
3 Katzenstein AL, Sale SR, Greenberger PA: Allergic Aspergillus sinusitis: a newly recognized form of sinusitis. J Allergy Clin Immunol 1983;72:89–93.
4 Manning SC, Schaefer SD, Close LG, Vuitch F: Culture-positive allergic fungal sinusitis. Arch Otolaryngol Head Neck Surg 1991;117:174–178.
5 Lawson W, Blitzer A: Fungal infections of the nose and paranasal sinuses. Part II. Otolaryngol Clin North Am 1993;26:1037–1068.
6 Lanza DC, Kennedy DW: Adult rhinosinusitis defined. Otolaryngol Head Neck Surg 1997;117(3 pt 2):S1–S7.
7 Ence BK, Gourley DS, Jorgensen NL, et al: Allergic fungal sinusitis. Am J Rhinol 1990;4:169–178.
8 Schubert MS: Allergic fungal sinusitis. Otolaryngol Clin N Am 2004;37:301–326.
9 Corey JP, Delsupehe KG, Ferguson BJ: Allergic fungal sinusitis: allergic, infectious, or both? Otolaryngol Head Neck Surg 1995;113:110–119.
10 Kuhn FA, Swain R Jr: Allergic fungal sinusitis: diagnosis and treatment. Curr Opin Otolaryngol Head Neck Surg 2003; 11:1–5.
11 Ryan MW, Marple BF: Allergic fungal rhinosinusitis: diagnosis and management. Curr Opin Otolaryngol Head Neck Surg 2007;15:18–22.
12 Marple BF: Allergic fungal rhinosinusitis: current theories and management strategies. Laryngoscope 2001;111: 1006–1019.
13 Wise SK, Ghegan MD, Gorham E, Schlosser RJ: Socioeconomic factors in the diagnosis of allergic fungal rhinosinusitis. Otolaryngol Head Neck Surg 2008;138:38–42.
14 Thahim K, Jawaid MA, Marfani MS: Presentation and management of allergic fungal sinusitis. J Coll Physicians Surg Pak 2007;17:23–27.
15 Miller JD, Deal AM, McKinney KA, et al: Markers of disease severity and socioeconomic factors in allergic fungal rhinosinusitis. Int Forum Allergy Rhinol 2014;4:272–279.
16 Lu-Myers Y, Deal AM, Miller JD, et al: Comparison of socioeconomic and demographic factors in patients with chronic rhinosinusitis and allergic fungal rhinosinusitis. Otolaryngol Head Neck Surg 2015;153:137–143.
17 Ferguson BJ, Barnes L, Bernstein JM, et al: Geographic variation in allergic fungal rhinosinusitis. Otolaryngol Clin North Am 2000;33:441–449.
18 Deshpande RB, Shukla A, Kirtane MV: Allergic fungal sinusitis: incidence and clinical and pathological features of seven cases. J Assoc Physicians India 1995; 43:98–100.
19 Bent JP 3rd, Kuhn FA: Diagnosis of allergic fungal sinusitis. Otolaryngol Head Neck Surg 1994;111:580–588.
20 Callejas CA, Douglas RG: Fungal rhinosinusitis: what every allergist should know. Clin Exp Allergy 2013;43:835–849.
21 Pant H, Kette FE, Smith WB, Wormald PJ, Macardle PJ: Fungal-specific humoral response in eosinophilic mucus chronic rhinosinusitis. Laryngoscope 2005;115:601–606.
22 deShazo RD, Swain RE: Diagnostic criteria for allergic fungal sinusitis. J Allergy Clin Immunol 1995;96:24–35.
23 Saravanan K, Panda NK, Chakrabarti A, Das A, Bapuraj RJ: Allergic fungal rhinosinusitis: an attempt to resolve the diagnostic dilemma. Arch Otolaryngol Head Neck Surg 2006;132:173–178.
24 Clark DW, Wenaas A, Luong A, Citardi MJ, Fakhri S: Staphylococcus aureus prevalence in allergic fungal rhinosinusitis vs other subsets of chronic rhinosinusitis with nasal polyps. Int Forum Allergy Rhinol 2013;3:89–93.

25 Bachert C, Gevaert P, Holtappels G, Johansson SG, van Cauwenberge P: Total and specific IgE in nasal polyps is related to local eosinophilic inflammation. J Allergy Clin Immunol 2001;107:607–614.
26 Wise SK, Ahn CN, Lathers DM, Mulligan RM, Schlosser RJ: Antigen-specific IgE in sinus mucosa of allergic fungal rhinosinusitis patients. Am J Rhinol 2008;22:451–456.
27 Chang YT, Fang SY: Tissue-specific immunoglobulin E in maxillary sinus mucosa of allergic fungal sinusitis. Rhinology 2008;46:226–230.
28 Collins M, Nair S, Smith W, Kette F, Gillis D, Wormald PJ: Role of local immunoglobulin E production in the pathophysiology of noninvasive fungal sinusitis. Laryngoscope 2004;114:1242–1246.
29 Chakrabarti A, Denning DW, Ferguson BJ, et al: Fungal rhinosinusitis: a categorization and definitional schema addressing current controversies. Laryngoscope 2009;119:1809–1818.
30 Ghegan MD, Lee FS, Schlosser RJ: Incidence of skull base and orbital erosion in allergic fungal rhinosinusitis (AFRS) and non-AFRS. Otolaryngol Head Neck Surg 2006;134:592–595.
31 Wise SK, Rogers GA, Ghegan MD, Harvey RJ, Delgaudio JM, Schlosser RJ: Radiologic staging system for allergic fungal rhinosinusitis (AFRS). Otolaryngol Head Neck Surg 2009;140:735–740.
32 Ghegan MD, Wise SK, Gorham E, Schlosser RJ: Socioeconomic factors in allergic fungal rhinosinusitis with bone erosion. Am J Rhinol 2007;21:560–563.
33 Manning SC, Merkel M, Kriesel K, Vuitch F, Marple B: Computed tomography and magnetic resonance diagnosis of allergic fungal sinusitis. Laryngoscope 1997;107:170–176.
34 Zinreich SJ, Kennedy DW, Malat J, et al: Fungal sinusitis: diagnosis with CT and MR imaging. Radiology 1988;169:439–444.
35 Chan Y, Kuhn FA: An update on the classifications, diagnosis, and treatment of rhinosinusitis. Curr Opin Otolaryngol Head Neck Surg 2009;17:204–208.
36 Ponikau JU, Sherris DA, Kern EB, et al: The diagnosis and incidence of allergic fungal sinusitis. Mayo Clin Proc 1999; 74:877–884.
37 Fokkens WJ, Lund VJ, Mullol J, et al: EPOS 2012: European position paper on rhinosinusitis and nasal polyps 2012. A summary for otorhinolaryngologists. Rhinology 2012;50:1–12.
38 Orlandi RR, Thibeault SL, Ferguson BJ: Microarray analysis of allergic fungal sinusitis and eosinophilic mucin rhinosinusitis. Otolaryngol Head Neck Surg 2007;136:707–713.
39 Schubert MS, Hutcheson PS, Graff RJ, Santiago L, Slavin RG: HLA-DQB1 *03 in allergic fungal sinusitis and other chronic hypertrophic rhinosinusitis disorders. J Allergy Clin Immunol 2004; 114:1376–1383.
40 Das S, Maeso PA, Becker AM, Prosser JD, Adam BL, Kountakis SE: Proteomics blood testing to distinguish chronic rhinosinusitis subtypes. Laryngoscope 2008;118:2231–2234.
41 Den Beste KA, Hoddeson EK, Parkos CA, Nusrat A, Wise SK: Epithelial permeability alterations in an in vitro air-liquid interface model of allergic fungal rhinosinusitis. Int Forum Allergy Rhinol 2013;3:19–25.
42 Ebert CS Jr, McKinney KA, Urrutia G, et al: Expression of protease-activated receptors in allergic fungal rhinosinusitis. Int Forum Allergy Rhinol 2014;4:266–271.
43 Ayers CM, Schlosser RJ, O'Connell BP, et al: Increased presence of dendritic cells and dendritic cell chemokines in the sinus mucosa of chronic rhinosinusitis with nasal polyps and allergic fungal rhinosinusitis. Int Forum Allergy Rhinol 2011;1:296–302.
44 Mulligan JK, Bleier BS, O'Connell B, Mulligan RM, Wagner C, Schlosser RJ: Vitamin D3 correlates inversely with systemic dendritic cell numbers and bone erosion in chronic rhinosinusitis with nasal polyps and allergic fungal rhinosinusitis. Clin Exp Immunol 2011; 164:312–320.
45 Laury AM, Hilgarth R, Nusrat A, Wise SK: Periostin and receptor activator of nuclear factor κ-B ligand expression in allergic fungal rhinosinusitis. Int Forum Allergy Rhinol 2014;4:716–724.
46 Patro SK, Verma RK, Panda NK, Chakrabarti A, Singh P: Efficacy of preoperative itraconazole in allergic fungal rhinosinusitis. Am J Rhinol Allergy 2015;29:299–304.
47 Rupa V, Jacob M, Mathews MS, Seshadri MS: A prospective, randomised, placebo-controlled trial of postoperative oral steroid in allergic fungal sinusitis. Eur Arch Otorhinolaryngol 2010;267:233–238.
48 Gan EC, Thamboo A, Rudmik L, Hwang PH, Ferguson BJ, Javer AR: Medical management of allergic fungal rhinosinusitis following endoscopic sinus surgery: an evidence-based review and recommendations. Int Forum Allergy Rhinol 2014;4:702–715.
49 Khalil Y, Tharwat A, Abdou AG, et al: The role of antifungal therapy in the prevention of recurrent allergic fungal rhinosinusitis after functional endoscopic sinus surgery: a randomized, controlled study. Ear Nose Throat J 2011;90:E1–E7.
50 Mabry RL, Mabry CS: Allergic fungal sinusitis: the role of immunotherapy. Otolaryngol Clin North Am 2000;33: 433–440.
51 Mabry RL, Manning SC, Mabry CS: Immunotherapy in the treatment of allergic fungal sinusitis. Otolaryngol Head Neck Surg 1997;116:31–35.
52 Hall AG, deShazo RD: Immunotherapy for allergic fungal sinusitis. Curr Opin Allergy Clin Immunol 2012;12:629–634.
53 Kupferberg SB, Bent JP 3rd, Kuhn FA: Prognosis for allergic fungal sinusitis. Otolaryngol Head Neck Surg 1997;117: 35–41.

Sarah K. Wise, MD, MSCR
Department of Otolaryngology, Head and Neck Surgery, Emory University
550 Peachtree Street, MOT 11th Floor
Atlanta, GA 30308 (USA)
E-Mail skmille@emory.edu

Woodworth BA, Poetker DM, Reh DD (eds): Rhinosinusitis with Nasal Polyposis.
Adv Otorhinolaryngol. Basel, Karger, 2016, vol 79, pp 21–28 (DOI: 10.1159/000445093)

Aspirin Exacerbated Respiratory Disease

Kai Fruth · Jan Gosepath

Department of Otorhinolaryngology, Head and Neck Surgery, HELIOS Dr. Horst Schmidt Kliniken, Wiesbaden, Germany

Abstract

Aspirin exacerbated respiratory disease (AERD) has been defined as a non-steroidal anti-inflammatory drug (NSAID)-triggered hypersensitivity, non-allergic bronchial asthma and chronic rhinosinusitis (CRS) with nasal polyps. The underlying pathophysiology of AERD is not completely understood so far. An altered arachidonic acid metabolism and dysregulated enzyme activity are regarded to be causal. AERD is characterized by recalcitrant CRS with recurrent nasal polyps after sinus surgery, accompanied by difficult to treat bronchial asthma and adverse reaction after NSAID ingestion such as nasal blockage, itching, laryngospasm and severe asthma attacks. Affected individuals suffer from poor quality of life. Besides functional endoscopic sinus surgery, the application of topical and systemic steroids and symptomatic therapy, aspirin desensitization is the only causative treatment option. The diagnostic approach to AERD, the ideal desensitization protocol and especially the following daily maintenance dose is part of an ongoing debate. This article summarizes the current knowledge about the pathophysiology, focuses on modern diagnostic approaches of AERD and discusses various aspirin desensitization protocols with respect to efficacy as well as to undesirable side effects.

Pathophysiology

Chronic rhinosinusitis (CRS) is frequently associated with nasal polyps, non-allergic bronchial asthma and non-steroidal anti-inflammatory drug (NSAID)-triggered hypersensitivity. This clinical picture has been described first by Widal et al. [1], later known as Samter triad and more recently defined as aspirin exacerbated respiratory disease (AERD) [2, 3]. The prevalence of aspirin hypersensitivity in the general population is estimated as 0.6–2.5%, and in asthmatics as 4.3–11%, depending on the country (in Finland 8.8% of asthmatics, in Poland 4.3% asthmatics, in Australia 10.5%) [4–7].

In a recent meta-analysis, the overall prevalence of AERD was 7% in typical adult asthmatic patients and twice that number in patients with severe asthma [8].

The manifestation of upper and lower airway complaints usually becomes apparent during the second and the fourth decade of life. However, the development up to the complete triad can take many years [9].

Ingestion of NSAIDs can result in a non–IgE-related acute reaction with moderate clinical symptoms such as rhinorrhea, nasal itching or sneezing and in life-threatening dyspnea with stridor and laryngospasm [10]. The eosinophilic chronic rhinosinusitis with nasal polyps related to AERD is characterized by high recurrence rates after sinus surgery and promotes a substantial restriction in quality of life of the affected individuals [11, 12]. This burden reflects the urgent need for a sufficient causal therapy to control CRS symptoms as well as the complaints of the lower airways. However, the etiology of AERD is still under controversial debate. Individuals with AERD are thought to be characterized by genetic polymorphisms that lead to a reduced activity of the constitutively expressed cyclooxygenase 1 (cox) isoenzyme as well as by an increased leukotriene receptor affinity and leukotriene synthase activity [13, 14].

Caused by a dysregulated arachidonic acid metabolism, the measurable prostaglandin (PG)/leukotrienes (LT) imbalance in affected patients has a decisive impact on the inflammatory changes of both the upper and lower airway [15, 16]. Besides a dysregulation of arachidonic acid metabolism, Staphylococcal superantigens are also discussed to be a crucial part of polyp formation within AERD [17–19].

It is known that leukotrienes can transcriptionally activate vascular epithelial growth factor (VEGF) production. This statement of Poulin et al. [20] is supported by the observation that in nasal tissue samples of aspirin-intolerant patients the expression of VEGF and its receptors can be dysregulated and increased [21]. As VEGF is known to influence substantial elements of tissue homoeostasis such as vascular permeability, cell proliferation and apoptosis, elevated VEGF levels in nasal polyps might activate VEGF receptors and downstream pathways resulting in pronounced tissue proliferation, edema and finally polyp formation [22–24]. Additionally, VEGF is able to increase survivin, a protein in the inhibitors of the apoptosis family, also proposed to be characteristically overexpressed in nasal polyps from individuals with AERD [25].

An altered immune barrier might be another contributing factor in CRS and AERD, which is assumed to be an underlying cause of the pronounced susceptibility of individuals with AERD to environmental factors and toxins [26, 27].

Within the clinical subgroups of CRS, individuals with AERD are characterized by the significant tissue eosinophilia [28]. The eosinophilic infiltration of the mucosal surfaces in both upper and lower airway is triggered predominately by the cellular release of cytokines and chemokines such as IL-5 and eotaxin [29]. The multifactorial pathophysiology of AERD consists of various genetic variations that are regarded to be casual factors to alter enzyme kinetics and receptor function and finally result in a derailed arachidonic acid metabolism with an imbalanced expression of LTs and PGs [29–35].

Diagnosis

As the complete clinical picture of AERD may develop over years, it can be difficult to identify patients with AERD among ordinary CRS patients [9].

The first hints about the manifestation of AERD are the occurrence of recurrent rhinitis after virus infection during the third decade of life, followed by nasal congestion, hyposmia, chronic rhinorrhea and CRS with aggressive growth of nasal polyps along with high rates of recurrence [36, 37]. Over the course of time, asthmatic complaints and hypersensitivity to NSAIDs become apparent too [4]. However, the intolerance can sporadically disappear and makes it even more challenging to diagnose AERD properly [38]. The decisive diagnostic information is provided by the clinical picture, and frequently an additional oral or nasal aspirin provocation test is performed to confirm the tentative diagnosis [39, 40]. However, during oral provocation tests, severe adverse bronchial reactions can occur and cases of 'silent' desensitization are sometimes difficult to identify [41, 42].

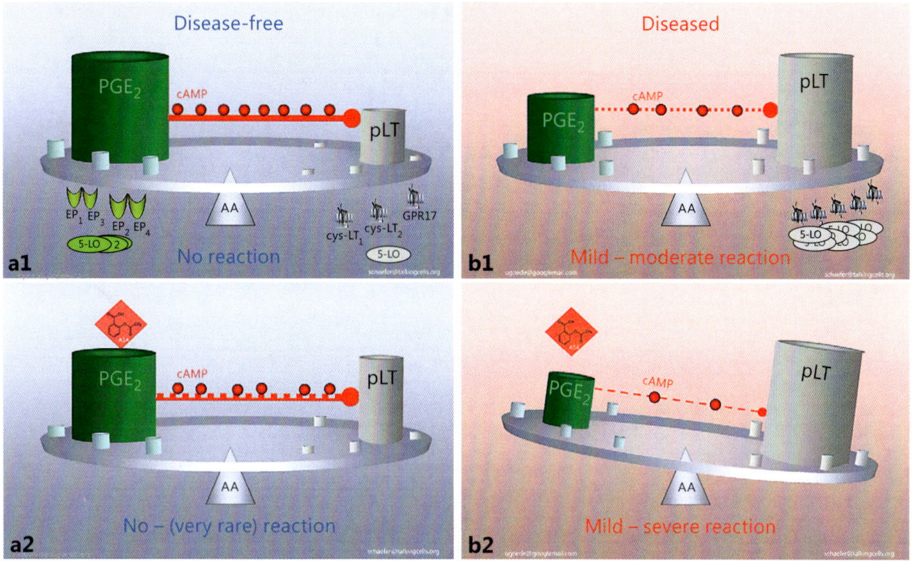

Fig. 1. Causal concept of NSAID-triggered eicosanoid imbalance for in vitro diagnosis of AERD. It is best allegorized as a tray balancing all parameters (which might be relevant for the pathway) on a needle. *Disease-free individuals:* housekeeping PGE_2 balances synthesis of pLT (e.g., by induction of endogenous cAMP, which inhibits synthesis of pLT); expression of enzymes or receptors is unremarkable (**a1**). Upon exposure to NSAIDs, the PGE_2 level is diminished but remains high enough ensuring 'uncritical' levels of pLT (even though cAMP might by diminished); expression of enzymes and/or receptors are not modified (**a2**). *Patients with AERD:* synthesis of housekeeping PGE_2 is diminished, but still balances synthesis of pLT (e.g., by reduced endogenous cAMP); expression of enzymes (upregulation of LTC_4 synthase) or receptors (upregulation of cysLT) can be mutated in some cases (**b1**). Exposure to NSAIDs/aspirin blocks the COX-pathway causing reduced synthesis of PGE_2 (and consequently further reduced cAMP level), and consequently the metabolism of arachidonic acid is shifted to the 5LO-pathway provoking elevated synthesis of pLT; expression of enzymes and/or receptors may by altered, but not modified by NSAIDs (**b2**). (With kind permission from Dirk Schaefer.)

The growing insight into the pathophysiology of AERD and the knowledge of downstream pathways and immunologic interactions have pushed the development of in vitro tests forward. Quite a few in vitro tests have been investigated in clinical trials and analysed regarding their sensitivity and specificity. Promising results demonstrated comparable validity to classic testing [41].The altered arachidonic acid metabolism and the disease defining PG/LT imbalance can be evaluated using the functional in vitro eicosanoid testing (FET) in the early and incomplete stage of AERD [14, 43, 44]. The resulting individualized dynamic eicosanoid pattern of the FET is classified in groups, which represent the severity of the disease and its symptoms. The so-called analgesic intolerance typing (AIT) value might be additionally used as a follow-up parameter to establish an individualized therapeutic desensitization protocol, which helps to increase efficacy since the maintenance aspirin dosage can be reduced when the AIT value indicates a normalization of the arachidonic metabolism [44]. The in vitro approach of this particular test is shown in figure 1 [44].

Table 1. Various studies investigated different application routes and maintenance aspirin doses

Study	Year	Application route	Maintenance aspirin dose
Stevenson et al.	1984	Oral	Up to 650 mg q.i.d., oral
Gosepath et al.	2001	Oral	100 mg daily, oral
Parikh and Scadding	2005	Intranasal	16 mg every 48 h, intranasal
Pfaar and Klimek	2006	Intravenous	300 mg daily, oral
Ogata et al.	2007	Intranasal	54 mg daily, intranasal
Lee et al.	2007	Oral	650 mg b.i.d, reduction to 325 mg b.i.d, oral
Rozsasi et al.	2008	Oral	300 mg daily, oral
Fruth et al.	2013	Oral	100 mg daily, oral

q.i.d. = Four times a day; b.i.d. = twice a day.

Taken together with patients' clinical symptoms, FET can be seen as a helpful diagnostic tool to confirm AERD adequately besides classic provocation testing.

Therapy

At present, besides the application of oral and topical steroids, functional endoscopic sinus surgery is the standard procedure in individuals with chronic rhinosinusitis suffering from AERD. However, these patients show recalcitrant nasal polyps with a high rate of recurrence after standard therapy and have to undergo sinus surgery frequently [11].

To overcome this dilemma for both, patients and physicians, there is the need for an additional causal therapeutic option, which helps to restore the dysregulated arachidonic metabolism in affected individuals [36, 45].

So far, aspirin desensitization represents the only causal treatment which fundamentally interacts with the arachidonic acid metabolism and its products. Stevenson et al. [46, 47] already described the clinical benefit of an escalated oral aspirin application followed by a daily maintenance dose in the past.

The clinical benefit and the sufficient control of CRS-related symptoms resulting from high-dose aspirin desensitization with up to more than 1,300 mg daily, come at the price of unfavorable, severe aspirin-related side effects. On the one hand, the authors observed a significant reduction of sinus infections, a decrease of indicated revision surgery per year and a reduction of nasal corticosteroids doses but on the other hand gastric bleeding and gastric pain were observed.

Therefore, the most suitable desensitization protocol with sufficient control of CRS symptoms and acceptable side effects has to be established, as does the optimal maintenance dose. To guarantee a long-lasting success with respect to a normalization of the prostaglandin/leukotriene index and the improvement of CRS-related symptoms, an aspirin intake for years, if not lifelong, is mandatory [45].

Several authors established numerous desensitization and maintenance protocols (table 1). Lee et al. [50] postulated a reduced maintenance dose of 325 mg twice a day for optimal symptom control, but current reports revealed that even aspirin doses of up to 325 mg daily entail the risk of gastrointestinal bleeding [48–50].

To avoid high dropout rates and side effects during desensitization, Gosepath et al. [45] investigated the clinical outcome using a low dose protocol with just 100 mg aspirin daily as maintenance dose in a prospective trial on 30 individuals with AERD and monitored consecutive changes of the arachidonic acid metabolism with the help of an in vitro analysis of eicosanoid release from mixed leukocyte cultures. The individuals included in this trial showed reduced recurrence rates of nasal polyposis, a reduction of the average incidence of purulent episodes of sinusitis, marked improvement in pulmonary function, impairment of nasal breathing, an increase of nasal patency and an improved sense of smell.

In 2013, the first double-blind placebo-controlled clinical trial using a low dose desensitization protocol was published. After sinus surgery, 70 individuals with AERD were allocated either to the placebo group or to the aspirin group with an initial challenge-dose reaching 800 mg aspirin followed by a maintenance dose of just 100 mg daily [51].

After 36 months, the evaluation of quality of life showed an obvious improvement in those patients who were allocated to the aspirin group ($p = 0.0324$), and typical CRS-related symptoms such as nasal obstruction, postnasal drip and cephalgia could be minimized ($p < 0.0001$). Nasal polyp relapse was additionally less pronounced with 28% in the aspirin group compared to 62% in the placebo group ($p = 0.0785$). As the occurrence of any recurrent polyp was regarded as relapse, the result failed to be statically significant; however, nasal polyp relapse occurred not only less frequently in the aspirin group but also at a later time point. Interestingly, none of the included participants dropped out due to aspirin-related side effects. An intensive supervision of patient's compliance and a close cooperation with general physicians involved in the treatment is recommended. The major conclusion of this study is the confirmation that low dose aspirin desensitization is an additional therapeutic option in patients with AERD that helps to reduce revision surgery and improves quality of life. In contrast, a study performed by Rozsasi et al. [53] failed to show satisfactory results when using a daily aspirin dose of 100 mg, but 300 mg seemed to be helpful to reduce nasal polyp recurrence and to improve sense of smell. However, this study was limited due to very few participants and contradictory to formerly reported results by others [45, 52].

Whereas most desensitization protocols use an oral application route, some prefer an intravenous scheme in the very beginning of the procedure. This is mainly for safety reasons, to be able to stop drug administration immediately [37, 51, 54].

As an alternative to oral or intravenous aspirin application, intranasal procedures have been described by several authors [55, 56]. The authors observed that intranasal lysine aspirin administration reduced nasal polyp volume with a maximum daily dose of 54 mg of lysine aspirin and CysLT1 downregulation in nasal tissue samples could be initiated by intranasal aspirin application [55–57].

It remains to be investigated to what extent an intranasal or moreover a gastrointestinal absorption of aspirin is the underlying mechanism of these promising results; however, it strengthens the assumption that low dose aspirin desensitization is clinically helpful and effective on cellular levels.

There is a great consensus in the literature that aspirin desensitization is helpful in individuals with AERD but the published data regarding the optimal maintenance are manifold and partially contradictory. There is a need for multicentre dose-finding trials in the future to define the optimal daily aspirin for an optimal long-lasting treatment success.

An uncertain issue is the upcoming question in clinical practise if an interruption of the maintenance dose of longer than 48 h subsequently necessitates a restart of the whole desensitization protocol. At present, we should recommend repeating the initialization of desensitizing as we do not exactly know when the clinically induced tolerance disappears [54].

In general, aspirin desensitization can be regarded as a fairly safe procedure but contraindications should be taken into account as well as home medication and potential interference with aspirin. Some authors suggest pregnancy, acute infection, partly or uncontrolled bronchial asthma, FEV1 <70% of the norm, local or systemic intake of β-blockers, intake of Marcumar® (phenprocoumon = warfarin) or other coumarin derivatives, severe cardiovascular, liver and kidney diseases, gastritis, gastroesophageal reflux, gastroduodenal ulcerations, mastocytosis, malcompliance and a high risk for injuries due to professional or personal lifestyle considerations as contraindications. However, these authors stress the fact that all contraindications have to be considered as relative and in the context of a precise individual evaluation of each patient [58]. Recently published data even suggest that potential side effects also depend on the individual genetic predisposition as well as on *H. pylori* infection status, which has to be taken into account [59, 60].

Future challenges include closer insight into AERDs pathophysiology in order to establish new therapeutic targets. Better understanding of the individual genetic profile and its clinical consequence could result in a personalized dose-adapted desensitization protocol and in vitro blood tests might help to regulate and adjust the individually needed maintenance dose for an optimal therapeutic success.

References

1 Widal F, Abrami P, Lermoyez J: Anaphylaxie et idiosyncrasie. 1992 [anaphylaxis and idiosyncrasy. 1992]. Allergy Proc 1993;14:373–376; discussion 371–372.

2 Stevenson DD, Sanchez-Borges M, Szczeklik A: Classification of allergic and pseudoallergic reactions to drugs that inhibit cyclooxygenase enzymes. Ann Allergy Asthma Immunol 2001;87:177–180.

3 Samter M, Beers RF Jr: Intolerance to aspirin. Clinical studies and consideration of its pathogenesis. Ann Intern Med 1968;68:975–983.

4 Szczeklik A, Sanak M, Nizankowska-Mogilnicka E, Kiełbasa B: Aspirin intolerance and the cyclooxygenase-leukotriene pathways. Curr Opin Pulm Med 2004;10:51–56.

5 Hedman J, Kaprio J, Poussa T, Nieminen MM: Prevalence of asthma, aspirin intolerance, nasal polyposis and chronic obstructive pulmonary disease in a population-based study. Int J Epidemiol 1999;28:717–722.

6 Kasper L, Sladek K, Duplaga M, Bochenek G, Liebhart J, Gladysz U, Malolepszy J, Szczeklik A: Prevalence of asthma with aspirin hypersensitivity in the adult population of Poland. Allergy 2003;58:1064–1066.

7 Vally H, Taylor ML, Thompson PJ: The prevalence of aspirin intolerant asthma (AIA) in Australian asthmatic patients. Thorax 2002;57:569–574.

8 Rajan JP, Wineinger NE, Stevenson DD, White AA: Prevalence of aspirin-exacerbated respiratory disease among asthmatic patients: a meta-analysis of the literature. J Allergy Clin Immunol 2015; 135:676–681.e1.

9 Berges-Gimeno MP, Simon RA, Stevenson DD: The natural history and clinical characteristics of aspirin-exacerbated respiratory disease. Ann Allergy Asthma Immunol 2002;89:474–478.

10 Stevenson DD: Aspirin and NSAID sensitivity. Immunol Allergy Clin North Am 2004;24:491–505.

11 Mendelsohn D, Jeremic G, Wright ED, Rotenberg BW: Revision rates after endoscopic sinus surgery: a recurrence analysis. Ann Otol Rhinol Laryngol 2011;120:162–166.

12 Ta V, White AA: Survey-defined patient experiences with aspirin-exacerbated respiratory disease. J Allergy Clin Immunol Pract 2015;3:711–718.

13 Kanaoka Y, Boyce JA: Cysteinyl leukotrienes and their receptors; emerging concepts. Allergy Asthma Immunol Res 2014;6:288–295.

14 Dobovišek A, Fajmut A, Brumen M: Role of expression of prostaglandin synthases 1 and 2 and leukotriene C4 synthase in aspirin-intolerant asthma: a theoretical study. J Pharmacokinet Pharmacodyn 2011;38:261–278.

15 Kowalski ML, Makowska JS, Blanca M, Bavbek S, Bochenek G, Bousquet J, Bousquet P, Celik G, Demoly P, Gomes ER, Niżankowska-Mogilnicka E, Romano A, Sanchez-Borges M, Sanz M, Torres MJ, De Weck A, Szczeklik A, Brockow K: Hypersensitivity to nonsteroidal anti-inflammatory drugs (NSAIDs) – classification, diagnosis and management: review of the EAACI/ENDA(#) and GA2LEN/HANNA*. Allergy 2011; 66:818–829.

16 Szczeklik A, Sanak M: The broken balance in aspirin hypersensitivity. Eur J Pharmacol 2006;533:145–155.

17 Pérez-Novo CA, Kowalski ML, Kuna P, Ptasinska A, Holtappels G, van Cauwenberge P, Gevaert P, Johannson S, Bachert C: Aspirin sensitivity and IgE antibodies to Staphylococcus aureus enterotoxins in nasal polyposis: studies on the relationship. Int Arch Allergy Immunol 2004;133:255–260.

18 Suh YJ, Yoon SH, Sampson AP, Kim HJ, Kim SH, Nahm DH, Suh CH, Park HS: Specific immunoglobulin E for staphylococcal enterotoxins in nasal polyps from patients with aspirin-intolerant asthma. Clin Exp Allergy 2004;34:1270–1275.
19 Juergens UR, Christiansen SC, Stevenson DD, Zuraw BL: Arachidonic acid metabolism in monocytes of aspirin-sensitive asthmatic patients before and after oral aspirin challenge. J Allergy Clin Immunol 1992;90(4 pt 1):636–645.
20 Poulin S, Thompson C, Thivierge M, Véronneau S, McMahon S, Dubois CM, Stankova J, Rola-Pleszczynski M: Cysteinyl-leukotrienes induce vascular endothelial growth factor production in human monocytes and bronchial smooth muscle cells. Clin Exp Allergy 2011;41: 204–217.
21 Fruth K, Zhu C, Schramek E, Angermair J, Kassem W, Haxel BR, Schneider A, Mann WJ, Brieger J: Vascular endothelial growth factor expression in nasal polyps of aspirin-intolerant patients. Arch Otolaryngol Head Neck Surg 2012; 138:286–293.
22 Yang J, Kong H, Dong Z: [Expression and significance of vascular permeability factor in nasal polyps]. Zhonghua Er Bi Yan Hou Ke Za Zhi 1998;33:297–298.
23 Coste A, Rateau JG, Roudot-Thoraval F, Chapelin C, Gilain L, Poron F, Peynegre R, Bernaudin JF, Escudier E: Increased epithelial cell proliferation in nasal polyps. Arch Otolaryngol Head Neck Surg 1996;122:432–436.
24 Lee HS, Myers A, Kim J: Vascular endothelial growth factor drives autocrine epithelial cell proliferation and survival in chronic rhinosinusitis with nasal polyposis. Am J Respir Crit Care Med 2009; 180:1056–1067.
25 Fruth K, Schramek E, Docter D, Haxel BR, Schneider A, Mann WJ, Brieger J: Dysregulated survivin expression in nasal polyps of individuals with aspirin exacerbated respiratory disease. Am J Rhinol Allergy 2012;26:380–384.
26 Fruth K, Goebel G, Koutsimpelas D, Gosepath J, Schmidtmann I, Mann WJ, Brieger J: Low SPINK5 expression in chronic rhinosinusitis. Laryngoscope 2012;122:1198–1204.
27 Kern RC, Conley DB, Walsh W, Chandra R, Kato A, Tripathi-Peters A, Grammer LC, Schleimer RP: Perspectives on the etiology of chronic rhinosinusitis: an immune barrier hypothesis. Am J Rhinol 2008;22:549–559.
28 Kaldenbach T, Schäfer D, Gosepath J, Bittinger F, Klimek L, Mann WJ: [Significance of eosinophilic granulocytes in relation to allergy and aspirin intolerance in patients with sinusitis polyposa]. Laryngorhinootologie 1999;78:429–434.
29 Choi JH, Kim MA, Park HS: An update on the pathogenesis of the upper airways in aspirin-exacerbated respiratory disease. Curr Opin Allergy Clin Immunol 2014;14:1–6.
30 Shin SW, Park BL, Chang H, Park JS, Bae DJ, Song HJ, Choi IS, Kim MK, Park HS, Kim LH, Namgoong S, Kim JO, Shin HD, Park CS: Exonic variants associated with development of aspirin exacerbated respiratory diseases. PLoS One 2014; 9:e111887.
31 Park SM, Park JS, Park HS, Park CS: Unraveling the genetic basis of aspirin hypersensitivity in asthma beyond arachidonate pathways. Allergy Asthma Immunol Res 2013;5:258–276.
32 Chang HS, Park JS, Shin HR, Park BL, Shin HD, Park CS: Association analysis of FABP1 gene polymorphisms with aspirin-exacerbated respiratory disease in asthma. Exp Lung Res 2014;40:485–494.
33 Chang HS, Shin SW, Lee TH, Bae DJ, Park JS, Kim YH, Uh ST, Choi BW, Kim MK, Choi IS, Park BL, Shin HD, Park CS: Development of a genetic marker set to diagnose aspirin-exacerbated respiratory disease in a genome-wide association study. Pharmacogenomics J 2015; 15:316–321.
34 Losol P, Kim SH, Shin YS, Ye YM, Park HS: A genetic effect of IL-5 receptor α polymorphism in patients with aspirin-exacerbated respiratory disease. Exp Mol Med 2013;45:e14.
35 Fruth K, Best N, Amro M, Ingel K, Gosepath J, Mann WJ, Brieger J: No evidence for a correlation of glutathione S-tranferase polymorphisms and chronic rhinosinusitis. Rhinology 2011;49: 180–184.
36 Stevenson DD: Aspirin sensitivity and desensitization for asthma and sinusitis. Curr Allergy Asthma Rep 2009;9:155–163.
37 Pfaar O, Klimek L: Eicosanoids, aspirin-intolerance and the upper airways – current standards and recent improvements of the desensitization therapy. J Physiol Pharmacol 2006;57(suppl 12):5–13.
38 Rosado A, Vives R, González R, Rodríguez J: Can NSAIDs intolerance disappear? A study of three cases. Allergy 2003;58:689–690.
39 Nizankowska-Mogilnicka E, Bochenek G, Mastalerz L, Swierczyńska M, Picado C, Scadding G, Kowalski ML, Setkowicz M, Ring J, Brockow K, Bachert C, Wöhrl S, Dahlén B, Szczeklik A: EAACI/GA2LEN guideline: aspirin provocation tests for diagnosis of aspirin hypersensitivity. Allergy 2007;62:1111–1118.
40 Lee RU, Stevenson DD: Aspirin-exacerbated respiratory disease: evaluation and management. Allergy Asthma Immunol Res 2011;3:3–10.
41 Baenkler HW: Salicylate intolerance: pathophysiology, clinical spectrum, diagnosis and treatment. Dtsch Arztebl Int 2008;105:137–142.
42 White AA, Bosso JV, Stevenson DD: The clinical dilemma of 'silent desensitization' in aspirin-exacerbated respiratory disease. Allergy Asthma Proc 2013;34: 378–382.
43 Schäfer D, Lindenthal U, Wagner M, Bölcskei PL, Baenkler HW: Effect of prostaglandin E2 on eicosanoid release by human bronchial biopsy specimens from normal and inflamed mucosa. Thorax 1996;51:919–923.
44 Schäfer D, Maune S: Pathogenic mechanisms and in vitro diagnosis of AERD. J Allergy (Cairo) 2012;2012:789232.
45 Gosepath J, Schaefer D, Amedee RG, Mann WJ: Individual monitoring of aspirin desensitization. Arch Otolaryngol Head Neck Surg 2001;127:316–321.
46 Stevenson DD, Pleskow WW, Simon RA, Mathison DA, Lumry WR, Schatz M, Zeiger RS: Aspirin-sensitive rhinosinusitis asthma: a double-blind crossover study of treatment with aspirin. J Allergy Clin Immunol 1984;73:500–507.
47 Stevenson DD, Hankammer MA, Mathison DA, Christiansen SC, Simon RA: Aspirin desensitization treatment of aspirin-sensitive patients with rhinosinusitis-asthma: long-term outcomes. J Allergy Clin Immunol 1996;98:751–758.
48 Lanas A, Wu P, Medin J, Mills EJ: Low doses of acetylsalicylic acid increase risk of gastrointestinal bleeding in a meta-analysis. Clin Gastroenterol Hepatol 2011;9:762–768.e6.

49 Moberg C, Naesdal J, Svedberg LE, Duchateau D, Harte N: Impact of gastrointestinal problems on adherence to low-dose acetylsalicylic acid: a quantitative study in patients with cardiovascular risk. Patient 2011;4:103–113.
50 Lee JY, Simon RA, Stevenson DD: Selection of aspirin dosages for aspirin desensitization treatment in patients with aspirin-exacerbated respiratory disease. J Allergy Clin Immunol 2007;119:157–164.
51 Fruth K, Pogorzelski B, Schmidtmann I, Springer J, Fennan N, Fraessdorf N, Boessert A, Schaefer D, Gosepath J, Mann WJ: Low-dose aspirin desensitization in individuals with aspirin-exacerbated respiratory disease. Allergy 2013; 68:659–665.
52 Gosepath J, Schäfer D, Mann WJ: [Aspirin sensitivity: long term follow-up after up to 3 years of adaptive desensitization using a maintenance dose of 100 mg of aspirin a day]. Laryngorhinootologie 2002;81:732–738.
53 Rozsasi A, Polzehl D, Deutschle T, Smith E, Wiesmiller K, Riechelmann H, Keck T: Long-term treatment with aspirin desensitization: a prospective clinical trial comparing 100 and 300 mg aspirin daily. Allergy 2008;63:1228–1234.
54 Macy E, Bernstein JA, Castells MC, Gawchik SM, Lee TH, Settipane RA, Simon RA, Wald J, Woessner KM: Aspirin challenge and desensitization for aspirin-exacerbated respiratory disease: a practice paper. Ann Allergy Asthma Immunol 2007;98:172–174.
55 Parikh AA, Scadding GK: Intranasal lysine-aspirin in aspirin-sensitive nasal polyposis: a controlled trial. Laryngoscope 2005;115:1385–1390.
56 Sousa AR, Parikh A, Scadding G, Corrigan CJ, Lee TH: Leukotriene-receptor expression on nasal mucosal inflammatory cells in aspirin-sensitive rhinosinusitis. N Engl J Med 2002;347:1493–1499.
57 Ogata N, Darby Y, Scadding G: Intranasal lysine-aspirin administration decreases polyp volume in patients with aspirin-intolerant asthma. J Laryngol Otol 2007;121:1156–1160.
58 Klimek L, Dollner R, Pfaar O, Mullol J: Aspirin desensitization: useful treatment for chronic rhinosinusitis with nasal polyps (CRSwNP) in aspirin-exacerbated respiratory disease (AERD)? Curr Allergy Asthma Rep 2014;14:441.
59 Shiotani A, Fujita Y, Nishio K: Low-dose aspirin-associated upper and mid gastrointestinal tract damage and gene polymorphism. Curr Pharm Des 2015; 21:5066–5072.
60 Iijima K, Shimosegawa T: Risk factors for upper GI damage in low-dose aspirin users and the interaction between H. pylori infection and low-dose aspirin use. Curr Pharm Des 2015;21:5056–5065.

Kai Fruth, MD, PhD
Department of Otorhinolaryngology, Head and Neck Surgery
HELIOS Dr. Horst Schmidt Kliniken
DE–65199 Wiesbaden (Germany)
E-Mail kai.fruth@helios-kliniken.de

Woodworth BA, Poetker DM, Reh DD (eds): Rhinosinusitis with Nasal Polyposis.
Adv Otorhinolaryngol. Basel, Karger, 2016, vol 79, pp 29–37 (DOI: 10.1159/000444959)

Cystic Fibrosis Sinusitis

Christopher Le • Hilary C. McCrary • Eugene Chang
Department of Otolaryngology – Head and Neck Surgery, The University of Arizona College of Medicine, Tucson, Ariz., USA

Abstract

Cystic fibrosis (CF) is an autosomal recessive genetic disorder caused by mutations in the *CF transmembrane conductance regulator gene (CFTR)* resulting in impaired ion transport. Nearly all people with CF will develop chronic rhino-sinusitis (CRS) and present with the characteristic viscous mucus, impaired mucociliary clearance and chronic inflammation/infection of the sinonasal cavity. While some individuals with CF can appear relatively asymptomatic in terms of their sinus disease, commonly reported symptoms include anosmia, headache, facial pain, nasal obstruction, chronic congestion and nasal discharge. Nasal endoscopy typically reveals mucosal edema, purulent discharge and nasal polyposis. Computed tomography (CT) imaging classically demonstrates the distinguishing findings of sinus hypoplasia or aplasia with generalized opacification, medial bulging of the lateral sinonasal sidewall and a demineralized uncinate process. Current treatment for CF sinusitis includes the use of hypertonic saline, topical and systemic steroids, antibiotics and endoscopic surgery. Research investigating novel therapies designed at targeting the primary defect of CF is showing promise for reversal of CF sinus disease, in addition to potential for disease prevention.

Introduction

Cystic fibrosis (CF) is an autosomal recessive genetic disorder caused by mutations in the *CF transmembrane conductance regulator gene (CFTR)*. Dorothy Anderson first described CF in 1938 based on the histopathology of the pancreas of affected children. The CF phenotype involves multiple organ systems including the intestine, lung, sweat gland, liver, gallbladder, male genital tract and the paranasal sinuses [1–3]. Recurrent infections of the respiratory tract are the leading cause of mortality in CF. However, improvements in medical care have increased the median age of survival from 33.4 years in 2003 to 40.7 years in 2013 [4]. Pertinent to otolaryngologists, nearly all individuals with CF will develop chronic sinusitis throughout the course of their disease [5, 6].

The association of impaired sodium chloride absorption and early death was made during the 18th century with the saying: 'The child will soon die whose brow taste salty when kissed.' However, it was not until 1989 when Drs. Collins, Riordan and Tsui identified the CF transmembrane conductance regulator *(CFTR)* gene responsible for the disease [7]. CFTR is an anion channel expressed on the cell surface that transports chloride (Cl^-) and bicarbonate (HCO_3^-) ions. There are close to 2000 mutations of *CFTR* associated with CF, which are classified by defects in protein production (Class I), protein processing (Class II), regulation (Class III), conduction (Class IV), reduced numbers of CFTR transcripts (Class V) and defective CFTR stability at the cell surface (Class VI) [7, 8]. The most common mutation is the *F508del-CFTR* mutation that accounts for 86.4% of all CFTR mutations [4]. This mutation represents the deletion of 3 nucleotides, which results in the absence of phenylalanine at position 508, ultimately leading to a misfolded protein that cannot be transported to the cell surface. The diagnosis of CF is based on clinical symptoms, the presence of 2 CFTR mutations and a sweat chloride >60 mM/l [9].

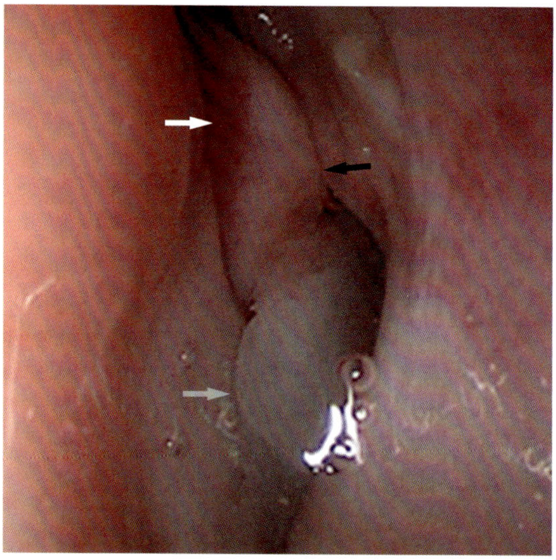

Fig. 1. Left sided nasal endoscopy of a 2-year old with CF. White arrow designates the middle turbinate. Black arrow indicates the prominent uncinate process. Grey arrow specifies a nasal polyp emanating from the middle meatus.

Presenting History and Symptoms

Due to widespread prenatal screening in the United States for the *CFTR* mutation, the diagnosis of CF is usually determined prior to referral to the otolaryngologist. However, the presence of nasal polyps in a young child should prompt a complete workup for CF (fig. 1). Loss of CFTR function in the sinonasal cavity results in thick mucus, impaired mucociliary clearance and chronic infection and inflammation that can be observed as early as 4 months of age. While nearly all CF patients have diseases that involve the nasal and sinus cavities, as few as 10% of patients report sinus symptoms [10]. Commonly, the severity of disease as demonstrated by endoscopy or computed tomography (CT) does not align with presenting symptoms, which could be attributed to the following: the congenital nature of the disease, inability to compare symptoms to a healthy baseline and increased focus on disease processes within the lung or gastrointestinal track [10–12]. When reported, symptoms most related to CF sinus disease include anosmia, headache, facial pain, nasal obstruction, chronic congestion and nasal discharge [13–16]. Bilateral nasal obstruction is the most common sinus symptom reported among patients with nasal polyps and affects approximately 81.3% of patients with CF-related sinus disease [17, 18]. Patients without nasal polyps may present with headache or facial pain [17]. CF sinusitis in the pediatric population can severely impact quality of life due to nasal obstruction, obstructive sleep apnea and developmental growth

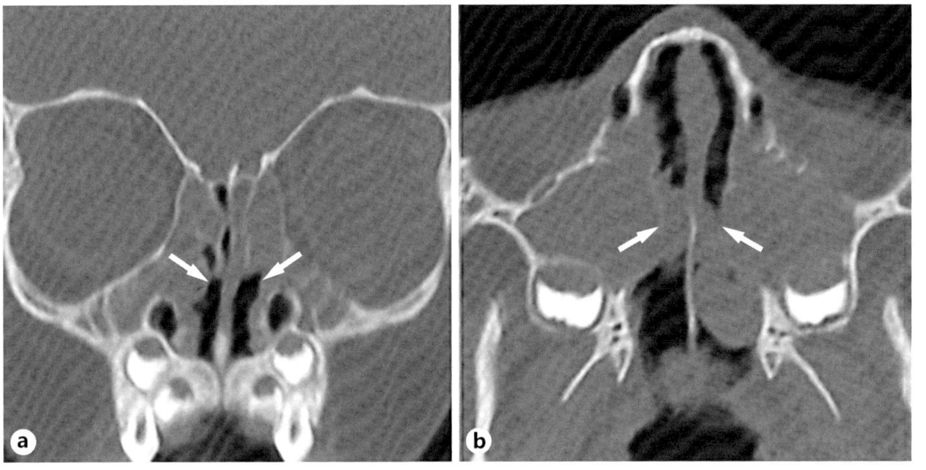

Fig. 2. a Coronal CT scan of a CF sinusitis patient showing hypoplastic maxillary sinus cavities. White arrows indicate demineralized uncinate process. **b** Axial CT scan of CF sinusitis patient with white arrows highlighting the medial bulging of the lateral sinonasal sidewall.

delay [19, 20]. The inconsistencies in sinus-related complaints make assessing the severity of sinus disease and response to treatment challenging.

Endoscopy

Rigid nasal endoscopy is an integral component of the physical examination for individuals with CF. The prevalence of nasal polyposis is present in up to 50% of CF patients and is found to increase with age [21]. Mucosal edema, inflammation and bulging of the sinonasal mucosa are characteristically discovered at the lateral wall middle meatus, but a small percentage of cases demonstrate an inflammatory process throughout the entire nasal cavity [13, 19, 22]. The finding of purulent nasal secretions is normally confined to the middle meatus, without extension into the sphenoethmoidal recess [18, 22]. The paranasal sinuses can become filled with thick viscous mucus that is culture positive for *Staphylococcus aureus* and *Haemophilus influenzae* in children and *Pseudomonas aeruginosa* among adults [23–26]. Correlating the data obtained from endoscopy with radiographic imaging provides key information in determining the best plan of treatment for CF nasal and sinus disease.

Imaging

CT imaging is a valuable tool to evaluate the extent of disease in CF sinusitis and to assess anatomy prior to any surgical interventions. Since individuals with CF show great anatomical variation of the sinuses, it is extremely important to carefully evaluate the CT scan before pursuing endoscopic sinus surgery. Patients with chronic rhinosinusitis and those with CF can both have findings of generalized sinus opacification and mucosal thickening on CT scans. However, one important finding on CT imaging that distinguishes patients with chronic rhinosinusitis from individuals with CF is the distinctive hypoplasia or even aplasia of the maxillary, ethmoid, frontal and sphenoid sinuses. The degree of sinus hypoplasia can be associated with the severity of the genotypic *CFTR* mutation [13, 27, 28]. Another typical CT imaging finding for CF patients is the medial bulging of the lateral sinonasal sidewall, with associated demineralization of the uncinate process (fig. 2) [13, 27, 28]. Other CT scan findings characteristic of CF include mucoceles and complete opacification of the sinuses, with the maxillary sinus carrying the largest burden of disease [18, 28]. While these findings assist with determining the extent nasal and sinus involvement, there is little correlation with CT imaging and the severity of CF disease [22].

Pathophysiology

Recent advances in electrophysiology, airway epithelial biology and animal model systems have shed light on the pathophysiology of CF in the airway. Although there is some controversy over the mechanism of impaired ion transport in CF, the end result of loss of CFTR results in viscous mucus, impaired mucociliary clearance and chronic infection and inflammation. Using a CFTR porcine knockout model, Stoltz et al. [29] found that CF pigs displayed a host defense defect against bacteria that contributed to airway inflammation. Pezzulo et al. [30] identified the impaired HCO_3^- transport and subsequent decreased pH in the CF airway epithelia as the cause of the innate immunity defect that resulted in chronic bacterial infection and inflammation of the upper and lower airway. These findings suggest that increasing the HCO_3^- delivery and pH to correct the innate immunity defect may be an effective approach to treat the chronic bacterial airway infections in CF.

Chang et al. [31] also used a porcine model to study the early pathogenesis of sinus disease in CF. They found that CF pigs have normal sinonasal epithelia but sinus hypoplasia at birth suggesting that the *CFTR* gene regulates sinus development. Additional findings showed that the CF pig sinus epithelia also had a defective anion transport similar to the defect identified by Chen et al. [32] in CF pig lung epithelia. Lastly, they demonstrated that CF pigs spontaneously developed sinus disease similar to humans with findings sinus opacification on CT imaging, thick viscous mucus and common CF pathogens.

To summarize, the loss of a functioning CFTR anion channel leads to upper and lower airway chronic bacterial infection, inflammation, impaired mucociliary clearance, and obstructive thick mucus, which complicate sinonasal and lung function in CF. The similar pathologic disease process that affects the airway epithelia in the sinonasal cavity and lung in CF support the unified airway model which suggests the health of the upper airway influences that of the lower airway and treatment of both areas synergistically improves the global CF airway disease state [2].

Current Treatment

The treatment of patients with CF requires a multidisciplinary team consisting of a primary care provider, pulmonologist, endocrinologist and otolaryngologist. In regards to CF sinus disease, patients require both preventative and therapeutic treatment methods (fig. 3). Preventative methods include routine use of isotonic or even hypertonic nasal saline to address the thick obstructing mucus caused by the impaired mucociliary clearance [33]. Therapeutic measures involve administration of both topical nasal steroids and use of systemic steroids to treat the chronic inflammation in the sinonasal cavity [34, 35].

There have been many studies investigating the similarities between the bacterial pathogens typically cultured in CF patients from the sinonasal cavity and in the lungs. In the early stages of CF disease, both the sinonasal cavity and lungs are commonly infected with *Staphylococcus aureus*, *Haemophilus influenza* and *Streptococcus pneumonia*. Therapeutic methods involve culture-directed antibiotic therapy to eliminate these common acute stage pathogens. The addition of low dose long-term macrolide therapy in multiple

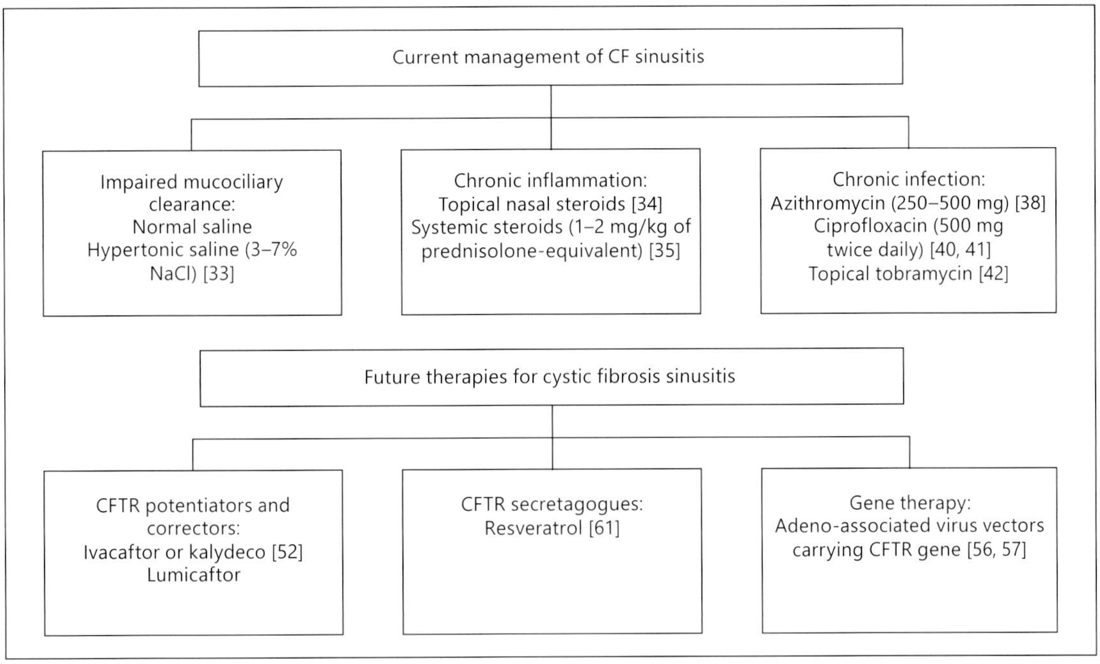

Fig. 3. Medical management of CF sinusitis.

studies has demonstrated modest improvement in lung function, weight gain and reduction in pulmonary exacerbations in CF patients due to the anti-inflammatory and immunomodulation activity of the antibiotic [36–39]. Antibiotics like ciprofloxacin and topical tobramycin also help decrease the severity of chronic infection [40–42].

In the later stages of CF disease, *Pseudomonas aeruginosa* is the predominant bacterial pathogen found in the sinonasal cavity and lungs [43, 44]. Early aggressive treatment of the lungs to eliminate *P. aeruginosa* has shown to be an important element in prolonging lifespan in CF. Unfortunately, the lungs eventually become recolonized with bacteria that adapt and become more drug-resistant and form biofilms that make them even more challenging to eliminate. The use of low dose long-term macrolide therapy in CF patients has been successful in treating the upper and lower airways of patients colonized with *P. aeruginosa* due to the macrolide-related function of decreasing sputum viscoelasticity and airway adhesion, and disrupting biofilm integrity [39, 45, 46].

In addition to treating CF medically, functional endoscopic sinus surgery also plays a role in disease management. However, since some CF patients exhibit very few signs and symptoms of sinus disease and function quite well from a sinonasal perspective, the presence of nasal polyps alone should not be an indication for sinus surgery. Those CF patients that undergo surgery have significant improvements in symptom relief. The primary risk factor of surgery in people with CF is associated with lung function. Therefore timing of the surgery should be performed when CF patients are at their best lung function, and in select cases can even be performed as outpatient procedures. The goal of surgery focuses on removing the obstructing nasal polyps, flushing out the thick obstructive mucus and widely opening the sinus cavities to permit aeration, drainage and postoperative nasal irrigation.

There are several studies documenting the various effect of endoscopic sinus surgery on reducing CF lung disease, especially in patients undergoing lung transplantation [47]. The improvement in lung function after reducing the sinonasal disease burden is likely associated with the finding of similar strains of *P. aeruginosa* in the lungs and sinonasal cavity after previous aggressive antibiotic treatment [43, 44]. These observational outcomes further suggest that the sinonasal cavity may serve as a reservoir for bacteria transmission to the lower airway and that aggressive treatment of CF-related infections within the sinuses may improve the health of the lungs [48, 49].

Future Therapies

Currently, there are no medical or surgical treatments that resulted in the reversal of the CT imaging findings of CF sinusitis. McMurphy et al. [50] evaluated 134 CF patients that underwent medical and surgical management and found no significant differences on CT imaging findings. Other studies actually demonstrated considerably worse outcomes after medical and surgical treatment of CF sinusitis, highlighting the likely inevitable progression of the disease [28].

The introduction of the drug VX-770, also known as ivacaftor or kalydeco marked a major advancement in CF medical therapy. Ivacaftor is the first US Food and Drug Administration (FDA) approved therapy to target the molecular defect in CF. It facilitates the opening of the defective CFTR channels, thus serving as a 'potentiator' of CFTR activity [51]. The initial randomized trial administrating ivacaftor to CF patients with the G551D mutation demonstrated clinical improvements in lung function and anion transport [52]. Another study showed reversal of chronic sinusitis based on nasal endoscopy and CT imaging in a CF patient treated with ivacaftor. The investigators speculated that the mechanism of CF sinusitis reversal due to CFTR modulation resulted from a decrease in mucus viscosity and an increase in sinonasal epithelia pH, which could potentiate the impaired host defense previously discussed [53]. The effect of ivacaftor is limited to CF patients with the G551D mutation (Class III mutation), where the CFTR protein is present but inactive due to defective regulation, which is unfortunately only present in 5% of the CF population [52]. An additional downside is the high cost of the medication and the possible need to be administered indefinitely [54]. Nonetheless, the discovery of ivacaftor opened doors to novel therapies investigating other small, organic molecules that could activate defective CFTR channels [51].

Recently, the FDA approved the first therapy that targets the most common CF mutation (ΔF508) and thus acts as a 'corrector' of the underlying genetic defect. The makeup of this drug is a combination of the CFTR potentiator (ivacaftor) and a CFTR corrector (lumacaftor), which functions by partially rescuing the ΔF508-CFTR trafficking to the membrane. In a phase III clinical trial, the combination therapy of ivacaftor and lumacaftor resulted in a modest improvement in lung function in CF patients homozygous for the ΔF508 mutation, and studies assessing the sinuses are pending [55].

The current research highlighted above illustrates why CF is a disease process that is an appealing candidate for gene therapy due to the genetic defect originating from a single gene. The implementation of topical gene therapy targeting the sinonasal cavity offers a potential treatment approach for CF sinus disease. Prior attempts to correct the *CFTR* defect in the sinuses of humans with topical delivery of an adeno-associated virus vector carrying the *CFTR* gene showed dose-dependent gene transfer and ion transport changes, but did not show a change in primary or secondary outcomes [56, 57]. However, these finding may be confounded due to advanced stage sinus disease and corresponding chronic inflammation in the adult human subjects.

Resveratrol is an organic polyphenol found in many plants and vegetables, including the skins of red fruits, flowers, peanuts and trees [58, 59]. Previous studies have demonstrated the immune modulator and anti-inflammatory properties of resveratrol [60]. Woodworth et al. [61] demonstrated in a mouse model that resveratrol is a robust CFTR channel potentiator of sinonasal epithelia due to its Cl^- secretagogue activity. The compound effectively activated the dysfunctional CFTR channel stimulating trans-epithelial anion secretion, which improved fluid and electrolyte transport, and increased hydration of airway surface liquid interface lining the sinonasal epithelium [62]. Activation of CFTR channels with resveratrol and other Cl^- secretagogues provides another innovative approach to treating CFTR defects in CF sinus disease.

Conclusion

Nearly all people with CF will develop CF sinusitis, characterized by thick mucus, impaired mucociliary clearance, chronic infection and inflammation of the sinonasal cavity and distinct radiographic CT findings of sinus hypoplasia or aplasia. Our current therapies are aimed at treating the symptoms of disease, and include sinonasal irrigations, topical and oral antibiotics and steroids, and endoscopic sinus surgery with improvements in outcomes. However, novel therapies designed at targeting the primary defect of CF are giving promise of reversing CF sinus disease and the potential for disease prevention.

References

1 Gysin C, Alothman GA, Papsin BC: Sinonasal disease in cystic fibrosis: clinical characteristics, diagnosis, and management. Pediatr Pulmonol 2000;30:481–489.
2 Quinton PM: Physiological basis of cystic fibrosis: a historical perspective. Physiol Rev 1999;79(1 suppl):S3–S22.
3 Welsh MJ, Ramsey BW, Accurso F, Cutting GR: Cystic Fibrosis. The Metabolic and Molecular Basis of Inherited Disease. New York, McGraw-Hill, 2001.
4 Cystic Fibrosis Foundation: Cystic Fibrosis Foundation Patient Registry: 2013 Annual Data Report. Bethesda, Cystic Fibrosis Foundation, 2013. https://www.cff.org/2013_CFF_Patient_Registry_Annual_Data_Report.pdf (accessed November 15, 2015).
5 Tos M: Distribution of mucus producing elements in the respiratory tract. Differences between upper and lower airway. Eur J Respir Dis Suppl 1983;128(pt 1):269–279.
6 Wine JJ, King VV, Lewiston NJ: Method for rapid evaluation of topically applied agents to cystic fibrosis airways. Am J Physiol 1991;261(2 pt 1):L218–L221.
7 Riordan JR, Rommens JM, Kerem B, Alon N, Rozmahel R, Grzelczak Z, Zielenski J, Lok S, Plavsic N, Chou JL, et al: Identification of the cystic fibrosis gene: cloning and characterization of complementary DNA. Science 1989;245:1066–1073.
8 Welsh MJ, Smith AE: Molecular mechanisms of CFTR chloride channel dysfunction in cystic fibrosis. Cell 1993;73:1251–1254.
9 Voter KZ, Ren CL: Diagnosis of cystic fibrosis. Clin Rev Allergy Immunol 2008;35:100–106.
10 King VV: Upper respiratory disease, sinusitis, and polyposis. Clin Rev Allergy 1991;9:143–157.
11 Nishioka GJ, Cook PR: Paranasal sinus disease in patients with cystic fibrosis. Otolaryngol Clin North Am 1996;29:193–205.
12 Robertson JM, Friedman EM, Rubin BK: Nasal and sinus disease in cystic fibrosis. Paediatr Respir Rev 2008;9:213–219.
13 Brihaye P, Jorissen M, Clement PA: Chronic rhinosinusitis in cystic fibrosis (mucoviscidosis). Acta Otorhinolaryngol Belg 1997;51:323–337.
14 Cepero R, Smith RJ, Catlin FI, Bressler KL, Furuta GT, Shandera KC: Cystic fibrosis – an otolaryngologic perspective. Otolaryngol Head Neck Surg 1987;97:356–360.
15 Cuyler JP, Monaghan AJ: Cystic fibrosis and sinusitis. J Otolaryngol 1989;18:173–175.
16 Duplechain JK, White JA, Miller RH: Pediatric sinusitis. The role of endoscopic sinus surgery in cystic fibrosis and other forms of sinonasal disease. Arch Otolaryngol Head Neck Surg 1991;117:422–426.
17 Gentile VG, Isaacson G: Patterns of sinusitis in cystic fibrosis. Laryngoscope 1996;106:1005–1009.
18 Coste A, Gilain L, Roger G, Sebbagh G, Lenoir G, Manach Y, Peynegre R: Endoscopic and CT-scan evaluation of rhinosinusitis in cystic fibrosis. Rhinology 1995;33:152–156.
19 Ramos RT, Salles C, Gregorio PB, Barros AT, Santana A, Araujo-Filho JB, Acosta AX: Evaluation of the upper airway in children and adolescents with cystic fibrosis and obstructive sleep apnea syndrome. Int J Pediatr Otorhinolaryngol 2009;73:1780–1785.

20 Scaparrotta A, Di Pillo S, Attanasi M, Consilvio NP, Cingolani A, Rapino D, Mohn A, Chiarelli F: Growth failure in children with cystic fibrosis. J Pediatr Endocrinol Metab 2012;25:393–405.
21 Mainz JG, Koitschev A: Pathogenesis and management of nasal polyposis in cystic fibrosis. Curr Allergy Asthma Rep 2012;12:163–174.
22 Sakano E, Ribeiro AF, Barth L, Condino Neto A, Ribeiro JD: Nasal and paranasal sinus endoscopy, computed tomography and microbiology of upper airways and the correlations with genotype and severity of cystic fibrosis. Int J Pediatr Otorhinolaryngol 2007;71:41–50.
23 Shapiro ED, Milmoe GJ, Wald ER, Rodnan JB, Bowen AD: Bacteriology of the maxillary sinuses in patients with cystic fibrosis. J Infect Dis 1982;146:589–593.
24 Muhlebach MS, Miller MB, Moore C, Wedd JP, Drake AF, Leigh MW: Are lower airway or throat cultures predictive of sinus bacteriology in cystic fibrosis? Pediatr Pulmonol 2006;41:445–451.
25 Moss RB, King VV: Management of sinusitis in cystic fibrosis by endoscopic surgery and serial antimicrobial lavage. Reduction in recurrence requiring surgery. Arch Otolaryngol Head Neck Surg 1995;121:566–572.
26 Wise SK, Kingdom TT, McKean L, DelGaudio JM, Venkatraman G: Presence of fungus in sinus cultures of cystic fibrosis patients. Am J Rhinol 2005;19:47–51.
27 Nishioka GJ, Cook PR, McKinsey JP, Rodriguez FJ: Paranasal sinus computed tomography scan findings in patients with cystic fibrosis. Otolaryngol Head Neck Surg 1996;114:394–399.
28 Eggesbo HB, Sovik S, Dolvik S, Kolmannskog F: CT characterization of inflammatory paranasal sinus disease in cystic fibrosis. Acta Radiol 2002;43:21–28.
29 Stoltz DA, Meyerholz DK, Pezzulo AA, Ramachandran S, Rogan MP, Davis GJ, Hanfland RA, Wohlford-Lenane C, Dohrn CL, Bartlett JA, Nelson GA 4th, Chang EH, Taft PJ, Ludwig PS, Estin M, Hornick EE, Launspach JL, Samuel M, Rokhlina T, Karp PH, Ostedgaard LS, Uc A, Starner TD, Horswill AR, Brogden KA, Prather RS, Richter SS, Shilyansky J, McCray PB Jr, Zabner J, Welsh MJ: Cystic fibrosis pigs develop lung disease and exhibit defective bacterial eradication at birth. Sci Transl Med 2010;2:29ra31.
30 Pezzulo AA, Tang XX, Hoegger MJ, Alaiwa MH, Ramachandran S, Moninger TO, Karp PH, Wohlford-Lenane CL, Haagsman HP, van Eijk M, Bánfi B, Horswill AR, Stoltz DA, McCray PB Jr, Welsh MJ, Zabner J: Reduced airway surface pH impairs bacterial killing in the porcine cystic fibrosis lung. Nature 2012;487:109–113.
31 Chang EH, Pezzulo AA, Meyerholz DK, Potash AE, Wallen TJ, Reznikov LR, Sieren JC, Karp PH, Ernst S, Moninger TO, Gansemer ND, McCray PB Jr, Stoltz DA, Welsh MJ, Zabner J: Sinus hypoplasia precedes sinus infection in a porcine model of cystic fibrosis. Laryngoscope 2012;122:1898–1905.
32 Chen JH, Stoltz DA, Karp PH, Ernst SE, Pezzulo AA, Moninger TO, Rector MV, Reznikov LR, Launspach JL, Chaloner K, Zabner J, Welsh MJ: Loss of anion transport without increased sodium absorption characterizes newborn porcine cystic fibrosis airway epithelia. Cell 2010; 143:911–923.
33 Reeves EP, Molloy K, Pohl K, McElvaney NG: Hypertonic saline in treatment of pulmonary disease in cystic fibrosis. ScientificWorldJournal 2012;2012: 465230.
34 Hadfield PJ, Rowe-Jones JM, Mackay IS: A prospective treatment trial of nasal polyps in adults with cystic fibrosis. Rhinology 2000;38:63–65.
35 Cheng K, Ashby D, Smyth RL: Oral steroids for long-term use in cystic fibrosis. Cochrane Database Syst Rev 2013; 6:CD000407.
36 Black PN: Anti-inflammatory effects of macrolide antibiotics. Eur Respir J 1997; 10:971–972.
37 Hansen CR, Pressler T, Koch C, Hoiby N: Long-term azitromycin treatment of cystic fibrosis patients with chronic Pseudomonas aeruginosa infection; an observational cohort study. J Cyst Fibros 2005;4:35–40.
38 Clement A, Tamalet A, Leroux E, Ravilly S, Fauroux B, Jais JP: Long term effects of azithromycin in patients with cystic fibrosis: a double blind, placebo controlled trial. Thorax 2006;61:895–902.
39 Yasuda H, Ajiki Y, Koga T, Kawada H, Yokota T: Interaction between biofilms formed by Pseudomonas aeruginosa and clarithromycin. Antimicrob Agents Chemother 1993;37:1749–1755.
40 Oomen KP, April MM: Sinonasal manifestations in cystic fibrosis. Int J Otolaryngol 2012;2012:789572.
41 Leung RS, Katial R: The diagnosis and management of acute and chronic sinusitis. Prim Care 2008;35:11–24.
42 Gysin C, Alothman GA, Papsin BC: Sinonasal disease in cystic fibrosis: clinical characteristics, diagnosis, and management. Pediatr Pulmonol 2000;30:481–489.
43 Burns JL, Gibson RL, McNamara S, Yim D, Emerson J, Rosenfeld M, Hiatt P, McCoy K, Castile R, Smith AL, Ramsey BW: Longitudinal assessment of Psuedomonas aeruginosa in young children with cystic fibrosis. J Infect Dis 2001;183: 444–452.
44 Koch C: Early infection and progression of cystic fibrosis lung disease. Pediatr Pulmonol 2002;34:232–236.
45 Hodge S, Hodge G, Brozyna S, Jersmann H, Holmes M, Reynolds PN: Azithromycin increases phagocytosis of apoptotic bronchial epithelial cells by alveolar macrophages. Eur Respir J 2006;28:486–495.
46 Tamaoki J: The effects of macrolides on inflammatory cells. Chest 2004;125(2 suppl):41S–50S; quiz 51S.
47 Holzmann D, Speich R, Kaufmann T, Laube I, Russi EW, Simmen D, Weder W, Boehler A: Effects of sinus surgery in patients with cystic fibrosis after lung transplantation: a 10-year experience. Transplantation 2004;77:134–136.
48 Jones JW, Parsons DS, Cuyler JP: The results of functional endoscopic sinus (FES) surgery on the symptoms of patients with cystic fibrosis. Int J Pediatr Otorhinolaryngol 1993;28:25–32.
49 Rosbe KW, Jones DT, Rahbar R, Lahiri T, Auerbach AD: Endoscopic sinus surgery in cystic fibrosis: do patients benefit from surgery? Int J Pediatr Otorhinolaryngol 2001;61:113–119.
50 McMurphy AB, Morriss C, Roberts DB, Friedman EM: The usefulness of computed tomography scans in cystic fibrosis patients with chronic sinusitis. Am J Rhinol 2007;21:706–710.
51 Chang EH: New insights into the pathogenesis of cystic fibrosis sinusitis. Int Forum Allergy Rhinol 2014;4:132–137.

52 Accurso FJ, Rowe SM, Clancy JP, Boyle MP, Dunitz JM, Durie PR, Sagel SD, Hornick DB, Konstan MW, Donaldson SH, Moss RB, Pilewski JM, Rubenstein RC, Uluer AZ, Aitken ML, Freedman SD, Rose LM, Mayer-Hamblett N, Dong Q, Zha J, Stone AJ, Olson ER, Ordoñez CL, Campbell PW, Ashlock MA, Ramsey BW: Effect of VX-770 in persons with cystic fibrosis and the G551D-CFTR mutation. N Engl J Med 2010;363:1991–2003.

53 Chang EH, Tang XX, Shah VS, Launspach JL, Ernst SE, Hilkin B, Karp PH, Abou Alaiwa MH, Graham SM, Hornick DB, Welsh MJ, Stoltz DA, Zabner J: Medical reversal of chronic sinusitis in a cystic fibrosis patient with ivacaftor. Int Forum Allergy Rhinol 2015;5:178–181.

54 Kaiser J: Personalized medicine. New cystic fibrosis drug offers hope, at a price. Science 2012;335:645.

55 Wainwright CE, Elborn JS, Ramsey BW: Lumacaftor-Ivacaftor in patients with cystic fibrosis homozygous for Phe508del CFTR. N Engl J Med 2015; 373:220–231.

56 Wagner JA, Moran ML, Messner AH, Daifuku R, Conrad CK, Reynolds T, Guggino WB, Moss RB, Carter BJ, Wine JJ, Flotte TR, Gardner P: A phase I/II study of tgAAV-CF for the treatment of chronic sinusitis in patients with cystic fibrosis. Hum Gene Ther 1998;9:889–909.

57 Wagner JA, Nepomuceno IB, Messner AH, Moran ML, Batson EP, Dimiceli S, Brown BW, Desch JK, Norbash AM, Conrad CK, Guggino WB, Flotte TR, Wine JJ, Carter BJ, Reynolds TC, Moss RB, Gardner P: A phase II, double-blind, randomized, placebo-controlled clinical trial of tgAAVCF using maxillary sinus delivery in patients with cystic fibrosis with antrostomies. Hum Gene Ther 2002;13:1349–1359.

58 Lee M, Kim S, Kwon OK, Oh SR, Lee HK, Ahn K: Anti-inflammatory and anti-asthmatic effects of resveratrol, a polyphenolic stilbene, in a mouse model of allergic asthma. Int Immunopharmacol 2009;9:418–424.

59 Donnelly LE, Newton R, Kennedy GE, Fenwick PS, Leung RH, Ito K, Russell RE, Barnes PJ: Anti-inflammatory effects of resveratrol in lung epithelial cells: molecular mechanisms. Am J Physiol Lung Cell Mol Physiol 2004; 287:L774–L783.

60 Manna SK, Mukhopadhyay A, Aggarwal BB: Resveratrol suppresses TNF-induced activation of nuclear transcription factors NF-kappa B, activator protein-1, and apoptosis: potential role of reactive oxygen intermediates and lipid peroxidation. J Immunol 2000;164: 6509–6519.

61 Woodworth BA: Resveratrol ameliorates abnormalities of fluid and electrolyte secretion in a hypoxia-induced model of acquired CFTR deficiency. Laryngoscope 2015;125(suppl 7):S1–S13.

62 Alexander NS, Hatch N, Zhang S, Skinner D, Fortenberry J, Sorscher EJ, Woodworth BA: Resveratrol has salutary effects on mucociliary transport and inflammation in sinonasal epithelium. Laryngoscope 2011;121:1313–1319.

Eugene Chang, MD
Department of Otolaryngology – Head and Neck Surgery
The University of Arizona College of Medicine
1501 N. Campbell Ave., PO Box 245074, Tucson, AZ 85724 (USA)
E-Mail echang@oto.arizona.edu

Woodworth BA, Poetker DM, Reh DD (eds): Rhinosinusitis with Nasal Polyposis.
Adv Otorhinolaryngol. Basel, Karger, 2016, vol 79, pp 38–47 (DOI: 10.1159/000445094)

Influence of P-Glycoprotein Function on Chronic Rhinosinusitis/Nasal Polyps Pathophysiology

Y. Song Cheng · Benjamin S. Bleier

Department of Otolaryngology – Head and Neck Surgery, Massachusetts Eye and Ear Infirmary, Boston, Mass., USA

Abstract

Permeability glycoprotein (P-gp) is an active efflux membrane transporter that has been researched extensively due to its ability to confer multidrug resistance in a wide range of cancers. P-gp has an impressively broad substrate specificity and is known to interact with hundreds of compounds, including drugs and toxins. This substrate promiscuity is the key to its physiological role, and P-gp is thought to be responsible for extruding xenobiotics and cellular metabolites, as well as maintaining tissue barriers at the blood–brain interface and gastrointestinal epithelium. In addition, P-gp is thought to be involved in regulating immune responses and is able to influence the secretion of cytokines and chemokines. This role as an immunomodulator links P-gp activity in the sinonasal epithelium with chronic rhinosinusitis (CRS), and a series of studies have provided evidence suggesting that P-gp may be a potential therapeutic target for treating CRS. Here, we highlight key knowledge about this intriguing protein, which may offer an important advancement in our understanding of CRS pathogenesis.

Introduction

Chronic rhinosinusitis (CRS) is an inflammatory disorder of the nose and paranasal sinuses. It is a common disease affecting about 12% of the U.S. population, but the pathogenesis of CRS is not well understood [1, 2]. Proposed etiologies can be broadly divided into exogenous insults (i.e., reaction to fungal antigen, superantigen, microbial biofilm or abnormal microbiome) and endogenous factors (i.e., dysregulation of epithelial barrier function, eicosanoid production or host immune response) [3]. It is widely accepted that exogenous factors can incite a host response and exacerbate CRS, but there is growing evidence that endogenous factors may be etiologic in the maintenance of the sustained inflammation that defines CRS [4].

Permeability glycoprotein (P-gp) is a membrane transporter that has been put forth recently as a potential player in the pathogenesis of CRS. P-gp is so named because it modulates the permeability of cell membranes to a broad range of chemically unrelated compounds including drugs, toxins, metabolites and even cytokines. This protein first intrigued researchers in the field of oncology because it was found to confer multidrug resistance (MDR) to cancer cell lines [5]. In attempting to manipulate P-gp activity to circumvent chemotherapy resistance, scientists revealed a central role in a wide range of physiological functions, including maintenance of the blood–brain barrier (BBB), preventing the accumulation of intracellular metabolite and xenobiotics and modulating immune responses through the regulation of cytokine secretion [6–8].

Clinically, P-gp has been shown to have a significant influence on drug bioavailability and therapeutic response to an astonishing range of drugs including anti-HIV agents, antiepileptics, antipsychotics, statins and glucocorticoids [7, 9–13]. Abnormal P-gp activity has also been implicated in the pathogenesis of several disorders including Alzheimer's disease, Parkinson's disease, inflammatory bowel diseases (IBD) and autoimmune diseases [14–18]. In the respiratory tract, polymorphisms in the P-gp gene are thought to influence the inflammatory response to environmental toxins such as cigarette smoke, and may have a role in the pathogenesis of lung cancer and chronic obstructive pulmonary disease [19, 20].

In 2012, the senior author's laboratory was the first to report on an association between P-gp expression and activity within the sinonasal mucosa and CRS-related inflammation [21–23]. Furthermore, our lab showed that P-gp is capable of modulating intracellular retention of corticosteroids within mucosal epithelial cells [24–26]. These features suggest that P-gp may offer a novel therapeutic target for managing CRS with multiple beneficial mechanisms of action. Here, we summarize briefly, the current knowledge on this interesting protein, and discuss recent studies exploring its role in perpetuating chronic inflammation in CRS.

Background

Discovery

In the mid-1970s, Ling and Thompson [5] reported that the expression of a membrane protein (later identified as P-gp) correlated proportionately to resistance to a wide range of drugs in Chinese hamster ovary mutants [27]. Further studies confirmed a causal link between the MDR phenotype and the expression of P-gp [28]. Detailed characterization of P-gp has revealed that it is an active efflux membrane transporter with very broad substrate specificity, thus explaining its ability to confer the MDR phenotype when overexpressed [29]. Since then, similar efflux pumps have been identified and are collectively classified as adenosine triphosphate (ATP)-binding cassette (ABC) transporters. The ABC transporter superfamily has a total of 7 subfamilies with 48 identified members in the human genome [30]. Within this large family, P-gp belongs to the 'B' subfamily and is sometimes referred to as ABCB1 protein.

Genetic Expression

The gene for P-gp, often referred to as *ABCB1* or *MDR1* gene, was identified in 1985 and is located on chromosome 7q21.12 [31]. In humans, this encodes for the 1280 amino acid forming the 170-kDa transmembrane glycoprotein transporter [32]. Polymorphisms and haplotypes for the *MDR1* gene have been identified and are associated with variations in P-gp function, but the clinical implications are currently unclear [7]. The expression and activity of P-gp is influenced by a wide range of extrinsic factors such as exposure to substrates, stress signals, heat shock, inflammation, hypoxia or UV irradiation, reflecting its role in protecting the cell [32]. Regulation of P-gp expression occurs at both the DNA and post-transcription level, and there are ongoing efforts to characterize these pathways with the hope of advancing treatment of MDR in cancer [33].

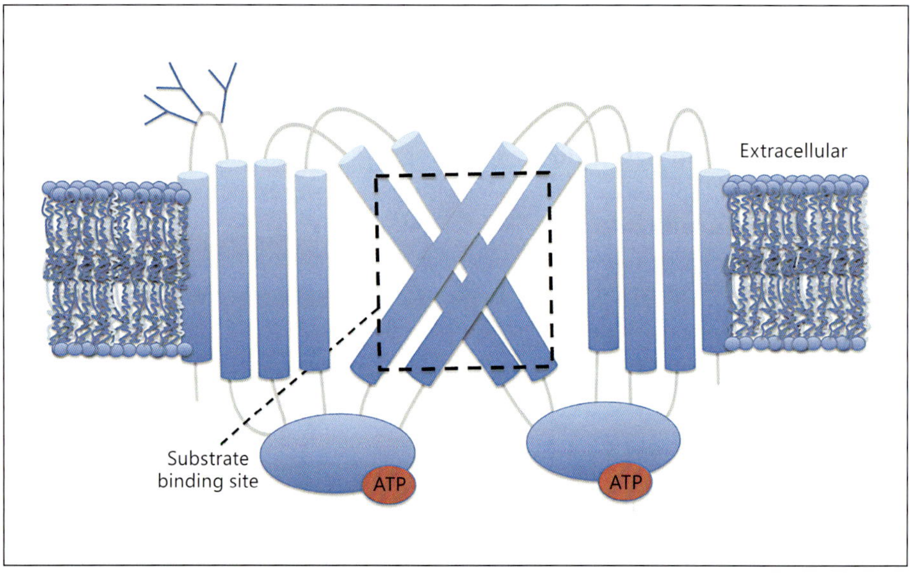

Fig. 1. Structure of human P-gp. Cylinders represent the 12 transmembrane domains. There are 2 intracytoplasmic ATP binding sites, which facilitate hydrolysis of ATP for active efflux of substrates. ATP = Adenosine triphosphate. Figure adapted from Loo and Clarke [99].

Structure

The P-gp transporter consists of 2 structurally identical halves, each with 6 transmembrane domains and a cytoplasmic ATP-binding site (fig. 1). X-ray crystal structures have revealed a highly flexible drug binding pocket with multiple sites of overlapping substrate specificity, which explains the promiscuity of P-gp [34–36]. This binding pocket is open to both the cytosol and cell membrane [29]. Substrates are transported via an alternate access mechanism that involves binding of substrate in the inward facing position, followed by a conformational change to an outward facing position that releases the substrate [37]. The hydrolysis of ATP resets the transporter to the inward facing position. P-gp has been described to function as a 'hydrophobic vacuum cleaner' by pumping substrates out into aqueous extracellular space [38]. Alternatively, P-gp has also been proposed to work as an outward-directed flippase, which constantly 'flips' substrates on the inner layer of the phospholipid bilayer to the outer layer, maintaining a high substrate concentration on the outer layer of the cell membrane [39, 40].

Anatomical Distribution

The anatomical distribution and polarized expression of P-gp is consistent with its role as an efflux pump involved in maintaining tissue barriers and extruding toxins. P-gp is constitutively expressed on the apical membrane of bile canaliculi in the liver, the ductal cells in the kidney and epithelial cells of the gastrointestinal tract [10, 41, 42]. It is also found in the endothelium of the BBB, the placenta and in the testis, where it is thought to protect these immune privileged sites from xenobiotics [43, 44]. Other anatomical areas that often express P-gp are the ductal cells of the breast, the pancreas and the adrenal cortex [42]. In the immune system, P-gp is expressed in adult hematopoietic stem cells, as well as in a range of leukocytes [45]. P-gp is also found within the respiratory tract including the sinonasal epithelium. P-gp expression in respiratory epithelium will be described in detail in the section titled *'P-gp in Chronic Rhinosinusitis'*.

Function of P-gp

P-gp as a Xenobiotic Efflux Pump

P-gp interacts with hundreds of compounds, which are generally amphipathic and have molecular masses ranging from 300 to 2,000 Da [35]. In the liver, it extrudes metabolites, toxins and drugs into the lumen of the biliary canaliculi [46]. In the gastrointestinal and respiratory tract, where epithelial cells are regularly in contact with the external environment, P-gp provides a barrier against lipophilic compounds, which could otherwise diffuse into cells with relative freedom [32]. As mentioned, P-gp also serves to provide a tissue barrier role at the BBB, the blood–testis barrier and placenta [43, 44]. Furthermore, the expression of P-gp on immune cells has pointed toward a role in hematopoietic stem cell development and immune response modulation [47, 48].

The Influence of P-gp on Multidrug Resistance and Corticosteroid Sensitivity

Cancers of tissue that intrinsically express P-gp such as colon, pancreatic, liver, adrenocortical and renal are associated with increased resistance to chemotherapy [49]. In cancers that do not usually have high P-gp activity (i.e., leukemia, lymphoma, breast, lung and ovarian cancers), overexpression of this membrane protein is associated with acquisition of the drug resistance phenotype [19, 50–52]. This link between P-gp activity and MDR phenotype in cancer led to the hypothesis that chemotherapy sensitivity can be restored by inhibiting P-gp activity, which has generated a great deal of interest in both cancer research and the pharmaceutical industry.

While P-gp inhibitors are generally well tolerated, the clinical use of these inhibitors in cancer has been hindered by complex drug–drug interactions [53]. Inhibition of P-gp influences gut absorption and drug permeability at the BBB resulting in unacceptable chemotherapy toxicity and severe central nervous system side effects [54]. Furthermore, P-gp has overlapping substrate specificity with cytochrome P450 (CYP3A4 isoform), which has an important role metabolizing drugs in the liver and therefore influences adverse reactions to a wide range of drugs [12].

Beyond cancer treatment, P-gp overexpression has also been linked to poor response to treatment in autoimmune and inflammatory disorders [13, 16, 18]. In IBD, overexpression of P-gp is independently associated with patients who require surgical intervention after failed glucocorticoid therapy [55]. Similar to chemotherapy resistance, it is hypothesized that P-gp overexpression induces steroid resistance by limiting intracellular retention [56–58]. Indeed, studies have found that P-gp is capable of transporting many steroids, including dexamethasone, prednisolone, budesonide, triamcinolone, cortisol, corticosterone and deoxycorticosterone, and intracellular corticosteroid activity can be potentiated by using P-gp inhibitors [59].

Corticosteroids are the mainstay of medical therapy for CRS but clinical response can be variable [60]. As in IBD, studies from our laboratory have demonstrated that retention of prednisone in nasal polyp explants can be regulated by P-gp [25]. This suggests that P-gp activity may influence the clinical response to steroids in CRS and overexpression may play a role in the development of steroid resistance. This finding raises the possibility that targeting P-gp activity could enhance intracellular steroid retention in CRS, thereby improving local efficacy while reducing systemic exposure.

P-gp as an Immunomodulator

Multiple lines of evidence suggest that P-gp is involved in modulating host immune reactions. P-gp is strongly expressed in CD56+ cells (natural killer cells) and is also found in CD4+, CD8+,

CD34+, CD15+, CD19+ and CD14+ cells in normal subjects [61–63]. The expression of P-gp is tightly regulated and thought to be important to the maturation of hematopoietic stem cells [45, 64]. P-gp-mediated secretion of cytokines and chemokines has been shown to be important in both T-cell activation and dendritic cell migration [65, 66]. As part of the complex network regulating immune response, P-gp expression is, in turn, influenced by inflammation [67]. However, studies characterizing this relationship have reported conflicting results, which may reflect differential regulation specific to cytokines and tissue types [6, 67, 68]. While the relationship between P-gp and inflammation requires further study, there is growing evidence that P-gp may play a primary role in local inflammation. This role as an immunomodulator provides a potential mechanism for its contribution to CRS pathogenesis.

P-gp in Chronic Rhinosinusitis

Sinonasal P-gp Expression and CRS Disease Severity

As previously mentioned, P-gp is expressed along the respiratory tract, where it is thought to participate in epithelial immune barrier function [20, 69]. In the lungs, P-gp is found on the apical membranes of tracheobronchial epithelial and alveolar epithelial type-1 cells. Within the upper respiratory tract, P-gp has been localized in both murine and bovine epithelial cells, nasal glands, vascular endothelium and olfactory mucosa [70], [71]. In human nasal mucosa, Henriksson et al. [72] demonstrated P-gp expression in both healthy mucosa as well as polypoid tissue. Wioland et al. [73] examined healthy human nasal turbinate mucosa and found intense expression of P-gp on both the apical and basolateral plasma membranes of ciliated cells.

To further characterize the local expression of P-gp in CRS, Bleier [21] performed quantitative fluorescent P-gp immunohistochemistry on sinus, septal and turbinate explants from patients with no sinonasal disease, CRS and CRS with nasal polyps (CRSwNP). P-gp expression was statistically different between all groups, with the greatest expression seen in the epithelium of patients with CRSwNP, and the least expression seen in healthy controls. Differences in expression within septal and inferior turbinate explants were not significant between the groups. This selective overexpression of P-gp in diseased tissue, but not in healthy tissue from adjacent sites, provided early evidence that P-gp may have a role in either the pathogenesis or maintenance of CRS.

Later studies found that known markers of CRS clinical severity predicted P-gp expression, further strengthening the link between P-gp and CRS pathogenesis [23, 74]. High P-gp expression was associated with significantly greater tissue eosinophil counts and Lund–Mackay scores (fig. 2) [23]. Similarly, P-gp overexpression was associated with increased osteitis burden as measured by the Kennedy Osteitis Score and the Global Osteitis Score [74].

P-gp as an Immunomodulator in CRS

Local overproduction of T-helper type 2 cells (Th2) skewing cytokines is a cardinal feature of eosinophilic CRS (eCRS) [75]. Multiple lines of evidence have demonstrated that the sinonasal epithelium is capable of independently orchestrating Th2 inflammation and eosinophil recruitment, but the mechanisms responsible for maintaining this over-secretion are not well understood [76, 77]. Non-classical pathways have been put forward because they may provide greater selectivity over microenvironmental cytokine release [78]. P-gp has been associated with cytokine release via these non-classical pathways, providing a potential mechanism through which the sinonasal epithelium can influence local cytokine environments [79, 80].

To investigate the physiologic role of P-gp as a sinonasal immunomodulator, P-gp expression and contribution to cytokine secretion were quantified in healthy primary nasal epithelial cell

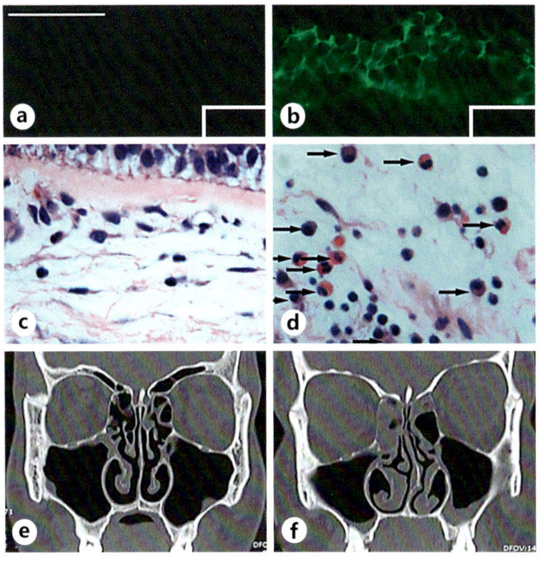

Fig. 2. Vertical columns depict findings from 2 distinct patients derived from the low (**a**, **c**, **e**) and high (**b**, **d**, **f**) P-gp expression groups [23]. **a**, **b** Fluorescent immunohistochemical images of mucosa depicting representative low (**a**) and high (**b**) expression of epithelial P-gp (bar = 50 μM, lower right inset represents negative control in which the primary antibody was omitted). **c**, **d** Matched high-powered (400×) H&E stromal images depicting the absence (**c**) and presence (**d**) of mucosal eosinophilia (black arrows denote individual eosinophils). Note the thickened basement membrane in (**c**) consistent with CRSsNP. **e**, **f** Coronal CT scans demonstrating increased radiographic inflammation in the patient with high P-gp expression (**f**) relative to the patient with low P-gp expression (**e**). CRSsNP = chronic rhinosinusitis without nasal polyps; H&E = hematoxylin and eosin. Figure reproduced from Feldman et al. [23].

cultures [81]. Stimulation of cells with lipopolysaccharide led to increased cytokine secretion as well as increased expression and activity of P-gp. Subsequent P-gp inhibition abrogated the secretion of IL-6, granulocyte macrophage colony-stimulating factor (GM-CSF) and thymic stromal lymphopoietin (TSLP), while IL-8 secretion was not affected. These findings pointed to P-gp as an active participant in epithelial derived inflammation which appeared to demonstrate a degree of cytokine selectivity.

In order to follow-up on these results, P-gp was next studied in nasal polyp-derived epithelial cultures. Here, inhibition of P-gp activity confirmed that the transporter is selectively involved in IL-6 and GM-CSF secretion, but not in IL-8 or IL-25 secretion [22]. Furthermore, the amount of cytokines released by the cell directly correlated with P-gp expression. To accurately replicate the complex immune environment of the sinonasal epithelium, which has multiple immune active cell populations, the influence of P-gp activity on IL-5, IL-8 and TSLP was next studied using organotypic explants derived from ethmoid mucosal from patients with CRS and CRSwNP [82]. Consistent with earlier studies, P-gp expression was significantly higher in CRSwNP than in CRS, and P-gp activity selectively influenced secretion of IL-5 and TSLP, but not IL-8 [22, 81, 83]. These findings were significant as they provided a link between the overexpression of P-gp previously described [21, 23, 74] and the supra-physiologic secretion of Th2 skewing cytokines such as IL-6, TSLP and GM-CSF within eCRS patients [75, 84].

P-gp Inhibition as a Therapeutic Strategy in CRS

The indication that P-gp may play a role in CRS pathogenesis raises the possibility of P-gp inhibition as a novel therapeutic strategy. Over the past decades, the search for a chemotherapy adjunct has led to the development of several generations of P-gp inhibitors, with the latest generation consisting of entirely new compounds with extremely high potency and P-gp selectivity. Verapamil was one of the first P-gp inhibitors identified [85]. It is an L-type calcium channel blocker that relaxes cardiac and vascular smooth muscle cells, and is commonly used to treat hypertension, angina and cardiac arrhythmias. Several studies, including our own [25], have reported that verapamil modulates inflammatory responses in human astrocytes and T cells, and even in animal models of asthma and hepatocyte inflammation [86–89]. To explore the possibility of verapamil as a therapeutic agent, Bleier et al. [83] compared the effect of verapamil and dexamethasone on sinonasal polyp explants. Verapamil demonstrated equivalent effects to the steroid in its ability to attenuate both IL-5 and IL-6 secretion. As verapamil has been safely used to treat cluster headache in otherwise healthy patients [90], this drug may represent a reasonable candidate to study clinically in patients with CRS.

Macrolide antibiotics and triazole antifungals are additional agents that are capable of inhibiting P-gp [91, 92]. Both macrolide antibiotics and triazole antifungals are effective in the treatment of CRS, but their effect appears to be independent of any obvious anti-microbial activity [93–95]. Macrolides have been shown to reduce pro-inflammatory cytokines in sinonasal mucosa [94, 96]. Azoles, too, have been shown to steer cytokine profiles away from Th2-biased pathways [97, 98]. To test whether these agents influence P-gp activity in the sinonasal epithelial cells, the senior author's lab quantified P-gp activity in the presence of these agents using a calcein acetoxymethyl ester assay [24]. The inhibitory dose response curves for both itraconazole and clarithromycin were found to be similar to that of Zosuquidar, a high affinity third generation P-gp inhibitor. This finding suggests that their anti-inflammatory properties in CRS may be derived in part from their influence on P-gp.

Conclusion

The development of targeted therapies for CRS is dependent on our evolving understanding of the etiopathogenesis of the disease. P-gp has emerged as a significant epithelial immunomodulator, which appears to play a key role in the orchestration and maintenance of CRS-related inflammation and the promotion of steroid resistance. Further studies are necessary to clarify its function. However, the existence of multiple candidate P-gp inhibitors suggests that P-gp targeted therapies may become an important addition to the clinical armamentarium for the management of patients with CRS.

Acknowledgment

The authors thank Sam Barber, MS, for his critical review of the manuscript.

References

1 Hamilos DL: Chronic rhinosinusitis: epidemiology and medical management. J Allergy Clin Immunol 2011;128:693–707; quiz 708–709.

2 Blackwell DL, Lucas JW, Clarke TC: Summary health statistics for U.S. adults: national health interview survey, 2012. Vital Health Stat 2014;10:1–161.

3 Lam K, Schleimer R, Kern RC: The Etiology and pathogenesis of chronic rhinosinusitis: a review of current hypotheses. Curr Allergy Asthma Rep 2015;15:41.

4 Hulse KE, Stevens WW, Tan BK, Schleimer RP: Pathogenesis of nasal polyposis. Clin Exp Allergy 2015;45:328–346.

5 Ling V, Thompson LH: Reduced permeability in CHO cells as a mechanism of resistance to colchicine. J Cell Physiol 1974;83:103–116.

6 Fernandez C, Buyse M, German-Fattal M, Gimenez F: Influence of the pro-inflammatory cytokines on P-glycoprotein expression and functionality. J Pharm Pharm Sci 2004;7:359–371.

7 Wolking S, Schaeffeler E, Lerche H, Schwab M, Nies AT: Impact of genetic polymorphisms of ABCB1 (MDR1, P-glycoprotein) on drug disposition and potential clinical implications: update of the literature. Clin Pharmacokinet 2015;54:709–735.

8 Nobili S, Landini I, Mazzei T, Mini E: Overcoming tumor multidrug resistance using drugs able to evade P-glycoprotein or to exploit its expression. Med Res Rev 2012;32:1220–1262.

9 Saneja A, Khare V, Alam N, Dubey RD, Gupta PN: Advances in P-glycoprotein-based approaches for delivering anticancer drugs: pharmacokinetic perspective and clinical relevance. Expert Opin Drug Deliv 2014;11:121–138.

10 Zakeri-Milani P, Valizadeh H: Intestinal transporters: enhanced absorption through P-glycoprotein-related drug interactions. Expert Opin Drug Metab Toxicol 2014;10:859–871.

11 Tempestilli M, Gentilotti E, Tommasi C, Nicastri E, Martini F, De Nardo P, Narciso P, Pucillo LP: Determination of P-glycoprotein surface expression and functional ability after in vitro treatment with darunavir or raltegravir in lymphocytes of healthy donors. Int Immunopharmacol 2013;16:492–497.

12 Burgess S, Partovi N, Yoshida EM, Erb SR, Azalgara VM, Hussaini T: Drug interactions with direct-acting antivirals for hepatitis C: implications for HIV and transplant patients. Ann Pharmacother 2015;49:674–687.

13 Barnes PJ, Adcock IM: Glucocorticoid resistance in inflammatory diseases. Lancet 2009;373:1905–1917.

14 Abuznait AH, Kaddoumi A: Role of ABC transporters in the pathogenesis of Alzheimer's disease. ACS Chem Neurosci 2012;3:820–831.

15 Narayan S, Sinsheimer JS, Paul KC, Liew Z, Cockburn M, Bronstein JM, Ritz B: Genetic variability in ABCB1, occupational pesticide exposure, and Parkinson's disease. Environ Res 2015;143(pt A):98–106.

16 Garcia-Carrasco M, Mendoza-Pinto C, Macias Diaz S, Vera-Recabarren M, Vazquez de Lara L, Mendez Martinez S, Soto-Santillan P, Gonzalez-Ramirez R, Ruiz-Arguelles A: P-glycoprotein in autoimmune rheumatic diseases. Autoimmun Rev 2015;14:594–600.

17 Tsujimura S, Saito K, Nakayamada S, Tanaka Y: Relevance of multidrug resistance 1 and P-glycoprotein to drug resistance in patients with systemic lupus erythematosus. Histol Histopathol 2007; 22:465–468.

18 De Iudicibus S, Franca R, Martelossi S, Ventura A, Decorti G: Molecular mechanism of glucocorticoid resistance in inflammatory bowel disease. World J Gastroenterol 2011;17:1095–1108.

19 Milojkovic M, Milacic N, Radovic J, Ljubisavljevic S: MDR1 gene polymorphisms and P-glycoprotein expression in respiratory diseases. Biomed Pap Med Fac Univ Palacky Olomouc Czech Repub 2015;159:341–346.

20 Scheffer GL, Pijnenborg AC, Smit EF, Müller M, Postma DS, Timens W, van der Valk P, de Vries EG, Scheper RJ: Multidrug resistance related molecules in human and murine lung. J Clin Pathol 2002;55:332–339.

21 Bleier BS: Regional expression of epithelial MDR1/P-glycoprotein in chronic rhinosinusitis with and without nasal polyposis. Int Forum Allergy Rhinol 2012;2:122–125.

22 Bleier BS, Nocera AL, Iqbal H, Hoang JD, Alvarez U, Feldman RE, Han X: P-glycoprotein promotes epithelial T helper 2-associated cytokine secretion in chronic sinusitis with nasal polyps. Int Forum Allergy Rhinol 2014;4:488–494.

23 Feldman RE, Lam AC, Sadow PM, Bleier BS: P-glycoprotein is a marker of tissue eosinophilia and radiographic inflammation in chronic rhinosinusitis without nasal polyps. Int Forum Allergy Rhinol 2013;3:684–687.

24 Lam A, Hoang JD, Singleton A, Han X, Bleier BS: Itraconazole and clarithromycin inhibit P-glycoprotein activity in primary human sinonasal epithelial cells. Int Forum Allergy Rhinol 2015;5: 477–480.

25 Kocharyan A, Feldman R, Singleton A, Han X, Bleier BS: P-glycoprotein inhibition promotes prednisone retention in human sinonasal polyp explants. Int Forum Allergy Rhinol 2014;4:734–738.

26 Bleier BS, Kocharyan A, Singleton A, Han X: Verapamil modulates interleukin-5 and interleukin-6 secretion in organotypic human sinonasal polyp explants. Int Forum Allergy Rhinol 2015;5: 10–13.

27 Juliano RL, Ling V: A surface glycoprotein modulating drug permeability in Chinese hamster ovary cell mutants. Biochim Biophys Acta 1976;455:152–162.

28 Debenham PG, Kartner N, Siminovitch L, Riordan JR, Ling V: DNA-mediated transfer of multiple drug resistance and plasma membrane glycoprotein expression. Mol Cell Biol 1982;2:881–889.

29 Aller SG, Yu J, Ward A, Weng Y, Chittaboina S, Zhuo R, Harrell PM, Trinh YT, Zhang Q, Urbatsch IL, Chang G: Structure of P-glycoprotein reveals a molecular basis for poly-specific drug binding. Science 2009;323:1718–1722.

30 Dean M, Rzhetsky A, Allikmets R: The human ATP-binding cassette (ABC) transporter superfamily. Genome Res 2001;11:1156–1166.

31 Riordan JR, Deuchars K, Kartner N, Alon N, Trent J, Ling V: Amplification of P-glycoprotein genes in multidrug-resistant mammalian cell lines. Nature 1985;316:817–819.

32 Sarkadi B, Homolya L, Szakacs G, Varadi A: Human multidrug resistance ABCB and ABCG transporters: participation in a chemoimmunity defense system. Physiol Rev 2006;86:1179–1236.

33 Fu D: Where is it and how does it get there – intracellular localization and traffic of P-glycoprotein. Front Oncol 2013;3:321.

34 Verhalen B, Ernst S, Borsch M, Wilkens S: Dynamic ligand-induced conformational rearrangements in P-glycoprotein as probed by fluorescence resonance energy transfer spectroscopy. J Biol Chem 2012;287:1112–1127.

35 Wen PC, Verhalen B, Wilkens S, Mchaourab HS, Tajkhorshid E: On the origin of large flexibility of P-glycoprotein in the inward-facing state. J Biol Chem 2013;288:19211–19220.

36 Martinez L, Arnaud O, Henin E, Tao H, Chaptal V, Doshi R, Andrieu T, Dussurgey S, Tod M, Di Pietro A, Zhang Q, Chang G, Falson P: Understanding polyspecificity within the substrate-binding cavity of the human multidrug resistance P-glycoprotein. FEBS J 2014;281: 673–682.

37 van Wonderen JH, McMahon RM, O'Mara ML, McDevitt CA, Thomson AJ, Kerr ID, MacMillan F, Callaghan R: The central cavity of ABCB1 undergoes alternating access during ATP hydrolysis. FEBS J 2014;281:2190–2201.

38 Higgins CF, Gottesman MM: Is the multidrug transporter a flippase? Trends Biochem Sci 1992;17:18–21.

39 Sharom FJ: Complex interplay between the P-glycoprotein multidrug efflux pump and the membrane: its role in modulating protein function. Front Oncol 2014;4:41.

40 Eytan GD: Mechanism of multidrug resistance in relation to passive membrane permeation. Biomed Pharmacother 2005;59:90–97.

41 Chu X, Bleasby K, Evers R: Species differences in drug transporters and implications for translating preclinical findings to humans. Expert Opin Drug Metab Toxicol 2013;9:237–252.

42 Cascorbi I: P-glycoprotein: tissue distribution, substrates, and functional consequences of genetic variations. Handb Exp Pharmacol 2011;201:261–283.

43 Miller DS: Regulation of ABC transporters blood-brain barrier: the good, the bad, and the ugly. Adv Cancer Res 2015; 125:43–70.

44 Huls M, Russel FG, Masereeuw R: The role of ATP binding cassette transporters in tissue defense and organ regeneration. J Pharmacol Exp Ther 2009;328: 3–9.
45 Chaudhary PM, Roninson IB: Expression and activity of P-glycoprotein, a multidrug efflux pump, in human hematopoietic stem cells. Cell 1991;66: 85–94.
46 Thiebaut F, Tsuruo T, Hamada H, Gottesman MM, Pastan I, Willingham MC: Cellular localization of the multidrug-resistance gene product P-glycoprotein in normal human tissues. Proc Natl Acad Sci U S A 1987;84:7735–7738.
47 Sigal N, Kaplan Zeevi M, Weinstein S, Peer D, Herskovits AA: The human P-glycoprotein transporter enhances the type I interferon response to Listeria monocytogenes infection. Infect Immun 2015;83:2358–2368.
48 Pilarski LM, Paine D, McElhaney JE, Cass CE, Belch AR: Multidrug transporter P-glycoprotein 170 as a differentiation antigen on normal human lymphocytes and thymocytes: modulation with differentiation stage and during aging. Am J Hematol 1995;49:323–335.
49 Gottesman MM, Pastan IH: The role of multidrug resistance efflux pumps in cancer: revisiting a JNCI publication exploring expression of the MDR1 (P-glycoprotein) gene. J Natl Cancer Inst 2015;107:pii:djv222.
50 Shaffer BC, Gillet JP, Patel C, Baer MR, Bates SE, Gottesman MM: Drug resistance: still a daunting challenge to the successful treatment of AML. Drug Resist Updat 2012;15:62–69.
51 van der Holt B, Lowenberg B, Burnett AK, Knauf WU, Shepherd J, Piccaluga PP, Ossenkoppele GJ, Verhoef GE, Ferrant A, Crump M, Selleslag D, Theobald M, Fey MF, Vellenga E, Dugan M, Sonneveld P: The value of the MDR1 reversal agent PSC-833 in addition to daunorubicin and cytarabine in the treatment of elderly patients with previously untreated acute myeloid leukemia (AML), in relation to MDR1 status at diagnosis. Blood 2005;106:2646–2654.
52 Trock BJ, Leonessa F, Clarke R: Multidrug resistance in breast cancer: a meta-analysis of MDR1/gp170 expression and its possible functional significance. J Natl Cancer Inst 1997;89:917–931.
53 Callaghan R, Luk F, Bebawy M: Inhibition of the multidrug resistance P-glycoprotein: time for a change of strategy? Drug Metab Dispos 2014;42:623–631.
54 Darby RA, Callaghan R, McMahon RM: P-glycoprotein inhibition: the past, the present and the future. Curr Drug Metab 2011;12:722–731.
55 Farrell RJ, Murphy A, Long A, Donnelly S, Cherikuri A, O'Toole D, Mahmud N, Keeling PW, Weir DG, Kelleher D: High multidrug resistance (P-glycoprotein 170) expression in inflammatory bowel disease patients who fail medical therapy. Gastroenterology 2000;118:279–288.
56 Sheng Y, Yang X, Pal D, Mitra AK: Prodrug approach to improve absorption of prednisolone. Int J Pharm 2015;487: 242–249.
57 Karssen AM, Meijer OC, van der Sandt IC, De Boer AG, De Lange EC, De Kloet ER: The role of the efflux transporter P-glycoprotein in brain penetration of prednisolone. J Endocrinol 2002;175:251–260.
58 Oka A, Oda M, Saitoh H, Nakayama A, Takada M, Aungst BJ: Secretory transport of methylprednisolone possibly mediated by P-glycoprotein in Caco-2 cells. Biol Pharm Bull 2002;25:393–396.
59 Webster JI, Carlstedt-Duke J: Involvement of multidrug resistance proteins (MDR) in the modulation of glucocorticoid response. J Steroid Biochem Mol Biol 2002;82:277–288.
60 Poetker DM, Jakubowski LA, Lal D, Hwang PH, Wright ED, Smith TL: Oral corticosteroids in the management of adult chronic rhinosinusitis with and without nasal polyps: an evidence-based review with recommendations. Int Forum Allergy Rhinol 2013;3:104–120.
61 Yamamoto T, Iwasaki T, Watanabe N, Oshimi K, Naito M, Tsuruo T, Kobayashi Y: Expression of multidrug resistance P-glycoprotein on peripheral blood mononuclear cells of patients with granular lymphocyte-proliferative disorders. Blood 1993;81:1342–1346.
62 Egashira M, Kawamata N, Sugimoto K, Kaneko T, Oshimi K: P-glycoprotein expression on normal and abnormally expanded natural killer cells and inhibition of P-glycoprotein function by cyclosporin A and its analogue, PSC833. Blood 1999;93:599–606.
63 Klimecki WT, Futscher BW, Grogan TM, Dalton WS: P-glycoprotein expression and function in circulating blood cells from normal volunteers. Blood 1994;83:2451–2458.
64 Kyle-Cezar F, Echevarria-Lima J, dos Santos Goldenberg RC, Rumjanek VM: Expression of c-kit and Sca-1 and their relationship with multidrug resistance protein 1 in mouse bone marrow mononuclear cells. Immunology 2007;121: 122–128.
65 Kooij G, Kroon J, Paul D, Reijerkerk A, Geerts D, van der Pol SM, van Het Hof B, Drexhage JA, van Vliet SJ, Hekking LH, van Buul JD, Pachter JS, de Vries HE: P-glycoprotein regulates trafficking of CD8(+) T cells to the brain parenchyma. Acta Neuropathol 2014;127:699–711.
66 Llaudo I, Cassis L, Torras J, Bestard O, Franquesa Ml, Cruzado JM, Cerezo G, Castano E, Petriz J, Herrero-Fresneda I, Grinyo JM, Lloberas N: Impact of small molecules immunosuppressants on P-glycoprotein activity and T-cell function. J Pharm Pharm Sci 2012;15:407–419.
67 Nakatsukasa H, Silverman JA, Gant TW, Evarts RP, Thorgeirsson SS: Expression of multidrug resistance genes in rat liver during regeneration and after carbon tetrachloride intoxication. Hepatology 1993;18:1202–1207.
68 Cherrington NJ, Slitt AL, Li N, Klaassen CD: Lipopolysaccharide-mediated regulation of hepatic transporter mRNA levels in rats. Drug Metab Dispos 2004;32: 734–741.
69 Campbell L, Abulrob AN, Kandalaft LE, Plummer S, Hollins AJ, Gibbs A, Gumbleton M: Constitutive expression of p-glycoprotein in normal lung alveolar epithelium and functionality in primary alveolar epithelial cultures. J Pharmacol Exp Ther 2003;304:441–452.
70 Kandimalla KK, Donovan MD: Localization and differential activity of P-glycoprotein in the bovine olfactory and nasal respiratory mucosae. Pharm Res 2005; 22:1121–1128.
71 Graff CL, Pollack GM: Functional evidence for P-glycoprotein at the nose-brain barrier. Pharm Res 2005;22:86–93.
72 Henriksson G, Norlander T, Zheng X, Stierna P, Westrin KM: Expression of P-glycoprotein 170 in nasal mucosa may be increased with topical steroids. Am J Rhinol 1997;11:317–321.
73 Wioland MA, Fleury-Feith J, Corlieu P, Commo F, Monceaux G, Lacau-St-Guily J, Bernaudin JF: CFTR, MDR1, and MRP1 immunolocalization in normal human nasal respiratory mucosa. J Histochem Cytochem 2000;48:1215–1222.

74 Gunel C, Feldman RE, Bleier BS: Osteitis is associated with P-glycoprotein overexpression in patients with chronic sinusitis without nasal polyps. Am J Rhinol Allergy 2014;28:99–102.
75 Kato A: Immunopathology of chronic rhinosinusitis. Allergol Int 2015;64:121–130.
76 Olze H, Forster U, Zuberbier T, Morawietz L, Luger EO: Eosinophilic nasal polyps are a rich source of eotaxin, eotaxin-2 and eotaxin-3. Rhinology 2006;44:145–150.
77 Van Crombruggen K, Zhang N, Gevaert P, Tomassen P, Bachert C: Pathogenesis of chronic rhinosinusitis: Inflammation. J Allergy Clin Immunol 2011;128:728–732.
78 Nickel W: The mystery of nonclassical protein secretion. A current view on cargo proteins and potential export routes. Eur J Biochem 2003;270:2109–2119.
79 Marty V, Medina C, Combe C, Parnet P, Amedee T: ATP binding cassette transporter ABC1 is required for the release of interleukin-1beta by P2X7-stimulated and lipopolysaccharide-primed mouse Schwann cells. Glia 2005;49:511–519.
80 Kooij G, Backer R, Koning JJ, Reijerkerk A, van Horssen J, van der Pol SM, Drexhage J, Schinkel A, Dijkstra CD, den Haan JM, Geijtenbeek TB, de Vries HE: P-glycoprotein acts as an immunomodulator during neuroinflammation. PLoS One 2009;4:e8212.
81 Bleier BS, Nocera AL, Iqbal H, Hoang JD, Feldman RE, Han X: P-glycoprotein functions as an immunomodulator in healthy human primary nasal epithelial cells. Int Forum Allergy Rhinol 2013;3:433–438.
82 Bleier BS, Singleton A, Nocera AL, Kocharyan A, Petkova V, Han X: P-glycoprotein regulates Staphylococcus aureus enterotoxin B-stimulated interleukin-5 and thymic stromal lymphopoietin secretion in organotypic mucosal explants. Int Forum Allergy Rhinol 2016;6:169–177.
83 Bleier BS, Kocharyan A, Singleton A, Han X: Verapamil modulates interleukin-5 and interleukin-6 secretion in organotypic human sinonasal polyp explants. Int Forum Allergy Rhinol 2015;5:10–13.
84 Peters AT, Kato A, Zhang N, Conley DB, Suh L, Tancowny B, Carter D, Carr T, Radtke M, Hulse KE, Seshadri S, Chandra R, Grammer LC, Harris KE, Kern R, Schleimer RP: Evidence for altered activity of the IL-6 pathway in chronic rhinosinusitis with nasal polyps. J Allergy Clin Immunol 2010;125:397–403.e10.
85 Tsuruo T, Iida H, Yamashiro M, Tsukagoshi S, Sakurai Y: Enhancement of vincristine- and adriamycin-induced cytotoxicity by verapamil in P388 leukemia and its sublines resistant to vincristine and adriamycin. Biochem Pharmacol 1982;31:3138–3140.
86 Hashioka S, Klegeris A, McGeer PL: Inhibition of human astrocyte and microglia neurotoxicity by calcium channel blockers. Neuropharmacology 2012;63:685–691.
87 Li G, Qi XP, Wu XY, Liu FK, Xu Z, Chen C, Yang XD, Sun Z, Li JS: Verapamil modulates LPS-induced cytokine production via inhibition of NF-kappa B activation in the liver. Inflamm Res 2006;55:108–113.
88 Matsumori A, Nishio R, Nose Y: Calcium channel blockers differentially modulate cytokine production by peripheral blood mononuclear cells. Circ J 2010;74:567–571.
89 Khakzad MR, Mirsadraee M, Mohammadpour A, Ghafarzadegan K, Hadi R, Saghari M, Meshkat M: Effect of verapamil on bronchial goblet cells of asthma: an experimental study on sensitized animals. Pulm Pharmacol Ther 2012;25:163–168.
90 Becker WJ: Cluster headache: conventional pharmacological management. Headache 2013;53:1191–1196.
91 Hughes J, Crowe A: Inhibition of P-glycoprotein-mediated efflux of digoxin and its metabolites by macrolide antibiotics. J Pharmacol Sci 2010;113:315–324.
92 Tapaninen T, Backman JT, Kurkinen KJ, Neuvonen PJ, Niemi M: Itraconazole, a P-glycoprotein and CYP3A4 inhibitor, markedly raises the plasma concentrations and enhances the renin-inhibiting effect of aliskiren. J Clin Pharmacol 2011;51:359–367.
93 Hashemi M, Fereidani A, Berjis N, Okhovat SA, Eshaghain A: Effectiveness of itraconazole on clinical symptoms and radiologic findings in patients with recurrent chronic rhinosinusitis and nasal polyposis. Adv Biomed Res 2014;3:162.
94 Peric A, Vojvodic D, Matkovic-Jozin S: Effect of long-term, low-dose clarithromycin on T helper 2 cytokines, eosinophilic cationic protein and the 'regulated on activation, normal T cell expressed and secreted' chemokine in the nasal secretions of patients with nasal polyposis. J Laryngol Otol 2012;126:495–502.
95 Wei CC, Adappa ND, Cohen NA: Use of topical nasal therapies in the management of chronic rhinosinusitis. Laryngoscope 2013;123:2347–2359.
96 Miyanohara T, Ushikai M, Matsune S, Ueno K, Katahira S, Kurono Y: Effects of clarithromycin on cultured human nasal epithelial cells and fibroblasts. Laryngoscope 2000;110:126–131.
97 Becker KL, Gresnigt MS, Smeekens SP, Jacobs CW, Magis-Escurra C, Jaeger M, Wang X, Lubbers R, Oosting M, Joosten LA, Netea MG, Reijers MH, van de Veerdonk FL: Pattern recognition pathways leading to a Th2 cytokine bias in allergic bronchopulmonary aspergillosis patients. Clin Exp Allergy 2015;45:423–437.
98 Agarwal R: What is the current place of azoles in allergic bronchopulmonary aspergillosis and severe asthma with fungal sensitization. Expert Rev Respir Med 2012;6:363–371.
99 Loo TW, Clarke DM: The transmission interfaces contribute asymmetrically to the assembly and activity of human P-glycoprotein. J Biol Chem 2015;290:16954–16963.

Benjamin S. Bleier, MD
Harvard Medical School, Massachusetts Eye and Ear Infirmary
Department of Otolaryngology – Head and Neck Surgery, 243 Charles Street
Boston, MA 02114 (USA)
E-Mail benjamin_bleier@meei.harvard.edu

Woodworth BA, Poetker DM, Reh DD (eds): Rhinosinusitis with Nasal Polyposis.
Adv Otorhinolaryngol. Basel, Karger, 2016, vol 79, pp 48–57 (DOI: 10.1159/000445129)

B-Cells and Antibody-Mediated Pathogenesis in Chronic Rhinosinusitis with Nasal Polyps

Jin-Young Min[a] • Kathryn E. Hulse[b] • Bruce K. Tan[a]

[a]Department of Otolaryngology, and [b]Division of Allergy-Immunology, Department of Medicine, Northwestern University Feinberg School of Medicine, Chicago, Ill., USA

Abstract

The sinonasal mucosa forms a dynamic immune barrier where epithelial cells and the immune system interact with the inhaled environment and nasal microbiome. Recent studies suggest that B-cells, plasma cells and antibody production are highly activated locally within the nasal mucosa of patients with chronic rhinosinusitis with nasal polyps (CRSwNP). Findings additionally suggest that polyp tissue contains elevated levels of cytokines, chemokines and complement that may drive this profound B-cell response. Currently, the data are conflicting on whether the B-cell response found in the CRSwNP nasal mucosa is antigen-specific, a superantigen response or an expansion of natural antibody responses. Indeed, investigations into the specificity of the mucosal antibody responses find increased production of class-switched antibodies that bind to aeroallergens, staphylococcus aureus as well as autoantigens. A continuation of these studies is needed to elucidate whether extrinsic factors, like the inhaled environment, or intrinsic factors, like the mucosal microbiome and host inflammatory response, are key to the pathogenesis of CRSwNP. This chapter will cover the current evidence regarding local B-cell responses in CRSwNP.

Overview of B-Cell Function and Pathways of Activation

B-cells are a subset of lymphocytes that contribute to the humoral adaptive immune response through their generation of antibodies. Antibodies are able to recognize a broad range of antigens through the tightly regulated process called V(D)J recombination and affinity maturation [1]. This process begins during development in the bone marrow or fetal liver, where a small number of genes recombine to generate a vast number of different antigen receptors. Because V(D)J recombination involves somatic gene rearrangement, all progeny of a particular B-cell clone will inherit the same receptor specificity [2]. Finally, human beings possess 5 isotypes of antibodies – IgM, IgD, IgG, IgA and IgE – that can exist both as cell surface receptors or secreted antibodies in the serum or in nasal secretions. The conjugation of a specific antibody with different isotypes does not alter its specific antigen recognition, but rather influences the nature of the biological response that will be triggered after the antibody binds to its cognate antigen.

In mice, there are 2 developmental pathways that lead to the generation of 2 distinct subsets of B-cells. While B1 B-cells develop in the fetal liver, B2 B-cells develop in the bone marrow, with each having distinct progenitor cells [3, 4]. B1 B-cells have been extensively studied in mice, but little is known about their function or identity in humans, in part due to difficulties in identifying them in humans [5]. Nonetheless, B1 B-cells journey to the pleural and peritoneal cavities, as well as to mucosal sites [3]. They produce large quantities of what are termed 'natural' antibodies, because they are polyreactive and recognize a variety of conserved microbial patterns that are critical for the control of infections at early time points. In contrast, B2 B-cells develop in the bone marrow, traffic to the periphery, where they undergo rapid differentiation through 2 transitional stages, generally in the spleen, and then become either marginal zone (MZ) or follicular B-cells [6, 7]. MZ B-cells, which, like B1 B-cells, are polyreactive and capable of T-dependent and independent activation, are located mainly in the marginal sinus of the spleen but possibly also in tonsils. Importantly, in humans, MZ B-cells can also recirculate through secondary lymphoid organs and are also found in blood [6, 8].

The proportion of B2 B-cells that develop into MZ B-cells is relatively small, and the majority of B2 B-cells will become follicular mature naïve B-cells [3, 8]. These B2 cells are activated in secondary lymphoid organs (e.g., lymph nodes, structures of the Waldeyer's ring) upon encounter with their cognate antigen (fig. 1). B-cell activation in secondary lymphoid organs leads to the development of a secondary follicle, which contains a germinal center where the B-cells interact with T-follicular helper (T_{FH}) cells to differentiate into either long-lived memory B-cells or plasma cells [9, 10]. Memory B2 cells continue to recirculate through the secondary lymphoid organs and can be rapidly reactivated upon secondary antigen encounter whereas plasma cells are terminally differentiated antibody-secreting cells. The B2 cells generated by a germinal center reaction have a high affinity for their antigen but significantly restricted antigen binding specificity. These cells can remain at the site of original antigen encounter for up to a week, or they can traffic to the bone marrow where they can survive and continue to secrete antibodies for decades [3].

Factors Promoting B-Cell Activation in CRSwNP

Nasal polyps from CRSwNP patients are characterized by elevations in a variety of inflammatory mediators. Interestingly, some of these mediators are known to play roles in the activation, survival and recruitment of B-cells in secondary lymphoid organs or the bone marrow (fig. 2). These factors include inflammatory cytokines and chemokines, and complement pathway products.

Cytokines

A variety of cytokines are known to be upregulated in CRSwNP [11]. Of these, B-cell activating factor of the TNF family (BAFF) is known to play a critical role in B-cell activation, differentiation and survival. It is thought that BAFF is mainly produced by activated epithelium and dendritic cells, but eosinophils in nasal polyp tissues are also reported to produce this cytokine [12]. BAFF signaling on B-cells promotes their activation and the induction of class switch recombination. Interestingly, the related molecule, a proliferation inducing ligand (APRIL) produced by eosinophils, has been shown to play a critical role in the survival of long-lived plasma cells in the bone marrow [13]. These data suggest that the significantly elevated levels of eosinophils in nasal polyps may play an important role in the survival and activation of B-cells in the tissue. Furthermore, overexpression of BAFF in murine models results in the development of autoimmunity that is similar to systemic lupus erythematosis (SLE) [14]. This also suggests that elevations in BAFF within

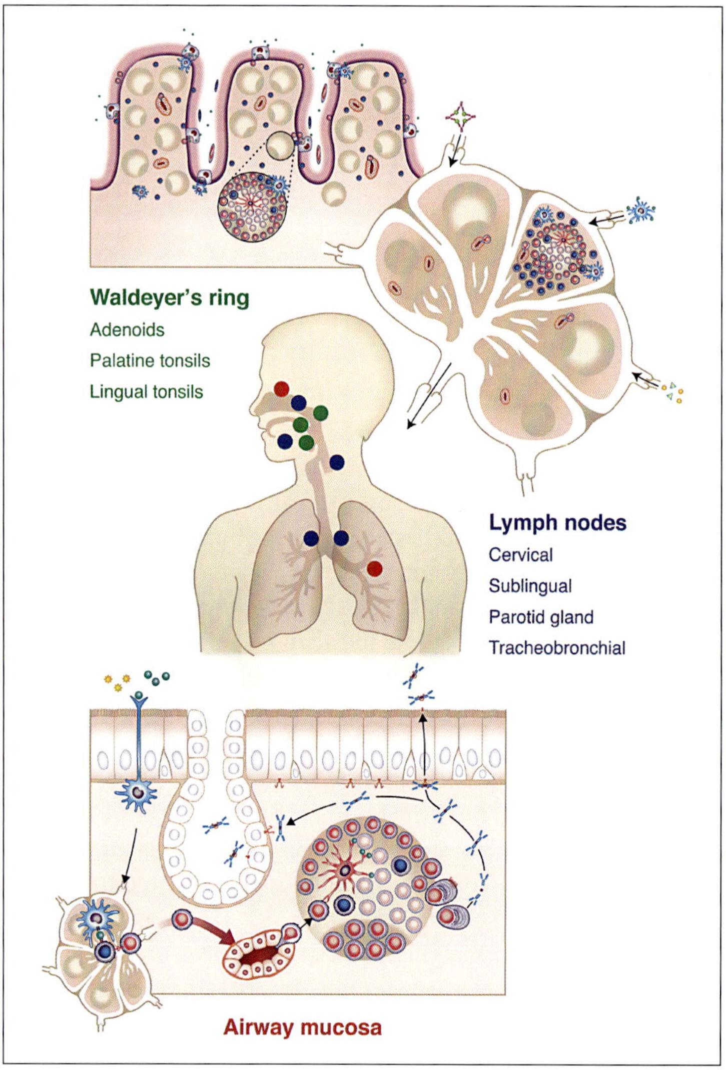

Fig. 1. Overview of the organization of tissues involved in the induction, elicitation and effector responses of B cells and plasma cells in the airways of humans. Secondary lymphoid organs like the Waldeyer's ring structures (green text and dots) and lymph nodes (blue text and dots) are important for generating high affinity B2 cell responses. The airway mucosa (red text and dots) also participates in B-cell responses using antibodies generated by the secondary lymphoid organs and by locally activated B-cells.

nasal polyps may play a role in the accumulation of local autoantibodies (see below).

IL-6 is another cytokine that is elevated in CRSwNP and plays an important role in B-cell activation [15]. IL-6 was originally named B-cell stimulation factor 2 (BSF-2) because of its ability to induce class switch recombination in B-cells [16]. It is also known to induce B-cell proliferation, and it can induce the differentiation of B-cells into plasma cells. Thus, IL-6 in nasal polyps may play a critical role in promoting significant increases in plasma cells and antibodies that have been reported in nasal polyps (see below).

The majority of nasal polyps from patients in the United States and Europe have been characterized by elevated expression of type 2 cytokines, particularly IL-5 and IL-13. While IL-5 has been shown to play a role in B-cell activation and differentiation in mice, it is not clear that IL-5 has the same direct effects on human B-cells [17]. However, it is well described that IL-5 does play a critical role in promoting the activation and sur-

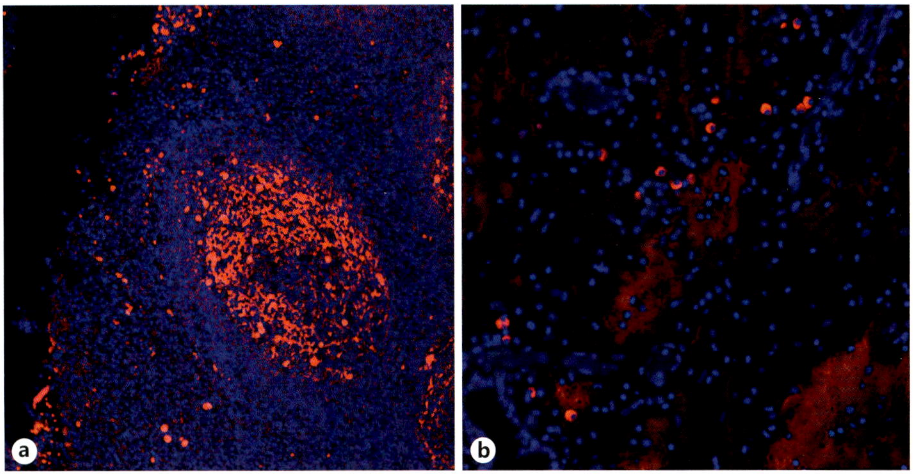

Fig. 2. Organization of IgM+ B-cells in (**a**) a classic lymphoid germinal center (tonsil) compared to (**b**) a less organized cluster of B-cells found typically in nasal polyp tissue.

vival of eosinophils, which may play a role in B-cell activation (see below). Thus, IL-5 may play an indirect role in B-cell activation in nasal polyps. IL-13 is also known to act directly on B-cells through the induction of class switching, particularly to IgE [18, 19]. We have also found elevated levels of both IgE and sterile transcripts for IgE in nasal polyps, suggesting that IL-13 may be an important factor for these events.

Chemokines
Chemokines are potent inducers of cell migration and play an important role in the recruitment of specific cell types to inflamed tissues. Many chemokines have been reported to be upregulated in nasal polyps, including 2 (CXCL12 and CXCL13) that specifically promote the influx of B-cells [11]. These chemokines are known to induce B-cell migration and localization within secondary lymphoid organs, by signaling through their receptors CXCR4 and CXCR5, respectively [20]. Given their important role in attracting B-cells into lymph nodes, it is reasonable to speculate that CXCL12 and CXCL13 play a similar role in the recruitment of B-cells into nasal polyps.

Another molecule that plays an important role in B-cell migration and localization is the receptor Epstein–Barr virus-induced protein 2 (EBI2) [21, 22]. While not a member of the chemokine receptor family, EBI2 is a 7 transmembrane G-protein coupled receptor that induces migration in response to its ligand, similar to traditional chemokine receptors. EBI2 expression on B-cells leads to their recruitment away from germinal centers, which facilitates their differentiation into what is termed extrafollicular plasmablasts, because they are activated outside of the germinal center follicle. We have found that EBI2 expression is highly elevated in nasal polyps, especially on plasmablasts [23]. Together, these data suggest that EBI2 may play a critical role in the localization of plasmablasts in nasal polyps.

Complement Pathway Products
Other mechanisms promoting the local activation of B-cells within nasal polyp tissue include findings that the complement cascade is highly activated in CRSwNP. Van Zele et al. [24] have previously demonstrated that the terminal complement complex (C5b-9), and the anaphylotoxins (C3a, C5a) are elevated in CRSwNP tissues.

Our own unpublished findings confirm these findings but further suggest that there is activation of the antibody-mediated and common complement activation cascades [25]. In addition to the well-described roles of anaphylotoxin-mediated recruitment and activation of mast cells and eosinophils [26, 27], the presence of C3 split products will likely activate B-cells. The C3 split product C3d, in particular, interacts with the complement receptor CD21 on B-cells to lower the threshold for activation. Interestingly, experimental studies also suggest that in the presence of C3d, B-cells with a 'natural' specificity can also be induced to activate cognate T-cells [28].

Evidence for B-Cell Activation in CRSwNP

Given the significant elevations in a variety of factors known to induce B-cell activation, differentiation and survival reported in nasal polyps, it is not surprising that B-cells and antibodies are also highly elevated in this tissue. Early studies evaluating the presence of B-cells in nasal polyps used immunohistochemical staining to identify CD20+ cells in tissue sections [29]. These semi-quantitative measures did not find elevations in CD20+ cells compared to control tissues. However, it is important to note that CD20 is one of the first markers to be lost from the B-cell surface during their differentiation into plasmablasts and plasma cells. More recently, studies using flow cytometry staining for CD19 and CD138 (a plasma cell marker) found significantly elevated levels of both B-cells and plasma cells in nasal polyps [23]. Moreover, these B-cells appear to be highly activated plasmablasts that express EBI2 and are proliferative (Hulse et al., unpublished observations). Some groups have reported evidence for the formation of tertiary lymphoid-like structures [30], and even T_{FH} cells [31], in nasal polyps. Tertiary lymphoid structures are similar to the follicular structures in secondary lymphoid organs where B-cells are normally activated, but they form at peripheral sites during inflammatory responses. However, we have also searched extensively for evidence of these structures and have not been able to confirm that they occur more frequently in nasal polyps than in control tissues (fig. 3, Hulse and Carter unpublished observations). Instead, we favor the hypothesis that local B-cell responses in nasal polyps are similar to extrafollicular B-cell responses, based on the elevated expression of EBI2 in nasal polyps (see above).

Antibody Specificities in CRS and Relationship to Pathogenesis and Disease Severity

To date, the antigen specificity of the majority of the antibody repertoire found in a nasal polyp is not known. Antibodies of almost every isotype, except IgD, have been found to be elevated in nasal polyp tissue, but not in sinus tissue from CRSsNP [32–34]. Studies aimed at characterizing the specificity of these antibodies will provide valuable information regarding the mechanisms that trigger their production. A robust, specific response against a microbe or allergen would result in antibodies with high affinity that are clonally closely related. In contrast, an antibody response driven by inflammation would result in more non-specific activation of a variety of unrelated B-cell clones and could result in autoreactivity. Such an antibody response would suggest a more generalized dysregulation of host mucosal immunity driven by unregulated B-cell activation. Studies regarding antibody specificity in CRSwNP are summarized here.

IgE to Aeroallergens, Concept of Entopy

Although IgE responses play a well-described role in allergic rhinitis, and atopy is found at higher prevalence in patients with CRSwNP, the centrality of atopy in the pathogenesis of CRSwNP remains unclear [35]. Interestingly, previous studies demonstrate that total IgE and tissue eosinophilia were similar between polyp tissue from atopic and

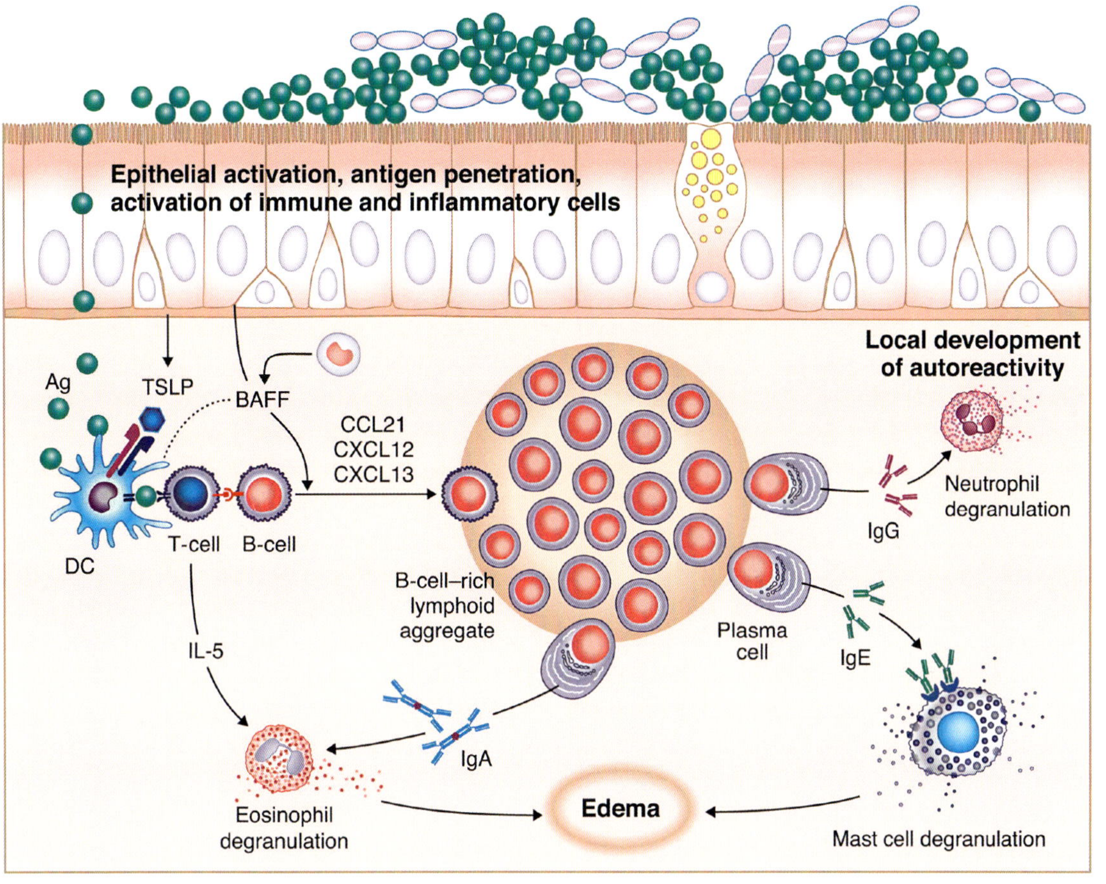

Fig. 3. Activation of B-cells and humoral responses in the inflammatory environment of a nasal polyp. Increased B-cell and plasma cell numbers are established in patients with CRSwNP and are accompanied by increased levels of the chemokines that attract them (including CXCL12 and CXCL13) and cytokines like BAFF. Although the specificity of the IgG, IgA, and IgE antibodies made in nasal polyp tissue is not completely known, recent evidence shows the presence of autoantibodies of the IgA and IgG isotypes. Cellular targets of immunoglobulins that are enriched in nasal polyps include eosinophils (which respond briskly to IgA activation), mast cells (which respond to IgE receptor cross-linking), and neutrophils (which respond to IgG ICs). Release of mediators by these cell types is likely to be important in the pathogenesis of the disease, including formation of nasal polyps. TSLP = Thymic Stromal Lymphopoietin.

non-atopic patients [36]. Other studies demonstrate equivalent skin-test sensitivity patterns and serum total IgE levels among patients with CRSwNP and CRSsNP [37]. Together, these studies suggest that local IgE production may be elevated in CRSwNP, regardless of atopic status. The term 'entopy' defines localized mucosal allergy in the absence of systemic responses for atopy [38]. Despite the absence of systemic sensitization in many patients with CRSwNP, studies by Zhang et al. [39] have demonstrated that the local IgE in nasal polyps was functional and could degranulate mast cells when exposed to grass allergens. Sabirov et al. also describe higher levels of Alternaria-specific IgE in NP tissue but not in serum [40]. They further found that the Alternaria IgE levels were positively correlated with tissue eosinophilic cationic protein (ECP), a marker of eosinophillia.

This study also found Alternaria-specific IgG and IgA in NPs tissue, with Alternaria-specific IgG response being more pronounced than the IgE response. Similarly, a more recent study by Porter et al. [41] found a high rate of airway fungal colonization among patients with CRSwNP and allergic fungal rhinosinusitis. Unlike the findings of Sabirov, they found that the presence of airway mycosis was significantly correlated with systemic responsiveness to Alternaria as measured by systemic production of IL-4 in an in vitro assay. Whether fungal IgE-mediated hypersensitivity plays a critical role in CRSwNP remains unclear, but enthusiasm for antifungal therapies in the condition have been tempered by the failure of topical amphotericin B treatment for improving clinical signs and symptoms in CRS patients [42].

Staphylococcus aureus

Staphylococcus aureus (S. aureus) secretes enterotoxins (SE) that can act as superantigens. Superantigens have the potential to directly activate T-cells by bypassing processing by antigen presenting cells (APCs) and directly crosslinking of the Vβ chain of T-cells to MHC class II on APCs. This produces an intense immune response that is distinct from T-cell activation induced by classical peptide antigens [43–45]. Indeed, experimental mouse models of airway inflammation find that airway stimulation with SEs can result in a pronounced eosinophilic inflammatory response [46]. Studies on the relevance of these responses in CRSwNP though have been conflicting. Although studies detect SEs in 50–80% of CRSwNP tissue, these rates do not appear higher than in control tissue [47, 48]. Studies evaluating the presence of *S. aureus* using cultures report a near universal prevalence of carriage in CRSwNP patients [49], while other studies found either modest elevations [50] or no elevations in prevalence compared to CRSsNP or control patients [47]. A more recent report utilized a highly sensitive detection method and found *S. aureus* prevalence was higher in patients with elevated total IgE, SE-specific IgE levels, IL-5 and ECP levels [51]. When considering the findings of these studies, it should be pointed out that intranasal carriage of *S. aureus* is prevalent in the general population with rates of 20–30% commonly reported.

Since SEs are present at minute concentrations and may be difficult to measure, the use of SE-specific IgE, has been advocated as a surrogate for SE effects on B-cell activation [33]. A recent meta-analysis of 12 related studies does demonstrate that Lund–Mackay CT scores, which measure CRS disease severity, were statistically higher in the SE-specific IgE-positive group than the IgE-negative group, suggesting that presence of SE could be considered as an index of CRSwNP severity [52]. Taken together, *S. aureus*-derived superantigens may be a disease modifier in CRSwNP, but given the high rate of endemic *S. aureus* colonization in the general population without CRS, and findings of a significant number of CRSwNP patients who do not have evidence for *S. aureus* carriage or enterotoxins, its role as etiologic factor is still under active investigation.

Autoantibodies

Studies in our laboratory have been focused on understanding findings that autoreactive, class switched antibodies are found at significantly higher levels in CRSwNP tissue. These findings are of pathogenic interest, as the autoreactive clones of B2 B-cells should normally be deleted in the bone marrow during B-cell development, and class-switched IgG autoantibodies are strongly implicated in the pathogenesis of autoimmune illness [53]. The expansion of autoreactive antibodies in CRS tissue may also drive persistent inflammation and help explain complement activation found in CRSwNP [54, 55]. Thus far, we find that the autoantibodies found in CRSwNP are reactive against nuclear antigens as best characterized by the anti-double stranded DNA (dsDNA) IgG, which are highly pathogenic in lupus [54]. The dsDNA autoantibodies were also found more commonly in patients with recurrent nasal polyps, suggesting a link between autoantibody generation and disease severity. We have also found locally elevated levels of anti-BP180 autoantibodies. BP180 (BPA2/collagen XVII) is a transmembrane glycoprotein that maintains adhesion of the stratified epithelia to the basement membrane, and this autoantibody may play a role in the loss of epithelial barrier function seen in nasal polyps [55].

A more recent report also describes the presence of local anti-cytokine autoantibodies in nasal secretions from CRS patients. They describe IgA autoantibodies against IL-1β, IL-2, IL-5, and IL-8 in nasal secretions from all CRS patients, whereas the highest levels of anti-IL-5 and anti-IL-17A autoantibodies were detected only in patients with CRSwNP [56]. Within CRSwNP patients, a positive correlation was found between secreted anti-IL-5 autoantibodies and IL-5, total IgE, and IgA. Since the antigenic targets of these autoantibodies have only begun to be characterized, their pathogenicity and role in activating complement or modulating inflammatory responses is under active investigation.

Summary

B-cells, plasma cells and antibodies are found at elevated levels in CRSwNP tissue, and studies indicate that B-cells are activated, switch isotypes and secrete antibodies locally within nasal polyps. Ongoing investigations are aimed at evaluating whether this B-cell activation occurs through antigen-specific activation, superantigen effects and/or B-cell dysregulation by the inflammation associated with CRSwNP. Nonetheless, the highly activated B-cell response may offer a novel target for more targeted treatment in CRS.

Acknowledgments

We extend our gratitude to Jacqi Schaffer in preparation of the figures in this review. Figures 1 and 5 are reprinted from Kato A, Hulse KE, Tan BK, Schleimer RP: B-lymphocyte lineage cells in the respiratory system. J Allergy Clin Immunol 2013;131:933–957.

References

1 Cobb RM, Oestreich KJ, Osipovich OA, Oltz EM: Accessibility control of V(D)J recombination. Adv Immunol 2006;91:45–109.

2 Hwang JK, Alt FW, Yeap LS: Related mechanisms of antibody somatic hypermutation and class switch recombination. Microbiol Spectr 2015;3:MDNA3-0037-2014.

3 Kato A, Hulse KE, Tan BK, Schleimer RP: B-lymphocyte lineage cells and the respiratory system. J Allergy Clin Immunol 2013;131:933–957; quiz 958.

4 Montecino-Rodriguez E, Leathers H, Dorshkind K: Identification of a B-1 B cell-specified progenitor. Nat Immunol 2006;7:293–301.

5 Griffin DO, Rothstein TL: Human B1 cell frequency: isolation and analysis of human B1 cells. Front Immunol 2012;3:122.

6 Weill JC, Weller S, Reynaud CA: Human marginal zone B cells. Annu Rev Immunol 2009;27:267–285.

7 Cerutti A, Cols M, Puga I: Marginal zone B cells: virtues of innate-like antibody-producing lymphocytes. Nat Rev Immunol 2013;13:118–132.

8 Pillai S, Cariappa A: The follicular versus marginal zone B lymphocyte cell fate decision. Nat Rev Immunol 2009;9:767–777.

9 Gatto D, Brink R: The germinal center reaction. J Allergy Clin Immunol 2010;126:898–907; quiz 908–909.

10 Vinuesa CG, Linterman MA, Goodnow CC, Randall KL: T cells and follicular dendritic cells in germinal center B-cell formation and selection. Immunol Rev 2010;237:72–89.

11 Hulse KE, Stevens WW, Tan BK, Schleimer RP: Pathogenesis of nasal polyposis. Clin Exp Allergy 2015;45:328–346.

12 Kato A, Peters A, Suh L, Carter R, Harris KE, Chandra R, et al: Evidence of a role for B cell-activating factor of the TNF family in the pathogenesis of chronic rhinosinusitis with nasal polyps. J Allergy Clin Immunol 2008;121:1385–1392, 1392.e1–e2.

13 Chu VT, Berek C: The establishment of the plasma cell survival niche in the bone marrow. Immunol Rev 2013;251:177–188.

14 Mackay F, Schneider P: Cracking the BAFF code. Nat Rev Immunol 2009;9:491–502.

15 Peters AT, Kato A, Zhang N, Conley DB, Suh L, Tancowny B, et al: Evidence for altered activity of the IL-6 pathway in chronic rhinosinusitis with nasal polyps. J Allergy Clin Immunol 2010;125:397–403.e10.

16 Vazquez MI, Catalan-Dibene J, Zlotnik A: B cells responses and cytokine production are regulated by their immune microenvironment. Cytokine 2015;74: 318–326.
17 Bertolini JN, Sanderson CJ, Benson EM: Human interleukin-5 induces staphylococcal A Cowan 1 strain-activated human B cells to secrete IgM. Eur J Immunol 1993;23:398–402.
18 Cocks BG, de Waal Malefyt R, Galizzi JP, de Vries JE, Aversa G: IL-13 induces proliferation and differentiation of human B cells activated by the CD40 ligand. Int Immunol 1993;5:657–663.
19 Oettgen HC: Regulation of the IgE isotype switch: new insights on cytokine signals and the functions of epsilon germline transcripts. Curr Opin Immunol 2000;12:618–623.
20 Patadia M, Dixon J, Conley D, Chandra R, Peters A, Suh LA, et al: Evaluation of the presence of B-cell attractant chemokines in chronic rhinosinusitis. Am J Rhinol Allergy 2010;24:11–16.
21 Hannedouche S, Zhang J, Yi T, Shen W, Nguyen D, Pereira JP, et al: Oxysterols direct immune cell migration via EBI2. Nature 2011;475:524–527.
22 Liu C, Yang XV, Wu J, Kuei C, Mani NS, Zhang L, et al: Oxysterols direct B-cell migration through EBI2. Nature 2011; 475:519–523.
23 Hulse KE, Norton JE, Suh L, Zhong Q, Mahdavinia M, Simon P, et al: Chronic rhinosinusitis with nasal polyps is characterized by B-cell inflammation and EBV-induced protein 2 expression. J Allergy Clin Immunol 2013;131:1075–1083.
24 Van Zele T, Coppieters F, Gevaert P, Holtappels G, Van Cauwenberge P, Bachert C: Local complement activation in nasal polyposis. Laryngoscope 2009; 119:1753–1758.
25 Van Roey GA, Vanison CC, Huang H, Kern RC, Chandra RK, Smith SS, et al: Complement activation in nasal tissue of patients with chronic rhinosinusitis. J Allergy Clin Immunol 2015; 135(suppl):AB237.
26 Erdei A, Andrásfalvy M, Péterfy H, Tóth G, Pecht I: Regulation of mast cell activation by complement-derived peptides. Immunol Lett 2004;92:39–42.
27 DiScipio RG, Schraufstatter IU: The role of the complement anaphylatoxins in the recruitment of eosinophils. Int Immunopharmacol 2007;7:1909–1923.
28 Nielsen CH, Leslie RG: Complement's participation in acquired immunity. J Leukoc Biol 2002;72:249–261.
29 Van Zele T, Claeys S, Gevaert P, Van Maele G, Holtappels G, Van Cauwenberge P, et al: Differentiation of chronic sinus diseases by measurement of inflammatory mediators. Allergy 2006;61: 1280–1289.
30 Gevaert P, Holtappels G, Johansson SG, Cuvelier C, Cauwenberge P, Bachert C: Organization of secondary lymphoid tissue and local IgE formation to Staphylococcus aureus enterotoxins in nasal polyp tissue. Allergy 2005;60:71–79.
31 Zhang YN, Song J, Wang H, Wang H, Zeng M, Zhai GT, et al: Nasal IL-4(+) CXCR5(+)CD4(+) T follicular helper cell counts correlate with local IgE production in eosinophilic nasal polyps. J Allergy Clin Immunol 2016;137:462–473.
32 Min JY, Kern RC, Hulse KE, Chandra R, Conley D, Suh L, et al: Evidence for immunoglobulin D in patients with chronic rhinosinusitis. J Allergy Clin Immunol 2014;133(suppl):AB236.
33 Van Zele T, Gevaert P, Holtappels G, van Cauwenberge P, Bachert C: Local immunoglobulin production in nasal polyposis is modulated by superantigens. Clin Exp Allergy 2007;37:1840–1847.
34 Hulse KE, Norton JE, Suh L, Zhong Q, Mahdavinia M, Simon P, et al: Chronic rhinosinusitis with nasal polyps is characterized by B-cell inflammation and EBV-induced protein 2 expression. J Allergy Clin Immunol 2013;131:1075–1083, 1083.e1–e7.
35 Tan BK, Chandra RK, Pollak J, Kato A, Conley DB, Peters AT, et al: Incidence and associated premorbid diagnoses of patients with chronic rhinosinusitis. J Allergy Clin Immunol 2013;131:1350–1360.
36 Bachert C, Gevaert P, Holtappels G, Johansson SG, van Cauwenberge P: Total and specific IgE in nasal polyps is related to local eosinophilic inflammation. J Allergy Clin Immunol 2001;107:607–614.
37 Tan BK, Zirkle W, Chandra RK, Lin D, Conley DB, Peters AT, et al: Atopic profile of patients failing medical therapy for chronic rhinosinusitis. Int Forum Allergy Rhinol 2011;1:88–94.
38 Powe DG, Bonnin AJ, Jones NS: 'Entopy': local allergy paradigm. Clin Exp Allergy 2010;40:987–997.
39 Zhang N, Holtappels G, Gevaert P, Patou J, Dhaliwal B, Gould H, et al: Mucosal tissue polyclonal IgE is functional in response to allergen and SEB. Allergy 2011;66:141–148.
40 Sabirov A, Hamilton RG, Jacobs JB, Hillman JB, Lebowitz, RA, Watts, JD: Role of local immunoglobulin E specific for Alternaria alternata in the pathogenesis of nasal polyposis. Laryngoscope 2008; 118:4–9.
41 Porter PC, Lim DJ, Maskatia ZK, Mak G, Tsai CL, Citardi MJ, et al: Airway surface mycosis in chronic TH2-associated airway disease. J Allergy Clin Immunol 2014;134:325–331.
42 Ebbens FA, Scadding GK, Badia L, Hellings PW, Jorissen M, Mullol J, et al: Amphotericin B nasal lavages: not a solution for patients with chronic rhinosinusitis. J Allergy Clin Immunol 2006; 118:1149–1156.
43 Conley DB, Tripathi A, Seiberling KA, Schleimer RP, Suh LA, Harris K, et al: Superantigens and chronic rhinosinusitis: skewing of T-cell receptor V beta-distributions in polyp-derived CD4+ and CD8+ T cells. Am J Rhinol 2006;20: 534–539.
44 Conley DB, Tripathi A, Seiberling KA, Suh LA, Harris KE, Paniagua MC, et al: Superantigens and chronic rhinosinusitis II: analysis of T-cell receptor V beta domains in nasal polyps. Am J Rhinol 2006;20:451–455.
45 Bachert C, Zhang N, Patou J, van Zele T, Gevaert P: Role of staphylococcal superantigens in upper airway disease. Curr Opin Allergy Clin Immunol 2008;8:34–38.
46 Rajagopalan G, Iijima K, Singh M, Kita H, Patel R, David CS: Intranasal exposure to bacterial superantigens induces airway inflammation in HLA class II transgenic mice. Infect Immun 2006;74: 1284–1296.
47 Heymans F, Fischer A, Stow NW, Girard M, Vourexakis Z, Des Courtis A, et al: Screening for staphylococcal superantigen genes shows no correlation with the presence or the severity of chronic rhinosinusitis and nasal polyposis. PLoS One 2010;5:e9525.
48 Seiberling KA, Conley DB, Tripathi A, Grammer LC, Shuh L, Haines GK 3rd, et al: Superantigens and chronic rhinosinusitis: detection of staphylococcal exotoxins in nasal polyps. Laryngoscope 2005;115:1580–1585.

49 Van Zele T, Gevaert P, Watelet JB, Claeys G, Holtappels G, Claeys C, et al: Staphylococcus aureus colonization and IgE antibody formation to enterotoxins is increased in nasal polyposis. J Allergy Clin Immunol 2004;114:981–983.
50 Zhang Z, Adappa ND, Doghramji LJ, Chiu AG, Cohen NA, Palmer JN: Different clinical factors associated with Staphylococcus aureus and Pseudomonas aeruginosa in chronic rhinosinusitis. Int Forum Allergy Rhinol 2015;5: 724–733.
51 Chalermwatanachai T, Zhang N, Holtappels G, Bachert C: Association of mucosal organisms with patterns of inflammation in chronic rhinosinusitis. PLoS One 2015;10:e0136068.
52 Ou J, Wang J, Xu Y, Tao ZZ, Kong YG, Chen SM, et al: Staphylococcus aureus superantigens are associated with chronic rhinosinusitis with nasal polyps: a meta-analysis. Eur Arch Otorhinolaryngol 2014;271:2729–2736.
53 Wardemann H, Nussenzweig MC: B-cell self-tolerance in humans. Adv Immunol 2007;95:83–110.
54 Tan BK, Li QZ, Suh L, Kato A, Conley DB, Chandra RK, et al: Evidence for intranasal antinuclear autoantibodies in patients with chronic rhinosinusitis with nasal polyps. J Allergy Clin Immunol 2011;128:1198–1206.e1.
55 Jeffe JS, Seshadri S, Hamill KJ, Huang JH, Carter R, Suh L, et al: A role for anti-BP180 autoantibodies in chronic rhinosinusitis. Laryngoscope 2013;123:2104–2111.
56 Tsybikov NN, Egorova EV, Kuznik BI, Fefelova EV, Magen E: Anticytokine autoantibodies in chronic rhinosinusitis. Allergy Asthma Proc 2015;36:473–480.

Bruce K. Tan, MD
Department of Otolaryngology, Northwestern University
Feinberg School of Medicine, 676 North St. Clair, Suite 1325
Chicago, IL 60611 (USA)
E-Mail b-tan@northwestern.edu

Woodworth BA, Poetker DM, Reh DD (eds): Rhinosinusitis with Nasal Polyposis.
Adv Otorhinolaryngol. Basel, Karger, 2016, vol 79, pp 58–68 (DOI: 10.1159/000445130)

Innate Lymphoid Cells: The Innate Counterpart to T Helper Cells

Caroline Padro Dietz[a, b] · Amber Luong[a, b]

[a]Department of Otolaryngology, Head and Neck Surgery, and [b]Center for Immunology and Autoimmune Diseases, Institute of Molecular Medicine, The University of Texas Medical School at Houston, Houston, Tex., USA

Abstract

Innate lymphoid cells (ILCs) are a recently discovered subset of innate immune cells that are capable of secreting great amounts of cytokines that have been found to influence effector cell activity. Chronic rhinosinusitis (CRS) in the absence (CRSsNP) or presence (CRSwNP) of nasal polyps has been characterized as type 1- and type 2-skewed, respectively, based on the presence of cytokines characteristic of type 1 and 2 immune responses. Based on the ability of type 1 ILCs to secrete interferon-γ, a type 1 cytokine found elevated in CRSsNP and type 2 ILCs to secrete IL-5 and IL-13, type 2 cytokines found elevated in CRSwNP, it is essential to examine the role that ILCs may play in the pathogenesis of CRS. This chapter introduces each subset of ILC (type 1–3) and the non-CRS pathologies they have been associated with in both mouse and human models. It will discuss the current research into ILCs in CRS, particularly ILC2s and NK cells in CRSwNP. Finally, the chapter will consider the therapeutic implications of ILC involvement in CRS and highlight the needs for future research into the role that ILCs play in CRS.

Introduction

Chronic rhinosinusitis (CRS) is a syndrome consisting of a heterogeneous group of diseases affecting the nasal and paranasal sinuses. Clinically, it describes chronic inflammation of sinonasal mucosa. Several clinical subtypes have been described primarily based on the absence (CRSsNP) and presence (CRSwNP) of nasal polyps. Within the CRSwNP phenotype, there are at least 3 defined and well-accepted subtypes including cystic fibrosis (CF), aspirin exacerbated respiratory disease (AERD) and allergic fungal rhinosinusitis (AFRS). These clinical subtypes of CRSwNP are defined by other factors, including defects in chloride channel (CF), association with aspirin sensitivity caused by biochemical defect(s) in the arachidonic acid metabolic pathway (AERD) and fungal sensitivity with heavy fungal load within eosinophilic mucin trapped within diseased sinuses (AFRS). However, a majority of CRS patients are categorized as only CRS with or without nasal polyps despite significant clinical differences in treatment responsiveness and disease presentation. This heterogeneity in clinical presentation suggests molecular differences and endotypes within CRS.

Given the inflammatory nature of CRS, groups began to evaluate the immunologic profiles of CRS patients with a focus on cytokines linked to adaptive immunity. Although the existence and critical role of the innate immune response was appreciated, the specificity to antigens/allergens associated with adaptive immunity elevated its priority over innate immunity. As such, cytokines were often associated with the adaptive immune response, and immunologic responses were characterized as T helper 1 (Th1) or T helper 2 (Th2) responses. For CRS, cytokine expression and levels were analyzed from tissue homogenates of inflamed sinonasal mucosa of CRSwNP and CRSsNP. From these studies, CRSwNP was considered a Th2-skewing disease with elevated levels of interleukin (IL)-4, IL-5 and IL-13, and CRSsNP was categorized as Th1 skewing with increased levels of interferon (IFN)-γ and TGF-β [1–3].

Over the last decade, studies focusing on the specific cellular sources of these critical immune driving cytokines identified innate lymphoid cells (ILCs), a novel subset of innate immune cells capable of secreting significant quantities of cytokines complementary to the Th subset of adaptive immune cells. ILCs are a distinct component of the innate immune system that coordinate both hematopoietic and non-hematopoietic cells. In addition, these cells respond to a variety of different signals including alarmins, neuropeptides, eicosanoids and cytokines. With this appreciation of ILCs' wide spectrum of cellular communication, recent studies highlight the central role of ILCs in coordinating the innate and adaptive immune response and as such, ILCs critical role in chronic inflammation. In this review on ILCs, the family of ILCs and the current understanding of their role in CRS are discussed.

Discovery of ILCs

Epithelial cells represent not only the physical barrier between an organism and its environment, but also serve as the initial immune defense. In this role, epithelial cells can detect various environmental threats such as bacteria, viruses, fungi, antigens and physical cellular damage and initiate a coordinated immune and wound healing response with a goal of re-establishing homeostasis through release of epithelial cell-derived cytokines. Significant interest recently has focused on three of these cytokines, IL-25, IL-33 and thymic stromal lymphopoietin protein (TSLP).

Several groups are credited with identifying what are now known as innate lymphoid cells. ILCs were once referred to as nuocytes, natural helper cells and innate helper cells. These cells were identified as a cell population that respond to IL-25, IL-33 and parasitic infections by releasing key type 2 cytokines, IL-5 and IL-13 in mice, but were not of B or T cell lineage [4–6]. Since then, these are described as innate lymphoid cells while other family members have been identified. ILCs are considered the innate counterpart to the adaptive T helper cells based on the cytokines they are capable of producing (fig. 1). As a group, ILCs express the IL-7Rα but lack the typical lineage markers including CD3, T cell receptors, CD11c, CD14, CD19, CD34 or CD123.

Subtypes of ILCs

ILCs are divided into type 1, 2 and 3 based on the cytokines they produce (fig. 1): Type 1 ILCs (ILC1) produce IFNγ, type 2 ILCs (ILC2) produce type 2 cytokines including IL-5 and IL-13, and type 3 ILCs (ILC3) produce IL-17 and IL-22.

Type 1 ILCs

Type I ILCs include both natural killer (NK) cells and ILC1s. NK cells were known prior to the discovery of ILCs. Similar to ILC1, NK cells produce

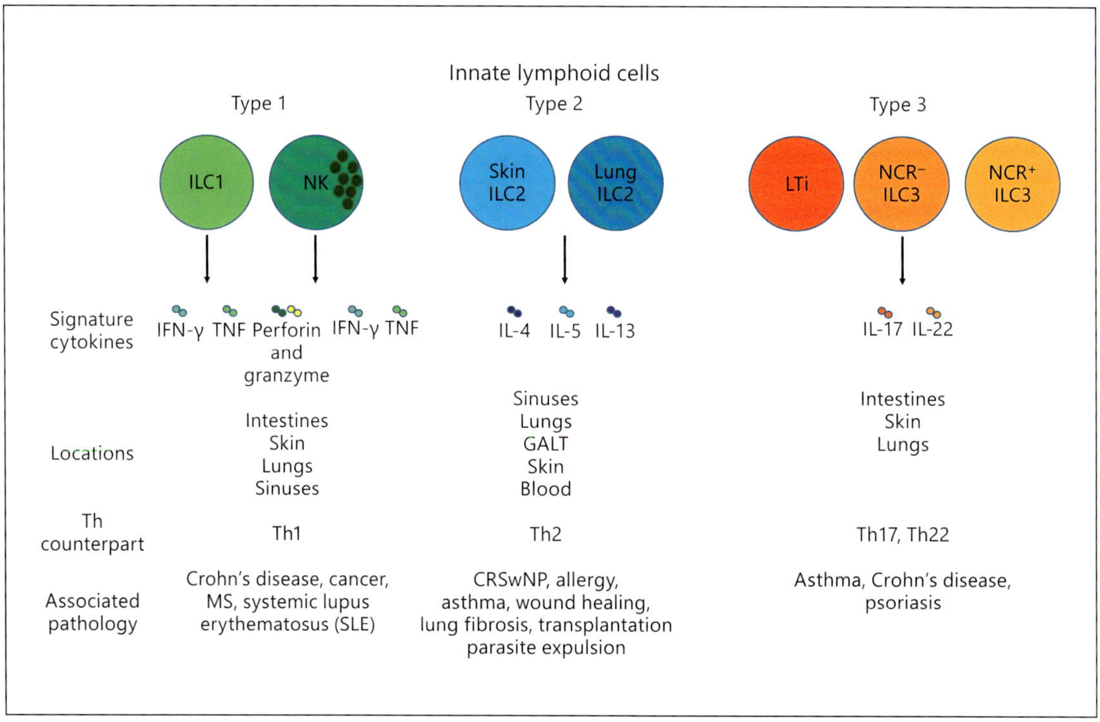

Fig. 1. ILC characteristics. Type 1–3 ILCs are defined by characteristic cytokine expression. Type 1 ILCs produce IFN-γ and TNF, type 2 ILCs produce IL-4, IL-5 and IL-13, and type 3 ILCs produce IL-17 and IL-22. There have been several subsets of type 1–3 ILCs identified. Additionally, each ILC has a corresponding Th cell counterpart based on signature cytokine production and transcriptional factor requirements for development. Type 1–3 ILCs are found at many mucosal interfaces including the intestines, skin, lungs and sinuses, and as such are implicated in many diseases associated with alterations in the immune system including CRSwNP, asthma, allergy, cancer, Crohn's disease, autoimmune diseases (MS, SLE), lung fibrosis and psoriasis. Type 2 ILCs are also important in non-pathological processes including wound healing, lung transplantation and parasite expulsion. CRTH2 = Chemoattractant receptor homologous molecule expressed on Th2 cells; GALT = gut-associated lymphoid tissue; NCR = natural cytotoxicity receptor.

type 1 cytokines such as IFN-γ and TNF, and thus are included in the Type 1 ILC category [7]. ILC1s and NK cells have been found in the intestine, skin, sinuses and lungs, indicating that they play an important role in innate immune defense against invading pathogens.

Several studies have investigated the role of Type 1 ILCs in human diseases including Crohn's disease, cancer and autoimmunity. Bernink et al. [8] described an abnormal accumulation of ILC1s in the inflamed intestines of people with Crohn's disease in comparison to non-inflamed controls. ILC1s from these patients expressed high levels of CXCR3 in comparison to ILC3 and NK cells and also expressed high levels of IFNγ mRNA. The role of ILC1s in intestinal pathology was confirmed in another study of patients with Crohn's disease and in a mouse model of colitis [9]. In addition, a number of studies have linked type 1 ILCs to autoimmune diseases. NK cells have been assigned a dual role in multiple sclerosis (MS). NK cells are capable of damaging myelin-producing oligodendrocytes, and are enhanced in lesions of MS patients [10, 11].

Additionally, they play a protective role by eliminating autoreactive T cells during IFN-β therapy [12]. In another autoimmune disease, systemic lupus erythematosus, NK cells are reduced and less effective, possibly contributing to the persistence of autoreactive T cells [13]. A reduction of NK cells was also observed in type II diabetes and correlated with reduced IFN-γ production [14]. Thus, while the study of non-NK ILC1s' role in disease is still early, it is apparent that the IFN-γ-producing subset of ILCs, whether they be NK or ILC1s, are important in autoimmune diseases.

Type 2 ILCs

Type 2 ILCs produce type 2 cytokines IL-4, IL-5 and IL-13. ILC2s were first described in studies attempting to uncover the cell type stimulated by IL-25 to produce IL-4, IL-5 and IL-13 leading ultimately to IgE production. These studies revealed a non-B, non-T cell population as the source [15]. This cell population was negative for lineage markers of macrophages, B cells, T cells, and eosinophils. Furthermore, in mice, the immune reaction stimulated by IL-25 in vivo was equivalent when comparing wild type (WT) and mice lacking B and T cells (RAG KO). This confirms in vitro studies indicating the existence of a non-B non-T cell population that could produce type 2 cytokines in response to IL-25 stimulation. Of note, these cells did not produce IL-4, and the RAG KO mice did not respond to IL-25 by increasing the antibody production [15], indicating a key difference between Th2 cells and the cells being observed. The existence and importance of this population of cells was confirmed in a study of mice lacking IL-25. IL-25-deficient mice were incapable of eliminating *N. brasiliensis*, a parasitic worm that is also the natural target of type 2 immune responses. Rescue of helminth expulsion was possible with the administration of exogenous IL-25 and the only cell population observed to be affected was a non-B non-T cell population that was c-kit$^+$ but FcεRI negative and produced IL-4, IL-5 and IL-13. In this study, basophils, eosinophils and mast cells were excluded as potential sources of these cytokines [16]. The presence of a non-B non-T cell subset that could produce IL-5 and IL-13 in response to IL-25 or IL-33 was confirmed by 3 subsequent studies [4, 5, 17] and they were termed type 2 ILCs. ILC2s have been identified in lymphoid-associated structures in the gut, peripheral blood, the skin, lungs and sinuses [18]. They require ROR-α and GATA3 [19–21] for development from Id2 precursors [20, 22, 23].

ILC2s are intimately involved in the pathogenesis of allergic diseases. ILC2s have been identified in healthy and asthmatic human lungs [24], indicating potential roles in both homeostasis and the allergic responses. In asthma, ILC2s were observed following allergen exposure, although the function of these cells was unclear at the time [24]. Migration of ILC2s into the lung during inflammation appears to be dependent on CRTH2 [25], a receptor for prostaglandin D2 and a commonly found receptor on ILC2s [26, 27]. In the context of allergic asthma, mouse studies have confirmed that ILC2s secrete IL-13 and IL-5 in an ovalbumin-induced allergic asthma model, but not IL-4 [28, 29]. Although Th2 cells are capable of producing IL-13 in this allergic asthma model, IL-13-deficient mice had reduced airway hyperresponsiveness, an effect reversed by the reintroduction of IL-13-secreting ILC2s. The ability of IL-13-secreting ILC2s to mediate airway hyperresponsiveness indicated that the IL-13 produced by ILC2s was important for the allergic asthma pathway in a mouse model [28, 29]. Collectively, these studies confirm the importance of ILC2s by demonstrating their role as a primary source of IL-13- and IL-5-mediated allergic airway response resulting from IL-25 and IL-33 administration [28–30].

Type 2 ILCs also seem to coordinate the innate and adaptive immune response. In allergic asthma, ILC2s directly communicate with CD4$^+$ T cells and mast cells. ILCs are found in close proximity to mast cells [26] in the lung, and the mast cell product, PGD_2 was found to interact with CRTH2 on ILC2 to enhance IL-13 production [26]. In vitro, lung ILC2s from naïve mice were capable of promoting Th2 differentiation and cytokine production. Furthermore, the combination of ILC2s and Th2 cells was required to rescue an antigen-specific allergic response and airway hyper-responsiveness that was lost when mice were deficient in IL-7Rα, indicating a key interplay between these 2 cell types despite similar cytokine production profiles [31]. Notably, this study identified IL-4 production by ILC2 and the costimulatory molecule OX40L as a key driver of the effects of ILC2s on Th2 cells.

In addition to its role in chronic inflammation, Type 2 ILCs seem to play a central role in re-establishing homeostasis after breaches in the epithelial cell barrier. ILC2s help repair the lung after influenza. When ILC2s are depleted, the damage from an influenza infection compromises epithelial integrity and is only restored when the ILC gene product, amphiregulin, is reintroduced [22], indicating a role of ILC2 in restoring the lung to homeostasis following sickness. ILC2s have also been found after lung transplantation [22] and in idiopathic pulmonary fibrosis [32]. In addition to its role in disease, ILCs may play a critical function in re-establishing homeostasis via wound healing effects.

Type 3 ILCs

Type 3 ILCs include lymphoid tissue inducer cells (LTi), natural cytotoxicity receptor $(NCR)^-$ and NCR^+ ILC3s that produce cytokines including IL-17 and IL-22. Based on LTi localization and studies in mice, these cells seem essential in lymphoid organogenesis and host defense in the skin, lungs and gut [33–35]. Interestingly, ILC3s have also been shown to exhibit considerable plasticity in vitro and are capable of converting to ILC1s [36]. Due to the signature production of IL-17 and IL-22, ILC3s are considered to be the innate immune counterpart to Th17 and Th22 cells. The convertibility of ILC3 to ILC1 directly parallels the observation that Th17 cells are capable of being converted to Th1 cells [37] and confirms the close relationship between ILCs and Th cells.

ILC3s are primarily found at mucosal interfaces and are implicated in psoriasis, Crohn's disease and asthma. In Crohn's disease, a decreased amount of an IL-22 producing ILC3 population and a concomitant increased level of IFN-γ producing ILC1 cells was found in the intestines in these patients, creating an ILC1/ICL3 imbalance [38]. It was subsequently demonstrated that cells from resected specimens of Crohn's disease patients were capable of interconverting between ILC1 and ILC3 depending on exposure to various cytokines produced by antigen presenting cells [36]. ILC3 plasticity in Crohn's is an example in which disease phenotype can be driven by the cellular make up within diseased tissue and the resultant cytokine milieu. Psoriasis is a non-atopic disease of the skin characterized by increased IL-17 and IL-22 levels in the blood [39–43]. Two separate mouse models have demonstrated that ILC3s are necessary and sufficient in the absence of functional T cells for development of psoriasis [44, 45]. Finally, asthma, which involves ILC2s, may also be influenced by ILC3s. Interestingly, ILC3s can function to limit as well as propagate airway inflammation and hyper-responsiveness. Its role in asthma seems dependent on whether it is an IL-22- or IL-17-producing ILC3 [46, 47]. Together, initial studies support central roles of ILC3s in several human diseases including Crohn's disease, psoriasis and asthma, but their specific function in these diseases remains to be further explored.

Despite the relative infancy of the field of ILC research, a substantial number of studies have demonstrated the relevance of ILCs in human disease. Based on the previously discussed cytokine profiles of CRSsNP and CRSwNP as type 1 and type 2-mediated diseases, respectively, it is essential to determine the involvement of ILCs in contributing to the pathogenesis of these diseases and the cytokines that characterize them.

Role of Type 2 ILCs in CRSwNP

CRSwNP has been described as a type 2-mediated disease based on elevated expression of IL-5 and IL-13 [1–3]. Prior to the discovery of ILCs, it was assumed that the initial and primary source of these cytokines were Th2 cells given the increased population of these cells in diseased sinonasal mucosa from CRSwNP patients. A study from our laboratory found increased memory Th2 cells in CRSwNP in comparison to CRSsNP and healthy controls (HC) [48]. Another study found increased numbers of Th2 cells in inflamed mucosa from CRSwNP compared to CRSsNP and HC [49]. However with the emerging appreciation for ILCs, we along with others began looking for ILCs in CRS patients and found increased ILC2s in the inflamed mucosa of patients with CRSwNP as compared to HC [50, 51] and to CRSsNP [27, 52–54]. As expected, these cells expressed CD117, c-kit and CD127, the α chain of the IL-7 receptor. In addition, they expressed the receptor for epithelial cell-derived cytokines IL-33, IL-25 and TSLP [51]. Increased levels of ILC2 are associated with clinical markers associated with more severe disease including eosinophilia, allergy and asthma status, nasal endoscopy score [52] and memory T cells [53]. Together, the increased presence of these cells and correlation with clinical markers along with surface expression of several key receptors suggested a key functional role of ILC2s in the pathophysiology of CRSwNP.

Given the expression of ST2, the IL-33 receptor, on these cells, we investigated the effects of IL-33 stimulation on ILC2 isolated from sinonasal mucosa of CRSwNP patients using flow cytometry analysis. In these studies, we found that ILC2s, and not mast cells or T cells, serve as the primary and initial source of IL-13 in response to IL-2/IL-33 stimulation (fig. 2) [27]. As mentioned, IL-33 is an epithelial cell-derived cytokine that is released in response to various environmental triggers including fungi, bacteria and viruses as well as to damage to the epithelial cells. It is one of several epithelial cell-derived cytokines that may initially orchestrate the type 2 immune response. As such, significant interest currently exists in targeting these cytokines for novel therapeutics.

Role of Other ILCs in CRS

Similar to CRSwNP, ILCs may be a significant source of type 1 cytokines found in diseased mucosa of CRS without nasal polyps and cystic fibrosis. To date, there are no studies that have examined the role of ILC1s and ILC3s in CRS subtypes. In other chronic inflammatory diseases such as asthma, elevated numbers of ILC3s have been found in the lungs of patients [47], and an altered ILC1:ILC3 ratio has been documented in Crohn's disease [36, 38]. In our studies of CRS patients, we observed overall fewer ILCs in CRSsNP [27] as compared to CRSwNP and there are less ILC1s and ILC3s in CRSsNP compared to CRSwNP (unpublished data), indicating that another cellular subtype most likely is responsible for the IFNγ-slanted cytokine profile. Indeed, we have observed a much larger proportion of IFNγ-producing Th1 cells within inflamed mucosa from CRSsNP in comparison to CRSwNP (unpublished data). It seems that CRSsNP and CRSwNP are not just separated by being type 1/2 skewed, but that the innate and adaptive immune arms may have differential contributions to the cytokine profile associated with these 2 diseases.

Although no published studies exist looking at ILC1 in CRS, NK cells have been examined. One study comparing CRSsNP to early stage CRSwNP found fewer, although not statistically significant, number of NK cells in the inflamed mucosa of

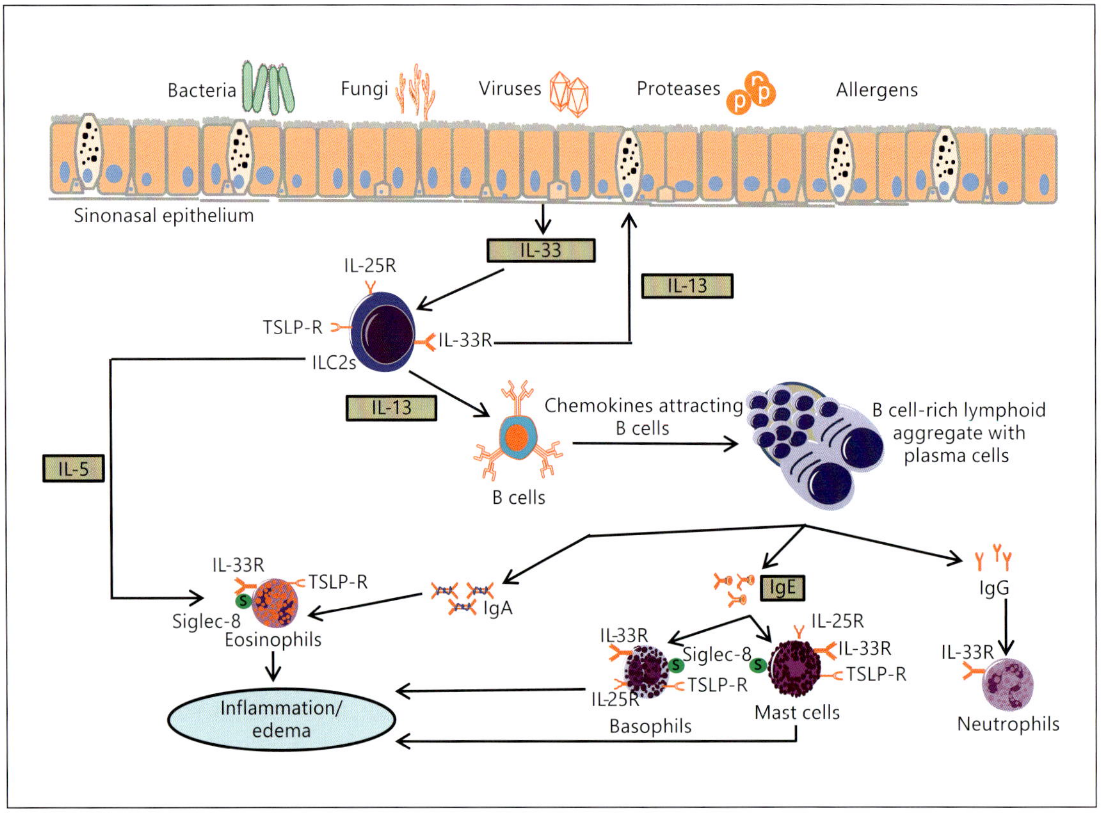

Fig. 2. Role of ILC2 in CRS in response to IL-33 stimulation. Upon release from respiratory epithelial cells, IL-33 can bind to ILC2 via ST2 receptor. ILC2s activated by IL-33 are the primary source of IL-13 in CRS. IL-13 drives class switching in B cells to promote IgE production. In addition, IL-13 stimulates mucus glands to increase mucus production in CRS. Both increased local production of IgE and increased mucus are associated with inflamed sinonasal mucosa of CRS.

CRSwNP patients [55]. In addition, functional studies of NK cells from CRSwNP patients suggest a defect in their intrinsic activity resulting in an impaired ability to degranulate and to produce IFNγ [56], Thus, the role that ILC1s and ILC3s play in the pathogenesis of CRS subtypes remains to be determined.

Consequence for Future Therapeutics

The increased appreciation for the role of innate immunity in disease processes has brought new therapeutic focus on this arm of the immune response. For CRS, oral and topical corticosteroids remain the primary therapy for the management of inflammation. With this new focus on innate immunity and ILCs, Walford et al. [54] investigated the effect of corticosteroids on ILC2s. They found that the presence of ILC2s were negatively associated with corticosteroid usage, suggesting that systemic steroids can affect the presence of ILC2s in nasal mucosa in CRSwNP. Another means of targeting ILCs is to target the receptors on these and other innate cells, for example, receptors for epithelial cell-derived cytokines such as TSLP and IL-33. Early studies characterizing the cellular distribution within inflamed mucosa from CRSwNP patients found increased numbers of $CD34^+$ hematopoietic progenitor cells [57, 58]. Follow-up studies suggested that some of these $CD34^+$ cells were ILC2 which increased IL-5 and IL-13 production when co-cultured with sinonasal explants, a source of epithelial cell-derived cytokines [24]. The enhancement in IL-5 and IL-13 production was found to be induced by both TSLP and IL-33. In addition, TSLP is a potent activator of mast cells [59, 60]. Thus, the discovery of ILC2s in CRSwNP has identified novel therapeutic targets, ones that may offer curative rather than just symptomatic benefits.

Future Research Needs

The family of CRS subtypes represents a large spectrum of immune diseases and the underlying mechanisms of these diseases are largely unexplored. Many studies have characterized the cytokine profile of the CRS subtypes, but few have clearly identified the key cellular sources of these inflammatory cytokines. In CRSsNP and CF, it remains unknown if ILC1 or NK cells are a significant contributor of IFNγ. In CF, IFNγ and IL-17 were found to be elevated in comparison to CRSwNP and CRSsNP [49] but no significant increase in Th17 cells was observed. The finding suggests the possibility that IL-17-producing ILC3 may be elevated in CF. Coupled with the reported interconvertibility of ILC1s to ILC3s, the increased IFNγ observed in CF may also be related to increased levels of ILC1. Thus, CF represents a CRS subtype where ILCs potentially play a large role in disease pathogenesis.

The increased presence of ILC2 in CRSwNP has been definitively shown by a large number of studies [27, 50–54]. What remains to be determined is if AFRS represents a more extreme version of CRSwNP. This has been postulated due to the increased IgE and presence of NP compared to CRSwNP and the fact that most CRSwNP patients have fungus present in their sinuses similar to AFRS patients [61]. Alternatively, AFRS may be an entirely different disease, potentially resulting from a defect of the innate immune system reflected by the inability to clear fungus from the sinuses that allows for subsequent colonization and growth. We have found equivalent levels of ILC2s in AFRS and a small trend toward increased Th2 cells (unpublished data), although Th2 cells are quite variable between patient samples. There is also the possibility of altered cytokine secretion profiles and receptor expression of ILC2s between AFRS and CRSwNP as has been described in dermal versus lung ILC2s [50, 62–65]. Dermal ILC2s are capable of producing IL-4 as opposed to lung ILC2s [50, 62], which produce IL-5 and IL-13, and some ILC2s have been found to express CRTH2, the receptor for PGD_2, while others have not [63–65]. Furthermore, some ILC2s are responsive to TSLP in an IL-33-dependent manner while others do not require IL-33 to produce cytokines [51, 66]. Since the field of ILC biology is still developing, it is entirely possible that ILC2s will be further subdivided and that the differences observed will underlie the differences we observe in CRSwNP and AFRS as well as other CRSwNP endotypes. Thus, there is a strong indication that ILCs are involved in the pathogenesis of CRS subtypes and there are many avenues of research that may lead to potential therapeutic targets in the treatment of CRS.

Conclusions

CRS and the characterization of CRS subtypes into endotypes based on cytokine signatures are a largely unexplored field of research. ILCs represent a potential cellular source of inflammatory cytokines. To date, ILC2s have been shown to be elevated in CRSwNP, a prototypical type 2 immune disease, and NK cells may serve as a significant source of type 1 cytokines characteristic of CRSsNP. Future research in this field will need to determine the role ILCs play in shaping the cytokine signature of each CRS endotype and to identify potentially novel therapeutic targets linked to ILCs in the pathogenesis of CRS.

Conflict of Interest

A.L. received consulting fees from Laurimed, LLC, Medtronic and ENTvantage and industry research funding from IntersectENT, Amgen and Mallinckrodt.

Financial Support

A.L. is supported by the Center for Clinical and Translational Sciences, which is funded by National Institutes of Health Clinical and Translational Award UL1 TR000371 and KL2 TR000370 from the National Center for Advancing Translational Science. The content is solely the responsibility of the authors and does not necessarily represent the official views of the National Center for Advancing Translational Science or the National Institutes of Health.

References

1 Cao PP, Li HB, Wang BF, Wang SB, You XJ, Cui YH, Wang DY, Desrosiers M, Liu Z: Distinct immunopathologic characteristics of various types of chronic rhinosinusitis in adult Chinese. J Allergy Clin Immunol 2009;124:478–484.
2 Van Bruaene N, Perez-Novo CA, Basinski TM, Van Zele T, Holtappels G, De Ruyck N, Schmidt-Weber C, Akdis C, Van Cauwenberge P, Bachert C, Gevaert P: T-cell regulation in chronic paranasal sinus disease. J Allergy Clin Immunol 2008;121:1435–1441.
3 Van Zele T, Claeys S, Gevaert P, Van Maele G, Holtappels G, Van Cauwenberge P, Bachert C: Differentiation of chronic sinus diseases by measurement of inflammatory mediators. Allergy 2006;61:1280–1289.
4 Moro K, Yamada T, Tanabe M, Takeuchi T, Ikawa T, Kawamoto H, Furusawa J, Ohtani M, Fujii H, Koyasu S: Innate production of T(H)2 cytokines by adipose tissue-associated c-Kit(+)Sca-1(+) lymphoid cells. Nature 2010;463:540–544.
5 Neill DR, Wong SH, Bellosi A, Flynn RJ, Daly M, Langford TK, Bucks C, Kane CM, Fallon PG, Pannell R, Jolin HE, McKenzie AN: Nuocytes represent a new innate effector leukocyte that mediates type-2 immunity. Nature 2010;464:1367–1370.
6 Price AE, Liang HE, Sullivan BM, Reinhardt RL, Eisley CJ, Erle DJ, Locksley RM: Systemically dispersed innate IL-13-expressing cells in type 2 immunity. Proc Natl Acad Sci U S A 2010;107:11489–11494.
7 Spits H, Artis D, Colonna M, Diefenbach A, Di Santo JP, Eberl G, Koyasu S, Locksley RM, McKenzie AN, Mebius RE, Powrie F, Vivier E: Innate lymphoid cells – a proposal for uniform nomenclature. Nat Rev Immunol 2013;13:145–149.
8 Bernink JH, Peters CP, Munneke M, te Velde AA, Meijer SL, Weijer K, Hreggvidsdottir HS, Heinsbroek SE, Legrand N, Buskens CJ, Bemelman WA, Mjosberg JM, Spits H: Human type 1 innate lymphoid cells accumulate in inflamed mucosal tissues. Nat Immunol 2013;14:221–229.
9 Fuchs A, Vermi W, Lee JS, Lonardi S, Gilfillan S, Newberry RD, Cella M, Colonna M: Intraepithelial type 1 innate lymphoid cells are a unique subset of IL-12- and IL-15-responsive IFN-γ-producing cells. Immunity 2013;38:769–781.
10 Benczur M, Petranyl GG, Palffy G, Varga M, Talas M, Kotsy B, Foldes I, Hollan SR: Dysfunction of natural killer cells in multiple sclerosis: a possible pathogenetic factor. Clin Exp Immunol 1980;39:657–662.
11 Kastrukoff LF, Lau A, Wee R, Zecchini D, White R, Paty DW: Clinical relapses of multiple sclerosis are associated with 'novel' valleys in natural killer cell functional activity. J Neuroimmunol 2003;145:103–114.
12 Saraste M, Irjala H, Airas L: Expansion of CD56Bright natural killer cells in the peripheral blood of multiple sclerosis patients treated with interferon-beta. Neurol Sci 2007;28:121–126.
13 Poggi A, Zocchi MR: NK cell autoreactivity and autoimmune diseases. Front Immunol 2014;5:27.
14 Rodacki M, Svoren B, Butty V, Besse W, Laffel L, Benoist C, Mathis D: Altered natural killer cells in type 1 diabetic patients. Diabetes 2007;56:177–185.
15 Fort MM, Cheung J, Yen D, Li J, Zurawski SM, Lo S, Menon S, Clifford T, Hunte B, Lesley R, Muchamuel T, Hurst SD, Zurawski G, Leach MW, Gorman DM, Rennick DM: IL-25 induces IL-4, IL-5, and IL-13 and Th2-associated pathologies in vivo. Immunity 2001;15:985–995.
16 Fallon PG, Ballantyne SJ, Mangan NE, Barlow JL, Dasvarma A, Hewett DR, McIlgorm A, Jolin HE, McKenzie AN: Identification of an interleukin (IL)-25-dependent cell population that provides IL-4, IL-5, and IL-13 at the onset of helminth expulsion. J Exp Med 2006;203:1105–1116.
17 Saenz SA, Siracusa MC, Perrigoue JG, Spencer SP, Urban JF Jr, Tocker JE, Budelsky AL, Kleinschek MA, Kastelein RA, Kambayashi T, Bhandoola A, Artis D: IL25 elicits a multipotent progenitor cell population that promotes T(H)2 cytokine responses. Nature 2010;464:1362–1366.
18 Hazenberg MD, Spits H: Human innate lymphoid cells. Blood 2014;124:700–709.
19 Halim TY, MacLaren A, Romanish MT, Gold MJ, McNagny KM, Takei F: Retinoic-acid-receptor-related orphan nuclear receptor alpha is required for natural helper cell development and allergic inflammation. Immunity 2012;37:463–474.

20 Wong SH, Walker JA, Jolin HE, Drynan LF, Hams E, Camelo A, Barlow JL, Neill DR, Panova V, Koch U, Radtke F, Hardman CS, Hwang YY, Fallon PG, McKenzie AN: Transcription factor RORα is critical for nuocyte development. Nat Immunol 2012;13:229–236.
21 Hoyler T, Klose CS, Souabni A, Turqueti-Neves A, Pfeifer D, Rawlins EL, Voehringer D, Busslinger M, Diefenbach A: The transcription factor GATA-3 controls cell fate and maintenance of type 2 innate lymphoid cells. Immunity 2012; 37:634–648.
22 Monticelli LA, Sonnenberg GF, Abt MC, Alenghat T, Ziegler CG, Doering TA, Angelosanto JM, Laidlaw BJ, Yang CY, Sathaliyawala T, Kubota M, Turner D, Diamond JM, Goldrath AW, Farber DL, Collman RG, Wherry EJ, Artis D: Innate lymphoid cells promote lung-tissue homeostasis after infection with influenza virus. Nat Immunol 2011;12:1045–1054.
23 Cherrier M, Sawa S, Eberl G: Notch, Id2, and RORγt sequentially orchestrate the fetal development of lymphoid tissue inducer cells. J Exp Med 2012;209:729–740.
24 Allakhverdi Z, Comeau MR, Smith DE, Toy D, Endam LM, Desrosiers M, Liu YJ, Howie KJ, Denburg JA, Gauvreau GM, Delespesse G: CD34+ hemopoietic progenitor cells are potent effectors of allergic inflammation. J Allergy Clin Immunol 2009;123:472–478.
25 Wojno ED, Monticelli LA, Tran SV, Alenghat T, Osborne LC, Thome JJ, Willis C, Budelsky A, Farber DL, Artis D: The prostaglandin D2 receptor CRTH2 regulates accumulation of group 2 innate lymphoid cells in the inflamed lung. Mucosal Immunol 2015;8:1313–1323.
26 Xue L, Salimi M, Panse I, Mjosberg JM, McKenzie AN, Spits H, Klenerman P, Ogg G: Prostaglandin D2 activates group 2 innate lymphoid cells through chemoattractant receptor-homologous molecule expressed on TH2 cells. J Allergy Clin Immunol 2014;133:1184–1194.
27 Shaw JL, Fakhri S, Citardi MJ, Porter PC, Corry DB, Kheradmand F, Liu YJ, Luong A: IL-33-responsive innate lymphoid cells are an important source of IL-13 in chronic rhinosinusitis with nasal polyps. Am J Respir Crit Care Med 2013;188: 432–439.
28 Barlow JL, Bellosi A, Hardman CS, Drynan LF, Wong SH, Cruickshank JP, McKenzie AN: Innate IL-13-producing nuocytes arise during allergic lung inflammation and contribute to airways hyperreactivity. J Allergy Clin Immunol 2012;129:191–198.e1–e4.
29 Klein Wolterink RG, Kleinjan A, van Nimwegen M, Bergen I, de Bruijn M, Levani Y, Hendriks RW: Pulmonary innate lymphoid cells are major producers of IL-5 and IL-13 in murine models of allergic asthma. Eur J Immunol 2012; 42:1106–1116.
30 Kim HY, Chang YJ, Subramanian S, Lee HH, Albacker LA, Matangkasombut P, Savage PB, McKenzie AN, Smith DE, Rottman JB, DeKruyff RH, Umetsu DT: Innate lymphoid cells responding to IL-33 mediate airway hyperreactivity independently of adaptive immunity. J Allergy Clin Immunol 2012;129:216–227.e1–e6.
31 Drake LY, Iijima K, Kita H: Group 2 innate lymphoid cells and CD4+ T cells cooperate to mediate type 2 immune response in mice. Allergy 2014;69:1300–1307.
32 Hams E, Armstrong ME, Barlow JL, Saunders SP, Schwartz C, Cooke G, Fahy RJ, Crotty TB, Hirani N, Flynn RJ, Voehringer D, McKenzie AN, Donnelly SC, Fallon PG: IL-25 and type 2 innate lymphoid cells induce pulmonary fibrosis. Proc Natl Acad Sci U S A 2014;111:367–372.
33 Mebius RE, Rennert P, Weissman IL: Developing lymph nodes collect CD4+CD3- LTbeta+ cells that can differentiate to APC, NK cells, and follicular cells but not T or B cells. Immunity 1997;7:493–504.
34 Yoshida H, Kawamoto H, Santee SM, Hashi H, Honda K, Nishikawa S, Ware CF, Katsura Y, Nishikawa SI: Expression of alpha(4)beta(7) integrin defines a distinct pathway of lymphoid progenitors committed to T cells, fetal intestinal lymphotoxin producer, NK, and dendritic cells. J Immunol 2001;167:2511–2521.
35 Sonnenberg GF, Monticelli LA, Elloso MM, Fouser LA, Artis D: CD4(+) lymphoid tissue-inducer cells promote innate immunity in the gut. Immunity 2011;34:122–134.
36 Bernink JH, Krabbendam L, Germar K, de Jong E, Gronke K, Kofoed-Nielsen M, Munneke JM, Hazenberg MD, Villaudy J, Buskens CJ, Bemelman WA, Diefenbach A, Blom B, Spits H: Interleukin-12 and -23 control plasticity of CD127(+) group 1 and group 3 innate lymphoid cells in the intestinal lamina propria. Immunity 2015;43:146–160.
37 Kurschus FC, Croxford AL, Heinen AP, Wortge S, Ielo D, Waisman A: Genetic proof for the transient nature of the Th17 phenotype. Eur J Immunol 2010; 40:3336–3346.
38 Takayama T, Kamada N, Chinen H, Okamoto S, Kitazume MT, Chang J, Matuzaki Y, Suzuki S, Sugita A, Koganei K, Hisamatsu T, Kanai T, Hibi T: Imbalance of NKp44(+)NKp46(–) and NKp44(–)NKp46(+) natural killer cells in the intestinal mucosa of patients with Crohn's disease. Gastroenterology 2010; 139:882–892, 892.e1–e3.
39 Ma HL, Liang S, Li J, Napierata L, Brown T, Benoit S, Senices M, Gill D, Dunussi-Joannopoulos K, Collins M, Nickerson-Nutter C, Fouser LA, Young DA: IL-22 is required for Th17 cell-mediated pathology in a mouse model of psoriasis-like skin inflammation. J Clin Invest 2008; 118:597–607.
40 Zheng Y, Danilenko DM, Valdez P, Kasman I, Eastham-Anderson J, Wu J, Ouyang W: Interleukin-22, a T(H)17 cytokine, mediates IL-23-induced dermal inflammation and acanthosis. Nature 2007;445:648–651.
41 Res PC, Piskin G, de Boer OJ, van der Loos CM, Teeling P, Bos JD, Teunissen MB: Overrepresentation of IL-17A and IL-22 producing CD8 T cells in lesional skin suggests their involvement in the pathogenesis of psoriasis. PLoS One 2010;5:e14108.
42 Hijnen D, Knol EF, Gent YY, Giovannone B, Beijn SJ, Kupper TS, Bruijnzeel-Koomen CA, Clark RA: CD8(+) T cells in the lesional skin of atopic dermatitis and psoriasis patients are an important source of IFN-γ, IL-13, IL-17, and IL-22. J Invest Dermatol 2013;133:973–979.
43 Wolk K, Witte E, Wallace E, Docke WD, Kunz S, Asadullah K, Volk HD, Sterry W, Sabat R: IL-22 regulates the expression of genes responsible for antimicrobial defense, cellular differentiation, and mobility in keratinocytes: a potential role in psoriasis. Eur J Immunol 2006; 36:1309–1323.

44 Hedrick MN, Lonsdorf AS, Shirakawa AK, Richard Lee CC, Liao F, Singh SP, Zhang HH, Grinberg A, Love PE, Hwang ST, Farber JM: CCR6 is required for IL-23-induced psoriasis-like inflammation in mice. J Clin Invest 2009;119:2317–2329.
45 Pantelyushin S, Haak S, Ingold B, Kulig P, Heppner FL, Navarini AA, Becher B: Rorγt+ innate lymphocytes and γδ T cells initiate psoriasiform plaque formation in mice. J Clin Invest 2012;122:2252–2256.
46 Taube C, Tertilt C, Gyulveszi G, Dehzad N, Kreymborg K, Schneeweiss K, Michel E, Reuter S, Renauld JC, Arnold-Schild D, Schild H, Buhl R, Becher B: IL-22 is produced by innate lymphoid cells and limits inflammation in allergic airway disease. PLoS One 2011;6:e21799.
47 Kim HY, Lee HJ, Chang YJ, Pichavant M, Shore SA, Fitzgerald KA, Iwakura Y, Israel E, Bolger K, Faul J, DeKruyff RH, Umetsu DT: Interleukin-17-producing innate lymphoid cells and the NLRP3 inflammasome facilitate obesity-associated airway hyperreactivity. Nat Med 2014;20:54–61.
48 Shaw JL, Ashoori F, Fakhri S, Citardi MJ, Luong A: Increased percentage of mast cells within sinonasal mucosa of chronic rhinosinusitis with nasal polyp patients independent of atopy. Int Forum Allergy Rhinol 2012;2:233–240.
49 Derycke L, Eyerich S, Van Crombruggen K, Perez-Novo C, Holtappels G, Deruyck N, Gevaert P, Bachert C: Mixed T helper cell signatures in chronic rhinosinusitis with and without polyps. PLoS One 2014;9:e97581.
50 Mjosberg JM, Trifari S, Crellin NK, Peters CP, van Drunen CM, Piet B, Fokkens WJ, Cupedo T, Spits H: Human IL-25- and IL-33-responsive type 2 innate lymphoid cells are defined by expression of CRTH2 and CD161. Nat Immunol 2011;12:1055–1062.
51 Mjosberg J, Bernink J, Golebski K, Karrich JJ, Peters CP, Blom B, te Velde AA, Fokkens WJ, van Drunen CM, Spits H: The transcription factor GATA3 is essential for the function of human type 2 innate lymphoid cells. Immunity 2012;37:649–659.
52 Ho J, Bailey M, Zaunders J, Mrad N, Sacks R, Sewell W, Harvey RJ: Group 2 innate lymphoid cells (ILC2s) are increased in chronic rhinosinusitis with nasal polyps or eosinophilia. Clin Exp Allergy 2015;45:394–403.
53 Miljkovic D, Bassiouni A, Cooksley C, Ou J, Hauben E, Wormald PJ, Vreugde S: Association between group 2 innate lymphoid cells enrichment, nasal polyps and allergy in chronic rhinosinusitis. Allergy 2014;69:1154–1161.
54 Walford HH, Lund SJ, Baum RE, White AA, Bergeron CM, Husseman J, Bethel KJ, Scott DR, Khorram N, Miller M, Broide DH, Doherty TA: Increased ILC2s in the eosinophilic nasal polyp endotype are associated with corticosteroid responsiveness. Clin Immunol 2014;155:126–135.
55 Polzehl D, Moeller P, Riechelmann H, Perner S: Distinct features of chronic rhinosinusitis with and without nasal polyps. Allergy 2006;61:1275–1279.
56 Kim JH, Kim GE, Cho GS, Kwon HJ, Joo CH, Kim HS, Jang YJ: Natural killer cells from patients with chronic rhinosinusitis have impaired effector functions. PLoS One 2013;8:e77177.
57 Otsuka H, Dolovich J, Richardson M, Bienenstock J, Denburg JA: Metachromatic cell progenitors and specific growth and differentiation factors in human nasal mucosa and polyps. Am Rev Respir Dis 1987;136:710–717.
58 Kim YK, Uno M, Hamilos DL, Beck L, Bochner B, Schleimer R, Denburg JA: Immunolocalization of CD34 in nasal polyposis. Effect of topical corticosteroids. Am J Respir Cell Mol Biol 1999;20:388–397.
59 Allakhverdi Z, Smith DE, Comeau MR, Delespesse G: Cutting edge: the ST2 ligand IL-33 potently activates and drives maturation of human mast cells. J Immunol 2007;179:2051–2054.
60 Nagarkar DR, Poposki JA, Tan BK, Comeau MR, Peters AT, Hulse KE, Suh LA, Norton J, Harris KE, Grammer LC, Chandra RK, Conley DB, Kern RC, Schleimer RP, Kato A: Thymic stromal lymphopoietin activity is increased in nasal polyps of patients with chronic rhinosinusitis. J Allergy Clin Immunol 2013;132:593–600.e12.
61 Porter PC, Lim DJ, Maskatia ZK, Mak G, Tsai CL, Citardi MJ, Fakhri S, Shaw JL, Fothergil A, Kheradmand F, Corry DB, Luong A: Airway surface mycosis in chronic TH2-associated airway disease. J Allergy Clin Immunol 2014;134:325–331.
62 Roediger B, Kyle R, Yip KH, Sumaria N, Guy TV, Kim BS, Mitchell AJ, Tay SS, Jain R, Forbes-Blom E, Chen X, Tong PL, Bolton HA, Artis D, Paul WE, Fazekas de St Groth B, Grimbaldeston MA, Le Gros G, Weninger W: Cutaneous immunosurveillance and regulation of inflammation by group 2 innate lymphoid cells. Nat Immunol 2013;14:564–573.
63 Kim BS, Siracusa MC, Saenz SA, Noti M, Monticelli LA, Sonnenberg GF, Hepworth MR, Van Voorhees AS, Comeau MR, Artis D: TSLP elicits IL-33-independent innate lymphoid cell responses to promote skin inflammation. Sci Transl Med 2013;5:170ra16.
64 Teunissen MB, Munneke JM, Bernink JH, Spuls PI, Res PC, Te Velde A, Cheuk S, Brouwer MW, Menting SP, Eidsmo L, Spits H, Hazenberg MD, Mjosberg J: Composition of innate lymphoid cell subsets in the human skin: enrichment of NCR(+) ILC3 in lesional skin and blood of psoriasis patients. J Invest Dermatol 2014;134:2351–2360.
65 Salimi M, Barlow JL, Saunders SP, Xue L, Gutowska-Owsiak D, Wang X, Huang LC, Johnson D, Scanlon ST, McKenzie AN, Fallon PG, Ogg GS: A role for IL-25 and IL-33-driven type-2 innate lymphoid cells in atopic dermatitis. J Exp Med 2013;210:2939–2950.
66 Shikotra A, Choy DF, Ohri CM, Doran E, Butler C, Hargadon B, Shelley M, Abbas AR, Austin CD, Jackman J, Wu LC, Heaney LG, Arron JR, Bradding P: Increased expression of immunoreactive thymic stromal lymphopoietin in patients with severe asthma. J Allergy Clin Immunol 2012;129:104–111.e1–e9.

Amber Luong, MD, PhD, FACS
Associate Professor of Otorhinolaryngology, Head and Neck Surgery
University of Texas Medical School at Houston, Texas Sinus Institute
6431 Fannin Street, MSB 5.036, Houston, TX 77030 (USA)
E-Mail amber.u.luong@uth.tmc.edu

Woodworth BA, Poetker DM, Reh DD (eds): Rhinosinusitis with Nasal Polyposis.
Adv Otorhinolaryngol. Basel, Karger, 2016, vol 79, pp 69–77 (DOI: 10.1159/000445132)

The Role of Innate Immunity and Aeroallergens in Chronic Rhinosinusitis

Nyall R. London Jr. • Anuj Tharakan • Murugappan Ramanathan Jr.
Johns Hopkins Department of Otolaryngology – Head and Neck Surgery, Baltimore, Md., USA

Abstract
Allergy has been inferred to contribute to the pathophysiology of chronic rhinosinusitis (CRS) although this role is controversial and the mechanism is debated. Furthermore, the role of aeroallergens in CRS is poorly defined and has been postulated to contribute to CRS through direct penetration in the sinuses or downstream systemic consequences. Common aeroallergens implicated in chronic rhinosinusitis include air pollution/second hand smoke, dust mite and pollen [1–3]. One emerging potential mechanism whereby aeroallergens contribute to CRS is through sinonasal epithelial barrier disruption (fig. 1). Characterization of cytokine disruption of sinonasal epithelial cell barrier has been described including interleukin (IL)-4 and IL-13, as well as aeroallergens such as house dust mite and cigarette smoke. Recent results have demonstrated severe barrier disruption in response to direct application of either particulate matter (PM) or house dust mite (HDM) to sinonasal epithelial cells. Sinonasal epithelial barrier disruption may contribute to CRS by enabling the perpetual and chronic exposure of inflammatory allergens and stimuli. The sinonasal epithelial barrier plays a significant role in innate immune host defense. Mechanisms of innate immune defense include pattern recognition receptors (PRRs), secreted endogenous antimicrobials and inflammatory cytokines that aid in repair mechanisms including IL-33. Here we discuss recent evidence implicating aeroallergens and dysregulated host innate immune responses in the development of CRS.

Introduction

Allergy is the abnormal IgE driven inflammatory reaction to a previously encountered allergen. Allergic reactions can range from systemic severe response or anaphylaxis characterized by airway edema, shock and death to localized rhinitis characterized by nasal congestion, rhinorrhea and sneezing. Aeroallergens are defined as inhaled agents, which can evoke an allergic inflammatory response and include seasonal sources such as pollens or perennial sources such as dust mites. Environmental components such as air pollution in the form of particulate

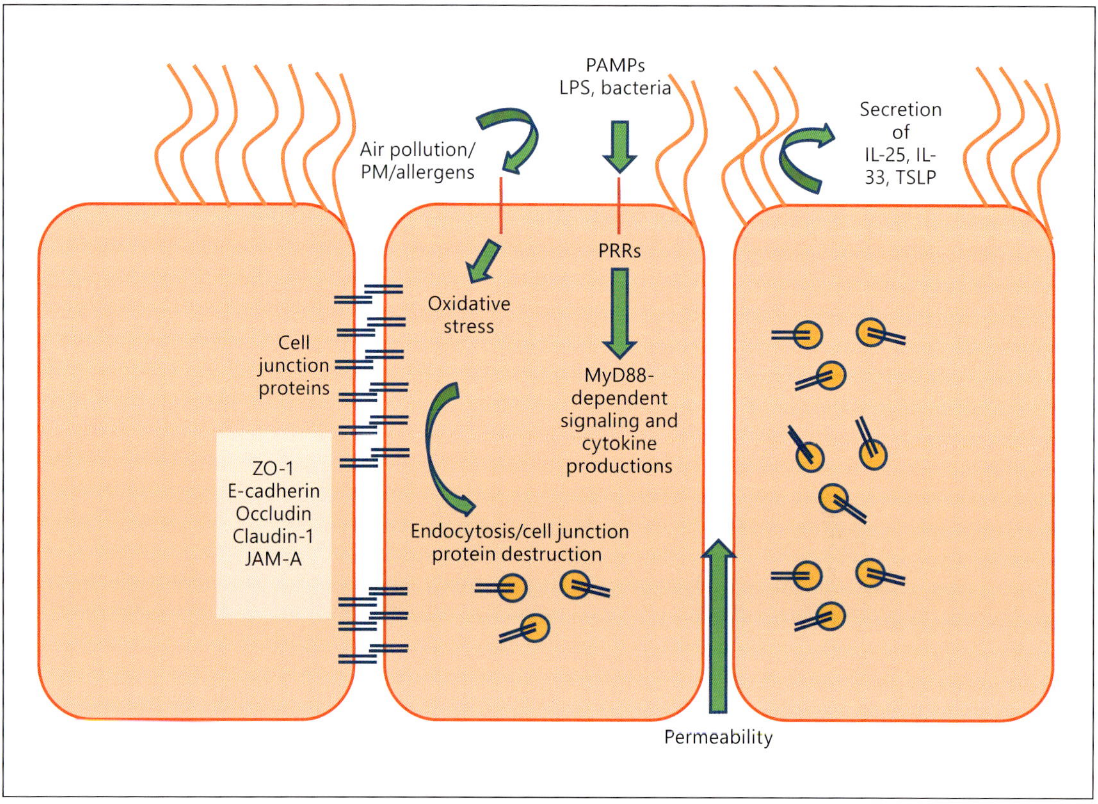

Fig. 1. Aeroallergens and inflammatory stimuli disrupt sinonasal epithelial barrier function. These agents act to destabilize the barrier through stimulating endocytosis and destruction of cell junction proteins via oxidative stress and MyD88-dependent mechanisms. Furthermore, aeroallergens and inflammatory stimuli induce secretion of IL-25, IL-33, and TSLP from sinonasal epithelial cells.

matter or second-hand smoke can also be exacerbating factors for allergic diseases. There has been significant interest in understanding whether allergy plays a role in chronic inflammatory disease such as chronic rhinosinusitis (CRS). Evidence supporting a role for allergy in CRS has largely demonstrated an association rather than causation. Indeed, the prevalence of allergic rhinitis has been reported between 40–84% in adults with CRS and 25–31% in acute sinusitis [4]. The prevalence of allergy in patients with acute and chronic sinusitis has been demonstrated to be higher than matched controls [5]. Furthermore, CT scans performed on patients with perennial allergic rhinitis found evidence of sinusitis in 67.5% of allergic patients compared to 33.4% of controls [6]. Patients with allergy and CRS have also been found to have worse symptoms than controls [5]. Lastly, data also suggest that patients with allergy who undergo sinus surgery do better when treated with immunotherapy [7].

Although a strong association between allergy and CRS has been suggested, the pathologic mechanism is unknown and controversial. Some aeroallergens may not be able to directly enter the sinuses in native settings as demonstrated by previous studies with radiolabelled ragweed particles and contrast media [8]. However, the ability for aeroallergens to directly enter the sinuses after functional endoscopic sinus surgery is likely increased due to removal of natural tissue barriers. Even if aeroallergens were not able to directly enter the sinuses, they may still worsen CRS through localized ostiomeatal complex mucosal edema or swelling which may predispose them to obstruction. An emerging model is that aeroallergens cause a systemic allergic response leading to sinusitis. This is supported by the finding that nasal allergen exposure increases inflammatory changes in the ipsilateral and contralateral maxillary sinus [9]. This systemic reaction is felt to be due to a coordinated interaction between the nasal airway, nasal associated lymphatic tissue, bone marrow and the sinuses [8, 9]. In this model, the nasal airway is exposed to allergens that stimulate local inflammatory cells such as dendritic cells, macrophages, lymphocytes, mast cells and eosinophils. The ensuing inflammatory response results not only in the release of cytokines but also migration of memory T cells to the bone marrow where the production of eosinophils is increased. Eosinophils are then recruited to distant inflamed tissue such as the sinonasal mucosa [8]. Regardless of the mechanism, allergy is likely a contributing factor or disease modifier to CRS pathology rather than a sole etiologic cause [9].

Inflammatory cytokines from the innate and adaptive immune response also contribute to CRS. Many of these cytokines arise from CD4+ helper T (Th) cells and have been subdivided into cytokines arising from a Th1 versus Th2 response. Th1 cytokines include tumor necrosis factor-alpha (TNF-α) and interferon-gamma (IFN-γ) which activate cytotoxic T cells and macrophages while Th2 cytokines include interleukin (IL)-4, IL-5 and IL-13 and enhance the eosinophil and mast cell response [10]. These inflammatory cytokines may also be released within the sinonasal microenvironment including sinonasal epithelial cells. Not only do Th1 and Th2 inflammatory cytokines enhance inflammatory cell activation but may also destabilize adjacent structures such as the sinonasal epithelial cell barrier.

Sinonasal Epithelial Barrier – A Potential Target in CRS

The sinonasal mucosa is lined by a layer of sinonasal epithelial cells that act as the initial barrier and interface with the air/environment. This interface serves to block outside allergens and inflammatory agents and regulate flow of fluid across the barrier. This tight barrier is formed by intercellular junction proteins including epithelial cadherin (E-cadherin), zonula occludens-1 (ZO-1), occludin, claudin-1 and junctional adhesion molecule A (JAM-A). Epithelial barrier dysfunction is a proposed pathogenic mechanism leading to persistent inflammation in diseases including Crohn's disease, asthma, atopic dermatitis and psoriasis [11]. While very less is known about the role of the sinonasal epithelial barrier in CRS, multiple recent studies have investigated the sinonasal epithelial cell barrier breakdown.

The presence of epithelial barrier disruption in sinonasal disease was first reported as alterations in tight junction protein expression in nasal polyposis [12]. In these studies, expression of claudin-1 and occludin was assessed in sections of nasal epithelium of polyposis and normal control patients. Immunofluorescence demonstrated a 79% and 64% decrease in the basal:apical staining density of claudin-1 and occludin, respectively, in nasal polyp epithelium compared to control. Human bronchial epithelial cells in vitro were exposed to IFN-γ and TNF-α. Although there was an initial increase on transient exposure, after exposure for a more chronic time point of 72 h, there was a 18% and 43% reduction in claudin-1 and occludin, respectively, as assessed by densitometric analysis of Western blots [9]. A similar result for occludin was observed as assessed by immunofluorescence. These preliminary studies paved the way for further analysis of sinonasal epithelial cell barrier breakdown.

Future studies evaluated whether the combination of IFN-γ and TNF-α, known to disrupt intercellular junction proteins, induced permeability. Using transepithelial resistance (TER) as a measurement of epithelial barrier disruption, a combination of IFN-γ and TNF-α reduced the TER by 64% at 24 h. IL-4 reduced TER by 51.6% while IL-13 reduced TER to 68.6% of baseline at 24 h. Next, tight junction protein expression after cytokine stimulation was assessed. While JAM-A expression and E-cadherin decreased 42 and 35% respectively with IL-4 exposure, JAM-A expression and E-cadherin decreased 37.5 and 32.9% respectively with IL-13. There were no changes in occludin, ZO-1 or claudin-1. Lastly, claudin-2, whose expression is known to increase rather than prevent barrier disruption, was found to have increased expression after IL-4 and IL-13 exposure [13]. Collectively, these data demonstrate that inflammatory cytokines selectively alter sinonasal epithelial cell tight junctions and are sufficient to induce permeability. Furthermore, these cytokines have been found to prevent the epithelial barrier from resealing which may contribute to the perpetuation of inflammation and exposure to inflammatory antigens. Although IL-13 did not prevent resealing, IL-4 was found to reduce sinonasal epithelial wound closure and decrease number of wounds closed compared to control [14].

Less is known about direct exposure of aeroallergens on sinonasal epithelial barrier disruption. One study did find that direct exposure of recombinant house dust mite antigen Der p 1 disrupted sinonasal epithelial cell barrier function [15]. In particular, exposure of Der p 1 decreased TER at 24 h. Western blot and immunofluorescence demonstrated decreased expression of claudin-1 and JAM-A in primary cultured sinonasal epithelial cells. Unpublished results from our research group also confirm these findings. Furthermore, we demonstrate that enhancement of the cytoprotective anti-oxidant transcription factor, Nrf2, is able to reverse HDM-induced sinonasal epithelial barrier dysfunction through restoration of ZO-1 and other tight junction proteins and restoration of TER (pending publication, fig. 2).

Sinonasal epithelial cells isolated from patients with allergic fungal rhinosinusitis (AFRS) were found at a baseline level to have less stability as assessed by TER as well as decreased expression of JAM-A, occludin and E-cadherin along with increased expression of claudin-2. This suggests that changes in the sinonasal epithelial cell barrier dysfunction may be chronic or persistent after exposure to the allergen.

In addition to disrupting the epithelial barrier, some aeroallergens such as cigarette smoke may directly damage the sinonasal epithelial cell. It is well known that tobacco smoke either through direct smoking or second-hand smoke contributes to CRS [16]. Cigarette condensate (the particulate phase of tobacco smoke) has been observed to decrease the epithelial production of IL-6 and IL-8 after bacterial stimulation [17]. Cigarette smoke condensate (CSC) also has been shown to decrease NF-kappa B activation. Furthermore, CSC impairs ciliogenesis in a dose dependent manner in mouse nasal septal epithelial cultures [18].

Innate Immunity

The sinonasal tract is constantly exposed to the external environment and as such relies on the innate immune system as an initial host defense [19]. The main roles of the innate immune response includes its role as a physical barrier, recruitment of appropriate inflammatory cells, activation of the complement system and initiation of the adaptive immune response [20]. Active areas of investigation in this respect include the sinonasal epithelial cell barrier for its role in barrier stability, mucociliary clearance and secretion of antimicrobials. Further areas of research include recognition of pathogens by the innate immune system via pathogen-associated molecular patterns (PAMPs) and pattern recognition receptors (PRRs). Of these PRRs, the most studied area includes toll-like receptors (TLRs) [10]. The initiation of an appropriate innate and adaptive immune response includes the

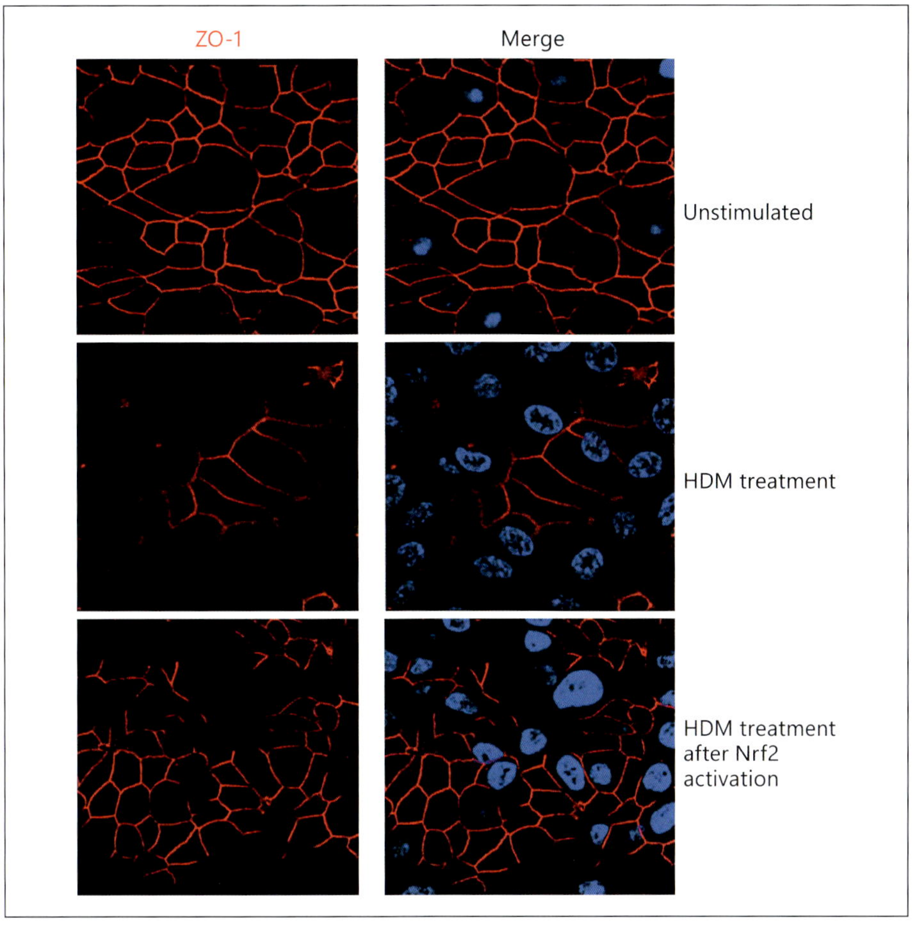

Fig. 2. House dust mite antigen disrupts sinonasal epithelial ZO-1 (red) as assessed by immunofluorescence (compare row 1 and 2). Nrf2 activation reduced HDM-induced disruption of ZO-1 (row 3). DAPI (blue).

secretion of inflammatory cytokines. Collectively, when these mechanisms become unbalanced through a failure to respond or through an exaggerated response, chronic inflammation and CRS may result.

Pattern Recognition Receptors

TLRs are a family of evolutionarily conserved proteins that recognize common pathogen associated molecules such as bacterial cell wall proteins, lipopolysaccharides (LPS) and unmethylated DNA [10]. There are 11 known mammalian TLRs [10]. These transmembrane receptors possess an extracellular leucine-rich domain and an intracellular signaling domain known as a TIR domain. Activation of these receptors induces a cascade of downstream signaling events and may be characterized by myeloid differentiation primary response gene 88 (MyD88) or TIR-containing adaptor-dependent pathways [19]. Activation of TLRs in sinonasal epithelial cells has been shown to increase expression of genes such as human β-defensin (HBD) 2 and IL-8, both important for initiating an innate immune response [21].

Expression of the TLR pathway has been heavily studied in CRS with conflicting results reported demonstrating the heterogeneity of this disease. In a Korean population of 214 subjects, 2 single-nucleotide polymorphisms (SNPs) in TLR2 showed significant differences with minor allele frequency and correlated with CRS risk [22]. RT-PCR analysis comparison of CRSwNP and CRSsNP compared to control demonstrated a significant increase in TLR2 expression in CRSwNP and CRSsNP [23, 24]. This is in contrast to another study which found a statistically significant decrease in the expression of TLR2 in CRSwNP and may represent the heterogeneity of this disease or the increased incidence of recalcitrant CRS in the study population [25]. Furthermore, expression of TLR2 and TLR4 has been found to be increased in nasal epithelial cells from CRS compared to normal controls [26]. Expression of TLR4 has been reported to be increased in CRSwNP and decreased in CRSsNP compared to control subjects [27]. Microarray gene analysis for 125 genes related to TLR signaling in tissue from patients with CRSwNP identified a greater than 2-fold increase in TLR9 [28]. These results are further solidified by another study reporting increased expression of TLR9 in CRSwNP but no significant change in CRSsNP [23]. Our group has demonstrated that sinonasal epithelial cells from CRSwNP are associated with decreased TLR9 expression as measured by intracellular flow cytometry [21] and furthermore that Th2 cytokines in vitro tend to lower epithelial cell TLR9 expression [29]. How these differential changes in gene expression support a role for TLR and innate immunity in CRS is controversial. Research from our group suggests that CRSwNP is a disease associated with a dysregulated innate immune response with cytokine polarity tilting more toward a Th2 picture. More recent work published in 2015 via association studies now suggest that expression of TLR2 and TLR4 correlate with neutrophil infiltration in CRSsNP, thus differential expression of TLR could potentially enhance chronic inflammation through a failure to respond or through an exaggerated response to TLR ligands [30].

A less well-studied group of PRR includes the nucleotide binding and oligomerization domain (NOD)-like receptors (NLRs) [19]. This family consists of 23 cytosolic receptor proteins in humans and is characterized by a NOD and C-terminal leucine-rich repeats [19]. Although there is little known regarding NLRs in CRS, polymorphisms in 2 members of the NLR family, NOD1 and NOD2, have been linked to allergy and asthma [31]. In the lung, NOD1 expression has been noted in lung epithelial cells and leukocytes while NOD2 expression has been reported in alveolar macrophages, neutrophils and bronchial epithelial cells [31]. One study found that in a model of human sinonasal mucosa explant, NOD2 expression increased when explants were exposed to Staphylococcus aureus in biofilm rather than planktonic form [32]. Another study reported significant NOD1 and NOD2 expression in nasal polyps which was decreased in response to topical steroid treatment indicating a potential role for NLR in CRSwNP [33]. Thus NLRs may play a role in CRS but requires further investigation.

Secreted Antimicrobials

Sinonasal epithelial cells secrete a variety of antimicrobial molecules including defensins, cathelicidins, lysozyme, lactoferrin and surfactant [10]. These secreted antimicrobials play a major role in the innate immune defense and inhibition of microbial growth. Inhibition of microbial growth allows time for additional mechanisms of host defense to take effect including mucociliary clearance, recruitment of inflammatory cells and initiation of an adaptive immune response. Therefore, a decrease in secretion or efficacy of these antimicrobials is hypothesized to potentially contribute to CRS through epithelial colonization [10, 29].

Defensins are a large family of secreted antimicrobial peptides and consist of the α-defensins and β-defensins 1–4. HBD have been found to be expressed in the lower airways and while HBD-1 is constitutively expressed, HBD-2 through -4 are induced in response to pro-inflammatory cytokines and endotoxins [10]. Similar to this are the cathelicidin family, of which the only known human cathelicidin whose post-enzymatic cleavage product is known as LL-37. There has been significant interest in using topical administration of defensins for disruption of biofilms as LL-37 has demonstrated efficacy against bacteria and fungus in vitro [19, 34]. LL-37 was used to treat rabbits in an animal model of biofilm Pseudomonas sinusitis and was found to in fact reduce CFU after 10 days of irrigation [34]. Unfortunately, however, LL-37 was found to cause mucosal inflammation as well as ciliotoxicity at concentrations necessary for biofilm eradication [34]. Further investigation is necessary to determine whether a similar approach with an alternate defensin may be effective without dose limiting toxicity.

Lysozyme is a secreted enzyme, which targets the peptidoglycan cell wall of bacteria causing cell lysis [10]. In addition to epithelial cells, lysozyme is also secreted by neutrophils, goblet cells, monocytes and macrophages [10, 19]. By itself lysozyme is minimally effective, but demonstrates increased efficacy in combination with additional antimicrobial agents [35]. One such agent is lactoferrin, an iron binding protein which functions to sequester iron. Concomitant addition of human apolactoferrin and lysozyme demonstrated synergistic destruction against a strain of pneumococcus [35]. Interestingly, there is a significant reduction in lactoferrin mRNA and protein expression reported in CRS [19]. Collectively, a reduction in secreted antimicrobials may result in inadequate removal of bacteria that may gain access to the sinonasal mucosa leading to colonization, potential biofilm formation and chronic inflammation.

Interleukin-33

IL-33 is an inflammatory cytokine whose role in CRS has gained recent interest. IL-33 has been shown to promote a Th2 response as IL-33 produces a Th2 type inflammatory response in Rag-deficient mice [36]. IL-33 acts through a heterodimeric receptor complex consisting of IL-1RL1 (ST2) and IL-1RacP [36]. One study found a significant increase in IL-33 expression in sinonasal epithelial cells derived from patients with CRSwNP that was recalcitrant to treatment compared to CRSwNP that was responsive to medical management [37]. Further supporting the importance of IL-33 in CRS was a report that found 5 SNPs in IL-1RL1 that were associated with a protective effect against CRS [38].

One hypothesis supported by recent data is that IL-33 is secreted by sinonasal epithelial cells in response to tissue damage [39]. As such, substances that signify nearby cell or tissue damage could act on sinonasal epithelial cells and cause the secretion of IL-33 as an attempt at tissue repair. If this response becomes dysregulated, a perpetuation of chronic inflammation could occur. Analogous to PAMPs are damage associated molecular patterns (DAMPs) that are believed to act as a signal of nearby injury and to initiate host repair [39]. A prototypical DAMP is constitutively expressed nuclear DNA-binding protein called high mobility group box-1 (HMGB-1) as well as purine metabolites such as ATP. In sinonasal epithelial cells isolated from CRSwNP recalcitrant to treatment, stimulation with HMGB-1 induced an exaggerated 2.8-fold increase in IL-33 mRNA as compared to a 1.2-fold increase after HMGB-1 stimulation in controls. A similar response was observed after stimulation with ATP, which induced an exaggerated 2.2-fold increase in IL-33 mRNA in sinonasal epithelial cells from recalcitrant CRSwNP [39]. These results suggest that there may be a dysregulation of IL-33 in recalcitrant CRSwNP that may contribute to persistent chronic inflammation and CRS.

Conclusion

Allergy has long been inferred to contribute to the pathophysiology of CRS although evidence has demonstrated an association rather than causation. The mechanism of how aeroallergens cause CRS is less well understood but may be through downstream systemic consequences, sinonasal epithelial barrier disruption or ostiomeatal complex obstruction. Th2 inflammatory cytokines such as IL-4 and IL-13 as well as house dust mite and cigarette smoke can disrupt normal sinonasal epithelial functions. Future studies will help us to better understand the role of the aeroallergen in the development of CRS.

References

1 Jang AS, Jun YJ, Park MK: Effects of air pollutants on upper airway disease. Curr Opin Allergy Clin Immunol 2016;16:13–17.
2 Hur K, Liang J, Lin SY: The role of secondhand smoke in sinusitis: a systematic review. Int Forum Allergy Rhinol 2014;4:22–28.
3 Higgins TS, Reh DD: Environmental pollutants and allergic rhinitis. Curr Opin Otolaryngol Head Neck Surg 2012;20:209–214.
4 Rosenfeld RM, et al: Clinical practice guideline (update): adult sinusitis executive summary. Otolaryngol Head Neck Surg 2015;152:598–609.
5 Krouse JH: Allergy and chronic rhinosinusitis. Otolaryngol Clin North Am 2005;38:1257–1266, ix–x.
6 Berrettini S, et al: Perennial allergic rhinitis and chronic sinusitis: correlation with rhinologic risk factors. Allergy 1999;54:242–248.
7 Nishioka GJ, et al: Immunotherapy in patients undergoing functional endoscopic sinus surgery. Otolaryngol Head Neck Surg 1994;110:406–412.
8 Kennedy JL, Borish L: Chronic sinusitis pathophysiology: the role of allergy. Am J Rhinol Allergy 2013;27:367–371.
9 Settipane RA, Borish L, Peters AT: Chapter 16: determining the role of allergy in sinonasal disease. Am J Rhinol Allergy 2013;27(suppl 1):S56–S58.
10 Ramanathan M Jr, Lane AP: Innate immunity of the sinonasal cavity and its role in chronic rhinosinusitis. Otolaryngol Head Neck Surg 2007;136:348–356.
11 Soyka MB, et al: Defective epithelial barrier in chronic rhinosinusitis: the regulation of tight junctions by IFN-γ and IL-4. J Allergy Clin Immunol 2012;130:1087–1096.e10.
12 Rogers GA, et al: Epithelial tight junction alterations in nasal polyposis. Int Forum Allergy Rhinol 2011;1:50–54.
13 Wise SK, et al: Interleukin-4 and interleukin-13 compromise the sinonasal epithelial barrier and perturb intercellular junction protein expression. Int Forum Allergy Rhinol 2014;4:361–370.
14 Wise SK, et al: Sinonasal epithelial wound resealing in an in vitro model: inhibition of wound closure with IL-4 exposure. Int Forum Allergy Rhinol 2013;3:439–449.
15 Henriquez OA, et al: House dust mite allergen Der p 1 effects on sinonasal epithelial tight junctions. Int Forum Allergy Rhinol 2013;3:630–635.
16 Reh DD, Higgins TS, Smith TL: Impact of tobacco smoke on chronic rhinosinusitis: a review of the literature. Int Forum Allergy Rhinol 2012;2:362–369.
17 Kulkarni R, et al: Cigarette smoke inhibits airway epithelial cell innate immune responses to bacteria. Infect Immun 2010;78:2146–2152.
18 Tamashiro E, et al: Cigarette smoke exposure impairs respiratory epithelial ciliogenesis. Am J Rhinol Allergy 2009;23:117–122.
19 Ooi EH, et al: Innate immunity. Otolaryngol Clin North Am 2010;43:473–487, vii.
20 van Drunen CM, et al: Role of innate immunity in the pathogenesis of chronic rhinosinusitis: progress and new avenues. Curr Allergy Asthma Rep 2012;12:120–126.
21 Ramanathan M Jr, et al: Sinonasal epithelial cell expression of toll-like receptor 9 is decreased in chronic rhinosinusitis with polyps. Am J Rhinol 2007;21:110–116.
22 Park CS, Cho JH, Park YJ: Toll-like receptor 2 gene polymorphisms in a Korean population: association with chronic rhinosinusitis. Otolaryngol Head Neck Surg 2011;144:96–100.
23 Hirschberg A, et al: Different activations of toll-like receptors and antimicrobial peptides in chronic rhinosinusitis with or without nasal polyposis. Eur Arch Otorhinolaryngol 2015, Epub ahead of print.
24 Lane AP, Truong-Tran QA, Schleimer RP: Altered expression of genes associated with innate immunity and inflammation in recalcitrant rhinosinusitis with polyps. Am J Rhinol 2006;20:138–144.
25 Detwiller KY, et al: Differential expression of innate immunity genes in chronic rhinosinusitis. Am J Rhinol Allergy 2014;28:374–377.
26 Dong Z, Yang Z, Wang C: Expression of TLR2 and TLR4 messenger RNA in the epithelial cells of the nasal airway. Am J Rhinol 2005;19:236–239.
27 Zhang Q, et al: Differential expression of toll-like receptor pathway genes in chronic rhinosinusitis with or without nasal polyps. Acta Otolaryngol 2013;133:165–173.
28 Zhao CY, et al: Microarray gene analysis of toll-like receptor signaling elements in chronic rhinosinusitis with nasal polyps. Int Arch Allergy Immunol 2011;156:297–304.
29 Ramanathan M Jr, et al: Th2 cytokines associated with chronic rhinosinusitis with polyps down-regulate the antimicrobial immune function of human sinonasal epithelial cells. Am J Rhinol 2008;22:115–121.

30 Wang X, et al: Relationship of TLR2, TLR4 and tissue remodeling in chronic rhinosinusitis. Int J Clin Exp Pathol 2015;8:1199–1212.
31 Chaput C, et al: NOD-like receptors in lung diseases. Front Immunol 2013;4: 393.
32 Cantero D, et al: Staphylococcus aureus biofilm activates the nucleotide-binding oligomerization domain containing 2 (Nod2) pathway and proinflammatory factors on a human sinonasal explant model. Int Forum Allergy Rhinol 2013; 3:877–884.
33 Månsson A, et al: NOD-like receptors in the human upper airways: a potential role in nasal polyposis. Allergy 2011;66: 621–628.
34 Chennupati SK, et al: Effects of an LL-37-derived antimicrobial peptide in an animal model of biofilm pseudomonas sinusitis. Am J Rhinol Allergy 2009;23: 46–51.
35 André GO, et al: Combined effects of lactoferrin and lysozyme on Streptococcus pneumoniae killing. Microb Pathog 2015;89:7–17.
36 Kato A: Immunopathology of chronic rhinosinusitis. Allergol Int 2015;64:121–130.
37 Reh DD, et al: Treatment-recalcitrant chronic rhinosinusitis with polyps is associated with altered epithelial cell expression of interleukin-33. Am J Rhinol Allergy 2010;24:105–109.
38 Castano R, et al: Evidence of association of interleukin-1 receptor-like 1 gene polymorphisms with chronic rhinosinusitis. Am J Rhinol Allergy 2009;23: 377–384.
39 Paris G, et al: Damage-associated molecular patterns stimulate interleukin-33 expression in nasal polyp epithelial cells. Int Forum Allergy Rhinol 2014;4:15–21.

Murugappan Ramanathan Jr., MD, FACS
Johns Hopkins Department of Otolaryngology – Head and Neck Surgery
601 N. Caroline Street, 6th Floor
Baltimore, MD 21287 (USA)
E-Mail mramana3@jhmi.edu

Woodworth BA, Poetker DM, Reh DD (eds): Rhinosinusitis with Nasal Polyposis.
Adv Otorhinolaryngol. Basel, Karger, 2016, vol 79, pp 78–85 (DOI: 10.1159/000445134)

Acquired Cystic Fibrosis Transmembrane Conductance Regulator Deficiency

Do-Yeon Cho[a, b] · Bradford A. Woodworth[a, b]

[a]Department of Otolaryngology and [b]Gregory Fleming James Cystic Fibrosis Research Center, University of Alabama at Birmingham, Birmingham, Ala., USA

Abstract

In the genetic airway disease cystic fibrosis (CF), deficiency or dysfunction of the cystic fibrosis membrane conductance regulator (CFTR) alters anion transport in respiratory epithelium and consequently disrupts mucociliary clearance. An enriched understanding of the role of CFTR in the maintenance of normal epithelial function has revealed that mild and variable CFTR mutations play a causative role in a number of diseases not classically associated with CF. Furthermore, recent evidence indicates that acquired defects in wild-type CFTR protein processing, endocytic recycling and function can contribute to the pathogenesis of airway diseases, such as chronic obstructive pulmonary disease. In this chapter, we discuss emerging findings implicating acquired CFTR dysfunction in the pathogenesis of chronic rhinosinusitis and propose a new and leading edge approach to future CRS therapy using CFTR potentiators.

The superficial lining of sinonasal epithelium is comprised of airway surface liquid (ASL) containing a low viscosity periciliary fluid layer (sol) around respiratory cilia and a superficial mucus (gel) layer, which function to trap and sweep inhaled particles into the digestive tract through coordinated mucociliary clearance (MCC) [1]. Ion transport channels located in the airway epithelial cell regulate hydration of airway mucosal surfaces. Therefore, altered ion transport disrupts MCC and plays a role in the pathogenesis of airway disease including rhinosinusitis [2, 3]. The cystic fibrosis transmembrane conductance regulator (CFTR) functions as a chloride (Cl^-) and bicarbonate (HCO_3) channel and is critical for maintaining the height of the ASL. In patients with cystic fibrosis (CF), loss of CFTR-mediated Cl^- secretion (genetic mutations) across the mucosal surface contributes to the development of airway disease by depleting ASL and increase the viscosity and adhesion of mucus leading to persistent infection and/or inflammation [4]. An enriched understanding of the role of CFTR in the maintenance of normal epithelial function has revealed that mild and variable CFTR mutations play a causative role in a number of diseases not classically associated with CF [5]. CFTR-related diseases encompass well-known pathological disorders that appear to be influenced by CFTR genotype, including allergic bronchopulmonary aspergillosis, idiopathic bronchiectasis and CRS [1]. In addition, recent evidence indicates that wild-type CFTR protein processing, endocytic recycling and function can also be markedly repressed by various environmental insults, including cigarette smoke exposure, high altitude/hypoxemia, inflammation and infectious agents and could contribute to the pathogenesis of CRS and other airway diseases, such as COPD [6–11]. In this chapter, we discuss emerging findings implicating acquired CFTR dysfunction in the pathogenesis of CRS and other chronic airway diseases, as well as the new treatments using Cl^- secretagogues.

Sinonasal Respiratory Epithelium in Health and Disease

Normal sinonasal MCC is a critical host defense mechanism that clears the upper airways of inhaled pathogens such as bacteria, dust and toxins [12]. Sinonasal respiratory epithelium is a highly regulated barrier, vital to the normal function of the mucociliary apparatus. MCC is dependent on inherent biological properties of intact respiratory epithelium, including proper ciliary beating and the ASL. Respiratory epithelium modifies the volume of the periciliary fluid layer and the viscoelastic properties of the mucus in a fashion that depends on vectorial transepithelial ion transport [13, 14]. Active and passive transport of electrolytes (primarily sodium [Na^+], Cl^- and HCO_3) regulate ASL, and significant alterations in ion transport can be detrimental to the airway, as clearly exemplified in CF, which affects approximately 30,000 persons in the United States (70,000 worldwide) and is the most common lethal inherited disease among Caucasians (fig. 1) [15]. In CF, mutations in the gene encoding CFTR result in decreased apical membrane chloride conductance and cause dysregulated Na^+ absorption (fig. 1) [15]. These abnormalities of fluid and electrolyte transport promote thick mucus formation and immobile exocrine secretions in multiple organ systems. In the sinuses of CF individuals, chronic stasis of inspissated mucus in combination with bacterial infection results in nearly universal inflammatory pan-sinusitis [1, 11, 16].

Importantly, less severe reductions in CFTR function may also be associated with CRS in the absence of classical CF disease [17]. It has been suggested that otherwise healthy patients heterozygous for the CFTR mutation have an increased likelihood of developing CRS with nasal polyposis [18–20]. Wang et al. [17]. performed genetic testing on 147 non-CF patients with severe CRS and discovered a 7% incidence of CFTR mutations compared to the presence of 2% in 123 healthy controls ($p = 0.04$). In another study of 58 children with CRS, 7 (12%) carried a single CF mutation, which was much higher than the expected frequency of 4% [21]. These data suggest that there is an increased occurrence of CFTR mutations in children who have CRS and do not meet diagnostic criteria for CF, usually in the setting of a normal sweat chloride. Together, the 2 genetic studies indicate that CFTR mutations predispose to CRS across different age groups and suggest that even with apparently 'normal' CFTR function, small derangements in CFTR conferred by a single mutated allele may impact the function of the upper airway.

Acquired CFTR Deficiency

Emerging evidence indicates that acquired CFTR deficiency may contribute to respiratory epithelial dysfunction in chronic airway diseases by increasing mucus viscosity via suppression of epithelial chloride (Cl^-) secretion [22–24]. While the pathogenesis of CRS is a heterogeneous disease process and secondary to multiple clinical, environmental and intrinsic factors, the presence of acquired ion transport deficiencies provides a more global, unifying mechanism for perpetuation of persistent CRS. For example, human sinonasal epithelial tissue freshly harvested from CRS patients exhibit markedly diminished CFTR-mediated Cl^- secretion compared to normal control tissue *despite the absence of mutations in the*

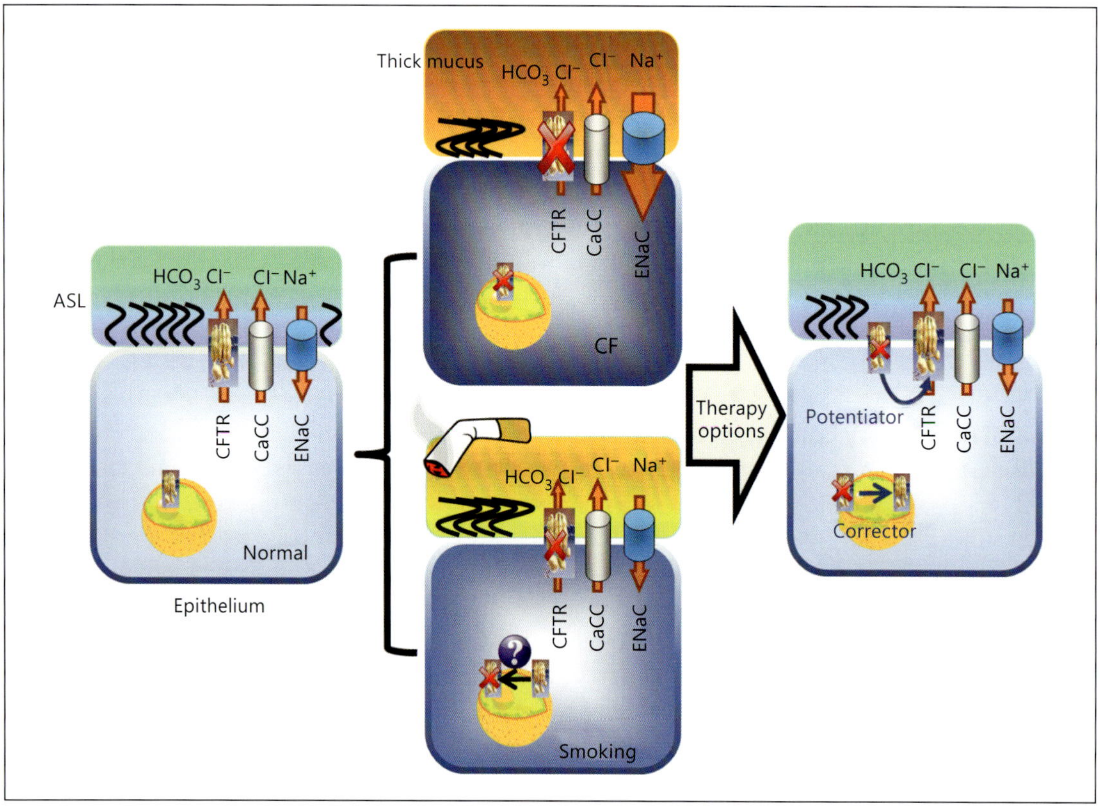

Fig. 1. Airway epithelium in health and disease. In normal airway epithelium, CFTR is expressed at the apical surface of epithelium with alternative Ca^{2+}-activated Cl^- channels (CaCC, also known as TMEM16A) and epithelial Na^+ channels (ENaC). Active and passive transport of electrolytes (primarily sodium [Na^+], Cl^- and HCO_3) regulate ASL, and significant alterations in ion transport can be detrimental to airway mucus clearance. In CF airway epithelia, CFTR dysfunction at the apical surface causes dehydration of the periciliary and mucus layers leading to mucociliary dysfunction and airway mucus plugging. Acquired CFTR dysfunction may hinder proper mucus hydration and put smokers at risk for mucus stasis and chronic airway disease. Current therapeutic strategies focus on the development of CFTR modulators that correct misprocessing of the most common mutation F508 (corrector) and enhance the function of CFTR (potentiator) to restore airway surface hydration and mucus clearance.

CFTR gene [2]. These findings indicate that abnormal ion transport is present in sinonasal epithelia of patients with CRS and likely contributes to airway surface dehydration and prolongation of mucostasis.

Tobacco Smoke

One such environmental perturbation that may lead to acquired CFTR deficiency in CRS and other chronic airway diseases is exposure to cigarette smoke. Children exposed to tobacco smoke require revision sinus surgery for persistent or recurrent rhinosinusitis substantially more often than children not exposed to tobacco smoke [25]. Critical analysis of a national cross-sectional health survey published in 2000 showed a higher prevalence of recurrent sinusitis and CRS in cigarette smokers as compared to non-smokers [26]. Furthermore, patients with COPD induced by smoking have histopathological similarities to patients with CF [27, 28]. The phenotypic similarity between COPD and CF is most pronounced in those with symptoms of chronic bronchitis in whom a relatively high incidence of bronchiectasis has been reported; however, the overproduction, poor clearance and accumulation of hyperviscous mucus within the small airways is also present in patients with an emphysema-dominant phenotype [29–31].

Studies analyzing the effect of cigarette smoke on airway ion transport demonstrated that cigarette smoke impairs CFTR expression and function in airway epithelia at various levels, ranging from reduced transcription to protein degradation, resulting in acquired CFTR dysfunction [10, 32–34]. Cigarette smoke has acute effects on CFTR activity in the airways of healthy nonsmokers causing ~60% inhibition of CFTR-mediated Cl^- secretion in vivo, as well as airway surface dehydration and reduced mucus transport in vitro. Cigarette smoke condensate has also been shown to inhibit transepithelial Cl^- secretion (through CFTR and the calcium-activated Cl^- channel TMEM16A) and ciliary beat frequencies in upper respiratory airway epithelial cells in vitro [9, 35]. Smokers who developed COPD exhibited reduced CFTR-mediated Cl^- secretion in the upper and lower airways associated with mucus depletion (dehydration) [33, 34]. Nasal MCC is also significantly slowed in humans with chronic cigarette smoke exposure [36]. In addition, subjects with COPD who no longer smoke have normal Cl^- transport as measured by nasal potential difference, suggesting that CFTR function in the upper airway can recover after smoking cessation perhaps because of rapid epithelial cell turnover or other mechanisms [10]. Recent data indicates that effects of cigarette smoke on CFTR are not limited to the airway, but that smoking causes systemic CFTR dysfunction, probably via a circulating agent, which may contribute to pancreatitis, male infertility and cachexia that have been linked to cigarette smoking and are also characteristic features of CF [32, 37–39]. In summary, these studies propose that reduced levels of functional CFTR in smokers may contribute to CRS pathogenesis and that drugs developed to improve mutant CFTR function in CF may also be beneficial in patients with chronic airway disease.

Hypoxia

It has been suggested that hypoxia does have considerable influence in the pathophysiology of CRS among non-CF individuals [40, 41]. Blockage of sinus ostia may lead to hypoxia, resulting in decreased MCC, elaboration of inflammatory mediators and bacterial colonization [42]. In addition, accumulated secretions and impacted mucus lead to poor oxygen delivery, resulting in near anaerobic tissue conditions that accelerate progression of disease [43]. Hypoxia in the sinuses of CRS patients could contribute to propagation of sinus disease by creating a localized CFTR-deficient environment where abnormalities of fluid and electrolyte transport persist [12]. In vitro experiments demonstrated that a low oxygen environment profoundly affected normal ion transport physiology in both murine and human sinonasal epithelium and leads to acquired defects in CFTR-mediated transport [12]. Importantly, human sinonasal epithelia developed a globally decreased transepithelial Cl^- secretion and *increased* Na^+ absorption in response to hypoxic conditions indicating that all major pathways necessary to maintain normal ASL hydration (Cl^- and HCO_3^- secretion through CFTR and TMEM16A pathways; Na^+ absorption through ENaC) are affected by tissue hypoxia. Thus, ion transport properties are consistent with CF airway pathophysiology (decreased Cl^- secretion and enhanced Na^+ absorption) resulting in dehydration of the ASL and, ultimately, disrupted mucociliary transport. ASL depth was also decreased under hypoxic conditions, providing direct evidence that altered ion transport in this culture model leads to ASL depletion (fig. 2). These findings suggest a strategy aimed at stimulating electrolyte secretion with drugs that target CFTR, therefore promoting mucus clearance, would furnish a valuable addition to the pharmacologic armamentarium available for treatment of sinusitis.

Targeting Acquired CFTR Dysfunction in CRS

Ivacaftor
Several small organic molecules that activate CFTR have been identified through high-throughput drug screening [12]. Pharmaceutical companies have pursued CFTR potentiators for therapy of diseases of mucus clearance, including both CF and COPD. Enhancing Cl^- secretion in sinus epithelia by CFTR potentiators represents a novel approach to treatment that has been shown to activate MCC in human subjects. Ivacaftor represents one of many drugs that enhance Cl^- transport and could provide significant therapeutic advantages in this regard. For example, recent studies have shown that Ivacaftor augments ASL depth, accelerates MCC and pharmacologically reverses acquired CFTR dysfunction due to cigarette smoke exposure [24, 44]. Given this precedent, the compound represents an excellent candidate for treatment of acquired Cl^- transport defects in human sinus disease based on an established safety profile, current FDA approval for a different clinical indication (CF) and oral bioavailability. Future clinical studies are necessary in subjects with non-CF CRS to test the efficacy of this exciting therapeutic.

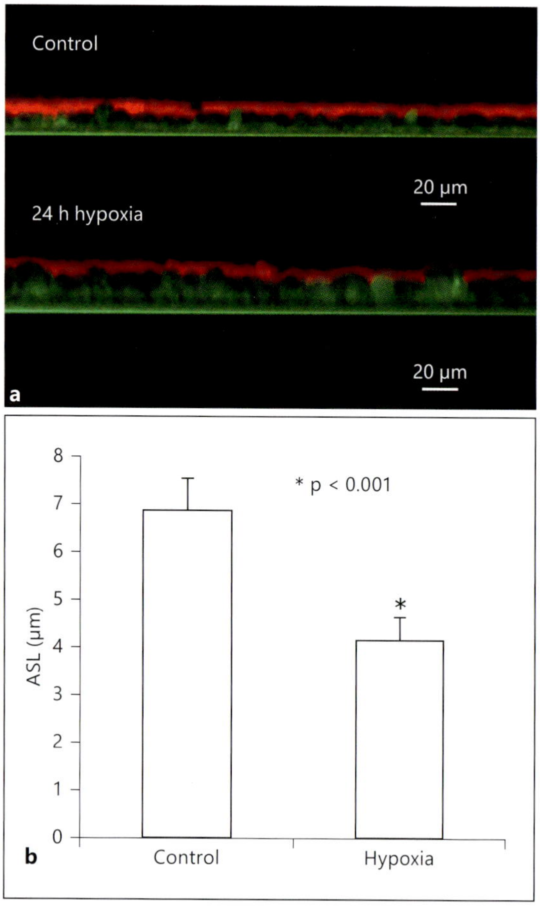

Fig. 2. ASL depth is decreased in cultured respiratory epithelium when incubated in a low oxygen environment. Because CFTR secretes Cl^- to regulate ASL depth, an important determinant of normal MCC, we evaluated whether hypoxic incubation for 24 h would induce ASL depletion by confocal microscopy (panel **a**). Incubation in 1% oxygen decreased ASL depth compared to control monolayers (panel **b**).

Resveratrol
Resveratrol is an organic polyphenol found in many plants and vegetables, including the skins of red fruits, trees, some flowering plants and peanuts [45, 46]. Broadly recognized for its immune-modulator activity attributable to inhibition of NF-κB signaling, resveratrol markedly reduces inflammatory pathways mediated by granulocyte macrophage colony-stimulating factor (GM-CSF), IL-8 (or the murine homologue KC), inducible nitric oxide synthase and COX-2 [47]. Resveratrol enhances CFTR-dependent Cl^- secretion in human sinonasal epithelium to an extent comparable to ivacaftor [12]. Cl^- transport across human sinonasal explants and in vivo murine nasal epithelium were also significantly increased by the drug. A 30-minute apical application of resveratrol increased ASL depth in normal epithelium and furthermore, hypoxia-induced

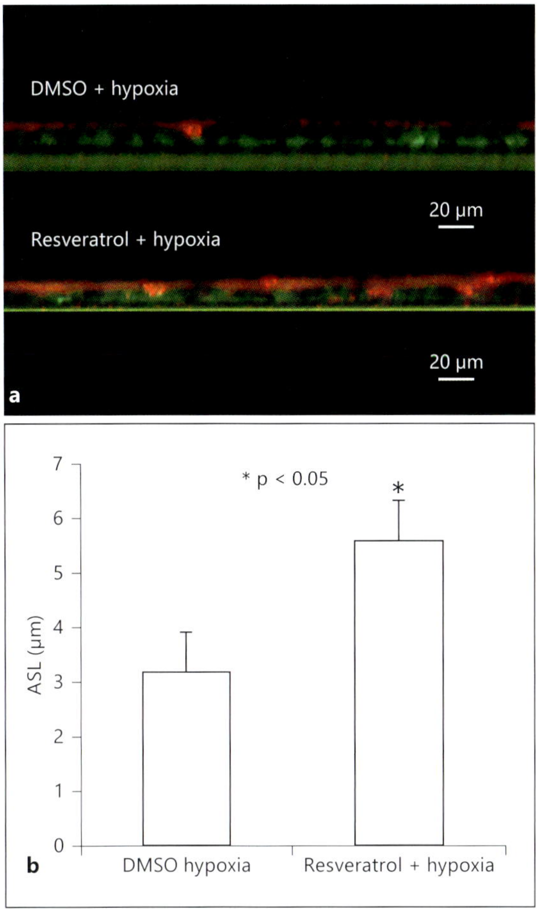

Fig. 3. Resveratrol restores hypoxia-depleted ASL. Because apical fluid is applied with resveratrol treatment, hypoxia controls require the corresponding control (DMSO) vehicle. Confocal images are demonstrated (panel **a**). Resveratrol treatment significantly mitigated hypoxia-induced reduction in ASL depth, reaching 91% of the ASL depth found in epithelial cultures incubated with DMSO (panel **b**). This indicates resveratrol could potentially be used as a topical treatment for ASL depleted sinus mucosa. DMSO = Dimethyl sulfoxide.

abnormalities of fluid and electrolyte secretion in sinonasal epithelium were restored with resveratrol treatment (fig. 3). CFTR activation with a leading edge Cl^- secretagogue such as resveratrol represents another innovative approach to overcoming acquired CFTR defects in sinus and nasal airway disease.

L-Ascorbate (Commonly Known as Vitamin C)

L-ascorbate is an essential nutrient most notable for its role as a powerful antioxidant working to lower oxidative stress on cells [48]. Application of L-ascorbate to the surface of freshly excised sinonasal tissue stimulated Cl^- secretion in a sustained fashion to 70% (in sinus epithelium from CRS) and 53.6% (in nasal epithelium from CRS) of maximally stimulated Cl^- currents [2]. Insufficient dietary intake of L-ascorbate, environmental pollutants and a number of inflammatory disorders of the airways are known to severely deplete the pools of this vitamin in ASL or plasma [49]. Because plasma concentration does not exceed to the level of CFTR stimulation even at higher oral doses, oral supplementation of vitamin C may not be sufficient to enhance transepithelial Cl^- secretion [50]. Topical delivery of L-ascorbate to the paranasal sinuses yields a higher concentration at the target tissues and may be an effective therapeutic modality for loosening thick mucus secretions and improving MCC within the paranasal sinuses [51].

Sinupret

Sinupret® has been utilized extensively throughout Europe for more than 70 years as treatment of airway diseases associated with inadequate MCC and has an excellent safety profile [10]. The medication is registered as a regulated phyto-pharmaceutical in Germany and has been available in the United States for 9 years where it is considered an herbal supplement (not regulated by the FDA) [10]. Several clinical trials have tested the effect of Sinupret either alone or in combination with antibiotics for rhinosinusitis. Significant improvement in radiologic outcomes and headache were demonstrated in a randomized, placebo-controlled trial [52]. Studies using upper airway epithelial cells demonstrated that Sinupret likely derives its clinical benefit, at least in part, through stimulating transepithelial Cl^- secretion, CBF and MCC [10, 53]. Given the clinical efficacy of the compound, these findings provide further rationale for using robust Cl^- secretagogue-based therapies as a treatment modality for common respiratory diseases of MCC including CRS.

Conclusions

The discovery of the CFTR gene 25 years ago has helped unravel the molecular and cellular pathogenesis of CF disease [24]. Basic and translational studies, multiple cell lines, human primary airway epithelia and animal models have led to a detailed and still growing understanding of the function and regulation of CFTR. Recent evidence that acquired CFTR dysfunction may contribute to CRS pathogenesis provides a new target for treatment that is distinct from current therapeutic strategies such as antibiotics and anti-inflammatories. Enhancing Cl^- secretion in sinus epithelia by CFTR potentiators represents a new and leading edge approach to future CRS therapy.

Conflict of Interest

Bradford A. Woodworth, MD, is a consultant for Olympus and Cook Medical which is not affiliated with this work.

References

1 Chaaban MR, Kejner A, Rowe SM, Woodworth BA: Cystic fibrosis chronic rhinosinusitis: a comprehensive review. Am J Rhinol Allergy 2013;27:387–395.
2 Cho DY, Hwang PH, Illek B: Effect of L-ascorbate on chloride transport in freshly excised sinonasal epithelia. Am J Rhinol Allergy 2009;23:294–299.
3 Dejima K, Randell SH, Stutts MJ, Senior BA, Boucher RC: Potential role of abnormal ion transport in the pathogenesis of chronic sinusitis. Arch Otolaryngol Head Neck Surg 2006;132:1352–1362.
4 Chaudhry AL, Chaaban MR, Ranganath NK, Woodworth BA: Topical triamcinolone acetonide/carboxymethylcellulose foam for acute exacerbations of chronic rhinosinusitis/nasal polyposis. Am J Rhinol Allergy 2014;28:341–344.
5 Knowles MR, Durie PR: What is cystic fibrosis? N Engl J Med 2002;347:439–442.
6 Alexander NS, Blount A, Zhang S, et al: Cystic fibrosis transmembrane conductance regulator modulation by the tobacco smoke toxin acrolein. Laryngoscope 2012;122:1193–1197.
7 Bebok Z, Varga K, Hicks JK, et al: Reactive oxygen nitrogen species decrease cystic fibrosis transmembrane conductance regulator expression and cAMP-mediated Cl- secretion in airway epithelia. J Biol Chem 2002;277:43041–43049.
8 Bomberger JM, Ye S, Maceachran DP, et al: A Pseudomonas aeruginosa toxin that hijacks the host ubiquitin proteolytic system. PLoS Pathog 2011;7:e1001325.
9 Cohen NA, Zhang S, Sharp DB, et al: Cigarette smoke condensate inhibits transepithelial chloride transport and ciliary beat frequency. Laryngoscope 2009;119:2269–2274.
10 Zhang S, Skinner D, Hicks SB, et al: Sinupret activates CFTR and TMEM16A-dependent transepithelial chloride transport and improves indicators of mucociliary clearance. PLoS One 2014;9:e104090.
11 Virgin FW, Rowe SM, Wade MB, et al: Extensive surgical and comprehensive postoperative medical management for cystic fibrosis chronic rhinosinusitis. Am J Rhinol Allergy 2012;26:70–75.
12 Woodworth BA: Resveratrol ameliorates abnormalities of fluid and electrolyte secretion in a hypoxia-Induced model of acquired CFTR deficiency. Laryngoscope 2015;125(suppl 7):S1–S13.
13 Phillips JE, Wong LB, Yeates DB: Bidirectional transepithelial water transport: measurement and governing mechanisms. Biophys J 1999;76:869–877.
14 Trout L, King M, Feng W, Inglis SK, Ballard ST: Inhibition of airway liquid secretion and its effect on the physical properties of airway mucus. Am J Physiol 1998;274(2 pt 1):L258–L263.
15 Knowles M, Gatzy J, Boucher R: Relative ion permeability of normal and cystic fibrosis nasal epithelium. J Clin Invest 1983;71:1410–1417.
16 Illing EA, Woodworth BA: Management of the upper airway in cystic fibrosis. Curr Opin Pulm Med 2014;20:623–631.
17 Wang X, Moylan B, Leopold DA, et al: Mutation in the gene responsible for cystic fibrosis and predisposition to chronic rhinosinusitis in the general population. JAMA 2000;284:1814–1819.
18 Burger J, Macek M Jr, Stuhrmann M, Reis A, Krawczak M, Schmidtke J: Genetic influences in the formation of nasal polyps. Lancet 1991;337:974.
19 Irving RM, McMahon R, Clark R, Jones NS: Cystic fibrosis transmembrane conductance regulator gene mutations in severe nasal polyposis. Clin Otolaryngol Allied Sci 1997;22:519–521.
20 Varon R, Magdorf K, Staab D, et al: Recurrent nasal polyps as a monosymptomatic form of cystic fibrosis associated with a novel in-frame deletion (591del18) in the CFTR gene. Hum Mol Genet 1995;4:1463–1464.
21 Raman V, Clary R, Siegrist KL, Zehnbauer B, Chatila TA: Increased prevalence of mutations in the cystic fibrosis transmembrane conductance regulator in children with chronic rhinosinusitis. Pediatrics 2002;109:E13.

22 Button B, Cai LH, Ehre C, et al: A periciliary brush promotes the lung health by separating the mucus layer from airway epithelia. Science 2012;337:937–941.
23 Dickey BF: Biochemistry. Walking on solid ground. Science 2012;337:924–925.
24 Sloane PA, Shastry S, Wilhelm A, et al: A pharmacologic approach to acquired cystic fibrosis transmembrane conductance regulator dysfunction in smoking related lung disease. PLoS One 2012; 7:e39809.
25 Ramadan HH, Hinerman RA: Smoke exposure and outcome of endoscopic sinus surgery in children. Otolaryngol Head Neck Surg 2002;127:546–548.
26 Lieu JE, Feinstein AR: Confirmations and surprises in the association of tobacco use with sinusitis. Arch Otolaryngol Head Neck Surg 2000;126:940–946.
27 Rowe SM, Miller S, Sorscher EJ: Cystic fibrosis. N Engl J Med 2005;352:1992–2001.
28 Sethi S, Maloney J, Grove L, Wrona C, Berenson CS: Airway inflammation and bronchial bacterial colonization in chronic obstructive pulmonary disease. Am J Respir Crit Care Med 2006;173: 991–998.
29 Hogg JC, Chu F, Utokaparch S, et al: The nature of small-airway obstruction in chronic obstructive pulmonary disease. N Engl J Med 2004;350:2645–2653.
30 Hogg JC, Chu FS, Tan WC, et al: Survival after lung volume reduction in chronic obstructive pulmonary disease: insights from small airway pathology. Am J Respir Crit Care Med 2007;176:454–459.
31 Martinez-Garcia MA, Soler-Cataluna JJ, Donat Sanz Y, et al: Factors associated with bronchiectasis in patients with COPD. Chest 2011;140:1130–1137.
32 Cantin AM, Hanrahan JW, Bilodeau G, et al: Cystic fibrosis transmembrane conductance regulator function is suppressed in cigarette smokers. Am J Respir Crit Care Med 2006;173:1139–1144.
33 Clunes LA, Davies CM, Coakley RD, et al: Cigarette smoke exposure induces CFTR internalization and insolubility, leading to airway surface liquid dehydration. FASEB J 2012;26:533–545.
34 Dransfield MT, Wilhelm AM, Flanagan B, et al: Acquired cystic fibrosis transmembrane conductance regulator dysfunction in the lower airways in COPD. Chest 2013;144:498–506.
35 Virgin FW, Azbell C, Schuster D, et al: Exposure to cigarette smoke condensate reduces calcium activated chloride channel transport in primary sinonasal epithelial cultures. Laryngoscope 2010; 120:1465–1469.
36 Stanley PJ, Wilson R, Greenstone MA, MacWilliam L, Cole PJ: Effect of cigarette smoking on nasal mucociliary clearance and ciliary beat frequency. Thorax 1986;41:519–523.
37 Rab A, Rowe SM, Raju SV, Bebok Z, Matalon S, Collawn JF: Cigarette smoke and CFTR: implications in the pathogenesis of COPD. Am J Physiol Lung Cell Mol Physiol 2013;305:L530–L541.
38 Raju SV, Jackson PL, Courville CA, et al: Cigarette smoke induces systemic defects in cystic fibrosis transmembrane conductance regulator function. Am J Respir Crit Care Med 2013;188:1321–1330.
39 Raju SV, Tate JH, Peacock SK, et al: Impact of heterozygote CFTR mutations in COPD patients with chronic bronchitis. Respir Res 2014;15:18.
40 Baroody FM: Mucociliary transport in chronic rhinosinusitis. Clin Allergy Immunol 2007;20:103–119.
41 Pahl A, Szelenyi S, Brune K: Hypoxia induced chemokine expression in nasal epithelial cells: development of an in vitro model for chronic rhinosinusitis. ALTEX 2006;23:59–63.
42 Steinke JW, Woodard CR, Borish L: Role of hypoxia in inflammatory upper airway disease. Curr Opin Allergy Clin Immunol 2008;8:16–20.
43 Worlitzsch D, Tarran R, Ulrich M, et al: Effects of reduced mucus oxygen concentration in airway Pseudomonas infections of cystic fibrosis patients. J Clin Invest 2002;109:317–325.
44 Conger BT, Zhang S, Skinner D, et al: Comparison of cystic fibrosis transmembrane conductance regulator (CFTR) and ciliary beat frequency activation by the CFTR modulators genistein, VRT-532, and UCCF-152 in primary sinonasal epithelial cultures. JAMA Otolaryngol Head Neck Surg 2013;139: 822–827.
45 Donnelly LE, Newton R, Kennedy GE, et al: Anti-inflammatory effects of resveratrol in lung epithelial cells: molecular mechanisms. Am J Physiol Lung Cell Mol Physiol 2004;287:L774–L783.
46 Lee M, Kim S, Kwon OK, Oh SR, Lee HK, Ahn K: Anti-inflammatory and anti-asthmatic effects of resveratrol, a polyphenolic stilbene, in a mouse model of allergic asthma. Int Immunopharmacol 2009;9:418–424.
47 Manna SK, Mukhopadhyay A, Aggarwal BB: Resveratrol suppresses TNF-induced activation of nuclear transcription factors NF-kappa B, activator protein-1, and apoptosis: potential role of reactive oxygen intermediates and lipid peroxidation. J Immunol 2000;164: 6509–6519.
48 Slade R, Crissman K, Norwood J, Hatch G: Comparison of antioxidant substances in bronchoalveolar lavage cells and fluid from humans, guinea pigs, and rats. Exp Lung Res 1993;19:469–484.
49 Kodavanti UP, Costa DL, Richards J, Crissman KM, Slade R, Hatch GE: Antioxidants in bronchoalveolar lavage fluid cells isolated from ozone – exposed normal and ascorbate-deficient guinea pigs. Exp Lung Res 1996;22:435–448.
50 Levine M, Conry-Cantilena C, Wang Y, et al: Vitamin C pharmacokinetics in healthy volunteers: evidence for a recommended dietary allowance. Proc Natl Acad Sci U S A 1996;93:3704–3709.
51 Fischer H, Schwarzer C, Illek B: Vitamin C controls the cystic fibrosis transmembrane conductance regulator chloride channel. Proc Natl Acad Sci U S A 2004; 101:3691–3696.
52 Richstein A, Mann W: [Treatment of chronic sinusitis with sinupret]. Ther Ggw 1980;119:1055–1060.
53 Virgin F, Zhang S, Schuster D, et al: The bioflavonoid compound, sinupret, stimulates transepithelial chloride transport in vitro and in vivo. Laryngoscope 2010; 120:1051–1056.

Bradford A. Woodworth, MD
Department of Otolaryngology – Head and Neck Surgery
University of Alabama at Birmingham
BDB 563, 1720 2nd Ave. S, Birmingham, AL 35294 (USA)
E-Mail bwoodwo@hotmail.com

Woodworth BA, Poetker DM, Reh DD (eds): Rhinosinusitis with Nasal Polyposis.
Adv Otorhinolaryngol. Basel, Karger, 2016, vol 79, pp 86–90 (DOI: 10.1159/000445136)

Role of Vitamin D in Pathogenesis of Chronic Sinusitis with Nasal Polyposis

Arash Shahangian · Rodney J. Schlosser

Medical University of South Carolina, Department of Otolaryngology/Head and Neck Surgery, Division of Rhinology, Charleston, S.C., USA

Abstract

Vitamin D3 (VD3) is a potent immunomodulatory steroid hormone involved in the regulation of numerous host immune cells. Additionally, it may have an important role in host immunity against chronic bacterial infections, as well as in chronic rhinosinusitis. Many factors modulate expression of various enzymes important for production of VD3, local concentration of which may be important for its complex and diverse functions. Here, we explore some of the contributions of VD3 to chronic rhinosinusitis with nasal polyposis and its role as a disease-modifying agent.

Introduction

Vitamin D3 (VD3) has long been known for its effects on calcium metabolism. However, in the recent years an increasing body of evidence suggests that this fat-soluble molecule is important in a variety of inflammatory and immune conditions. VD3 is produced via a photo-catalysed reaction in the skin. It undergoes 25-hydroxylation in the liver and then 1-hydroxylation in the kidneys to become 1,25VD3 [1]. This active form of VD3 has antibacterial and anti-inflammatory actions that have spurred interest in its contribution to chronic rhinosinusitis (CRS). In this chapter, we will review the current evidence in the field of rhinology with regards to VD3's contribution to CRS with nasal polyposis (CRSwNP).

Clinical Studies

Polyp Status

VD3 deficiency has been noted in patients with CRSwNP and allergic fungal rhinosinusitis (AFRS), but not CRS without nasal polyposis (CRSsNP). Mulligan et al. [2] found that patients with CRSwNP and AFRS, but not CRSsNP, have decreased levels of systemic 25VD3 compared with controls. Blood samples from these patients had increased levels of circulating mature den-

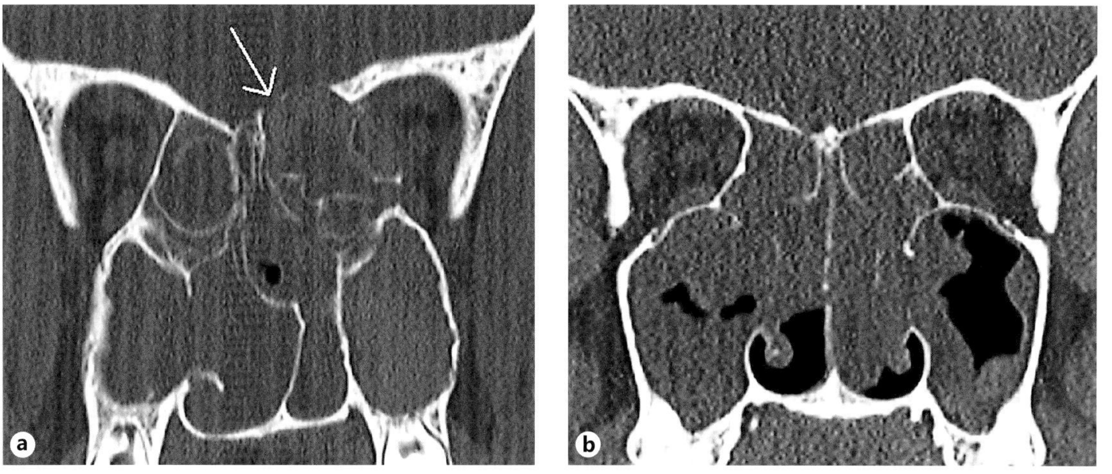

Fig. 1. (**a**) Sinus CT demonstrates bone erosion with differential densities in a typical AFRS patient with vitamin D deficiency, compared to (**b**) typical CT scan of a patient with AERD.

dritic cells expressing co-stimulatory molecules which correlated inversely with levels of 25VD3. It is likely that 25VD3 deficiency in polypoid variants of CRS contributes to the pathophysiology of disease by allowing increased activation of dendritic cells.

Recently, in a retrospective analysis of 70 CRSwNP patients, Schlosser et al. [3] found that greater than 85% of patients were 25VD3 insufficient or deficient (<30 ng/ml). African-American patients were particularly affected, approaching an 80% insufficiency rate. Interestingly, severity of sinonasal mucosal disease as defined by Lund–Mackay (LM) score on computed tomography (CT) scan inversely correlated with $25VD_3$ level in these patients. These findings were corroborated by Wang et al. [4] who found that patients with CRSwNP had lower levels of 25VD3 as compared with those with CRSsNP. This study also found that polyp grade and LM CT scores inversely correlated with 25VD3 levels.

Bone Erosion

VD3 deficiency has been correlated with bony erosion observed on CT scans in patients with CRSwNP (fig. 1). This phenomenon is particularly evident in patients with AFRS, which also are patients with the lowest levels of 25VD3 [2]. Possible mechanistic explanation were alluded to in a study by Sugimoto et al. [5] that showed ethmoid osteoblasts produced more TGFβ when cultured in the presence of VD3 (type was not described). Under these conditions, cultured osteoblasts produced higher levels of bone mineralization and osteocalcin, a marker for osteoclast activity.

Pediatric Patients

In pediatric patients, 25VD3 deficiency has been described in patients with CRSwNP and AFRS, but not CRSsNP. [6]. Systemic 25VD3 levels did not seem to be related to asthma status, gender, atopic status or age. In patients with CRSwNP and AFRS, there is impaired expression of 1-α-hydroxylase. This may explain lower levels of 1,25VD3 in sinonasal epithelium. Despite this, no differences in circulating levels of 1,25VD3 were detected suggesting that this is likely a local phenomenon. Interestingly, 1-α-hydoxylase expression was inversely correlated with symptoms scores in patients with CRSwNP. These data largely corroborate the findings in adult patients.

Tobacco Smoke
Effect of smoking on VD3 deficiency has been studied in the context of CRS and asthma. Environmental tobacco exposure has been shown to increase severity of both upper and lower respiratory inflammatory conditions. Exposure to tobacco increases inflammatory markers in human nasal mucosa and is linked to worsening nasal congestion and irritation. It appears that tobacco exposure at least in part inhibits production of 1,25VD3, thereby increasing the inflammatory milieu of the sinonasal cavity. Specifically, it appears that tobacco smoke inhibits expression of 1-α-hydroxylase and is associated with reduced 25VD3. Addition of 1,25VD3 to tobacco smoke-treated cells has been shown to inhibit production of inflammatory cytokines [7].

Inflammatory Response
Given the clinical findings of systemic 25VD3 deficiency and impaired local activation of 25VD3, more detailed immunologic studies have been conducted.

Epithelial Cells
Human sinonasal epithelial cells have been shown to express 1-α- hydroxylase [8]. This enzyme plays a role in production of 1,25VD3 in the sinonasal mucosa, which has putative anti-inflammatory and antibacterial action. The levels of this enzyme are reduced in CRSwNP when compared with normal and CRSsNP patients. Treatment of epithelial cells with 25VD3 leads to conversion to 1,25VD3 and production of the defensin-Like antibacterial peptide cathelicidin. Interestingly, this process has been shown to be impaired in patient with CRSwNP [7]. 1,25VD3 is in turn a potent inhibitor of nasal polyp fibroblast proliferation and production of pro-inflammatory cytokines RANTES, IL-6 and IL-8 [9]. Sansoni et al. [10] showed that lower plasma 25VD3 levels were associated with higher levels of RANTES and bFGF in the mucous from patients with CRSwNP, but not with CRSsNP. This study showed that 25VD3 levels were lower in CRSwNP patients as compared to those with CRSsNP, corroborating earlier data by Schlosser's group. Local deficiency of 1,25VD3 likely contributes the overactive inflammatory but impaired antibacterial phenotype observed in these patients.

Fibroblasts
Nasal polyp fibroblasts proliferation is potently inhibited by addition of 1,25VD3-analogue tacalcitol. This inhibition was potentiated by addition of the topical steroid budesonide (DR1) [9]. Furthermore, 1,25VD3 can inhibit production of RANTES and IL-1β-induced eotaxin in these cells [11]. Relative low levels of 1,25VD3 in patients with polypoid CRS likely contributes to proliferation of nasal polyp fibroblasts promoting polyp formation and inflammation.

Monocytes
VD3 has recently been found to be an important player in the host innate immune responses. In human monocytes, both 1-α-hydroxylase and vitamin D receptor (VDR) expression is markedly upregulated after stimulation of toll-like receptors (TLRs), leading to augmentation of local 1,25VD3 production and activity. In humans, it has been shown that 1,25VD3 is a potent inducer of cathelicidin, a defensin-like peptide produced by humans with activity against a myriad of bacterial pathogens. Furthermore, it has been shown that individuals with reduced levels of 1,25VD3 have decreased production of cathelicidin in response to TLR stimulation. Monocytes from VD3-deficient patients have reduced innate bactericidal activity and they are systemically more sensitive to bacterial infections [12]. VD3 has been shown to be important for autophagy, an important immune surveillance mechanisms by which various cytoplasmic contents including organelles are combined with lysosomes [13].

The effect of VD3 on sinonasal monocytes and macrophages is an area of interest for future studies.

Dendritic Cells

In the case of dendritic cells the picture is somewhat more complex. This is in part due to the fact that dendritic cells partake in both innate and adaptive arms of the immune system. In human dendritic cells (DCs), VD3 is important for maturation and antigen presentation upon stimulation of TLRs. It also is important for production of cathelicidin, which is again critical for innate antibacterial responses [12]. Moreover, 1,25VD3 is thought to play a tolerogenic role in dendritic cells. DCs can differentiate into myeloid or plasmacytoid dendritic cells. The former is a potent activator of T cell responses, while the latter plays a tolerogenic role. 25VD3 inhibits formation of myeloid DC, which results in attenuation of T cell responses [13]. Overall, CRSwNP patients have increased numbers of systemic and local dendritic cells, which may explain some of the TH-2 skewing, observed in these patients.

T and B Cells

Human T cells express increasing levels of VDR as they mature in the thymus. However once development is complete, VDR expression is turned off. Naïve B and T cells do not express any VDR; however, its expression is turned on upon activation by mitogens. It appears that 1,25VD3 potently inhibits proliferation of T lymphocytes. Via modulation of antigen presenting cells, as well direct effects on T cells, 1,25VD3 induces formation of regulatory T cells, which are important for peripheral tolerance [13]. The effect of 1,25VD3 on B cells is somewhat similar. Proliferation of isotype-switched B cell and plasma cell differentiation are both inhibited by 1,25VD3 [13]. Effects of VD3 deficiency on B and T cells from patients with CRS would be an area of interest for future research.

Vitamin D Supplementation

Given the increased prevalence of VD3 deficiency and its noted association with various inflammatory conditions, interest has emerged in using VD3 supplementation for treatment of inflammatory and infectious conditions. Randomized controlled trials have shown that VD3 supplementation can effectively reduce rates of influenza infection in children and patients prone to recurrent respiratory tract infections [14], [15]. Despite this, the vitamin D Add-on Therapy Enhances Corticosteroid Responsiveness in Asthma trial failed to show a significant reduction in asthma exacerbations or treatment failures based on oral supplementation with VD3 [16].

Conclusions

VD3 deficiency is problematic worldwide. Increased use of sunscreen, reduced time spent outdoors, rise of obesity and increased population in northern latitudes have been implicated as contributing factors. Besides its well-described role in calcium homeostasis, VD3 appears to play a role in modulation of the immune system by activating innate antibacterial responses while generally having a tolerogenic effect with respect to adaptive immunity. Its role in pathogenesis of CRSwNP is now just beginning to be better understood. It appears that sinonasal epithelial cells express 1-α-hydroxylase and can produce 1,25VD3 locally. Absence of this molecule likely leads to reduced antibacterial responses, increased elaboration of inflammatory cytokines and increased fibroblast proliferation in patients with CRSwNP. While it remains unclear whether 25VD3 deficiency is causational in this disease, there is likely a role for its use as a disease-modifying agent in treatment of patients with recalcitrant CRSwNP and AFRS.

References

1 Christakos S, Ajibade DV, Dhawan P, Fechner AJ, Mady LJ: Vitamin D: metabolism. Endocrinol Metab Clin North Am 2010;39:243–253.

2 Mulligan JK, Bleier BS, O'Connell B, Mulligan RM, Wagner C, Schlosser RJ: Vitamin D3 correlates inversely with systemic dendritic cell numbers and bone erosion in chronic rhinosinusitis with nasal polyps and allergic fungal rhinosinusitis. Clin Exp Immunol 2011; 164:312–320.

3 Schlosser RJ, Soler ZM, Schmedes GW, Storck K, Mulligan JK: Impact of vitamin D deficiency upon clinical presentation in nasal polyposis. Int Forum Allergy Rhinol 2014;4:196–199.

4 Wang LF, Lee CH, Chien CY, Chen JY, Chiang FY, Tai CF: Serum 25-hydroxyvitamin D levels are lower in chronic rhinosinusitis with nasal polyposis and are correlated with disease severity in Taiwanese patients. Am J Rhinol Allergy 2013;27:e162–e165.

5 Sugimoto I, Hirakawa K, Ishino T, Takeno S, Yajin K: Vitamin D3, vitamin K2, and warfarin regulate bone metabolism in human paranasal sinus bones. Rhinology 2007;45:208–213.

6 Mulligan JK, White DR, Wang EW, Sansoni SR, Moses H, Yawn RJ, Wagner C, Casey SE, Mulligan RM, Schlosser RJ: Vitamin D3 deficiency increases sinus mucosa dendritic cells in pediatric chronic rhinosinusitis with nasal polyps. Otolaryngol Head Neck Surg 2012;147: 773–781.

7 Mulligan JK, Nagel W, O'Connell BP, Wentzel J, Atkinson C, Schlosser RJ: Cigarette smoke exposure is associated with vitamin D3 deficiencies in patients with chronic rhinosinusitis. J Allergy Clin Immunol 2014;134:342–349.

8 Sultan B, Ramanathan M Jr, Lee J, May L, Lane AP: Sinonasal epithelial cells synthesize active vitamin D, augmenting host innate immune function. Int Forum Allergy Rhinol 2013;3:26–30.

9 Rostkowska-Nadolska B, Fraczek M, Gawron W, Latocha M: Influence of vitamin D(3) analogues in combination with budesonid R on proliferation of nasal polyp fibroblasts. Acta Biochim Pol 2009;56:235–242.

10 Sansoni ER, Sautter NB, Mace JC, Smith TL, Yawn JR, Lawrence LA, Schlosser RJ, Soler ZM, Mulligan JK: Vitamin D3 as a novel regulator of basic fibroblast growth factor in chronic rhinosinusitis with nasal polyposis. Int Forum Allergy Rhinol 2015;5:191–196.

11 Wang LF, Chien CY, Tai CF, Chiang FY, Chen JY: Vitamin D decreases the secretion of eotaxin and RANTES in nasal polyp fibroblasts derived from Taiwanese patients with chronic rhinosinusitis with nasal polyps. Kaohsiung J Med Sci 2015;31:63–69.

12 Liu PT: Toll-like receptor triggering of a vitamin D-mediated human antimicrobial response. Science 2006;311:1770.

13 Chun RF, Liu PT, Modlin RL, Adams JS, Hewison M: Impact of vitamin D on immune function: lessons learned from genome-wide analysis. Front Physiol 2014;5:151.

14 Bergman P, Norlin AC, Hansen S, Rekha RS, Agerberth B, Björkhem-Bergman L, Ekström L, Lindh JD, Andersson J: Vitamin D3 supplementation in patients with frequent respiratory tract infections: a randomised and double-blind intervention study. BMJ Open 2012;pii:e001663.

15 Urashima M, Segawa T, Okazaki M, Kurihara M, Wada Y, Ida H: Randomized trial of vitamin D supplementation to prevent seasonal influenza A in schoolchildren. Am J Clin Nutr 2010;91: 1255–1260.

16 Castro M, King TS, Kunselman SJ, Cabana MD, Denlinger L, Holguin F, Kazani SD, Moore WC, Moy J, Sorkness CA, Avila P, Bacharier LB, Bleecker E, Boushey HA, Chmiel J, Fitzpatrick AM, Gentile D, Hundal M, Israel E, Kraft M, Krishnan JA, LaForce C, Lazarus SC, Lemanske R, Lugogo N, Martin RJ, Mauger DT, Naureckas E, Peters SP, Phipatanakul W, Que LG, Sheshadri A, Smith L, Solway J, Sullivan-Vedder L, Sumino K, Wechsler ME, Wenzel S, White SR, Sutherland ER: Effect of vitamin D3 on asthma treatment failures in adults with symptomatic asthma and lower vitamin D levels: the VIDA randomized clinical trial. JAMA 2014;311: 2083–2091.

Rodney J. Schlosser, MD
135 Rutledge Ave., MSC 550
Charleston, SC 29425 (USA)
E-Mail schlossr@musc.edu

Woodworth BA, Poetker DM, Reh DD (eds): Rhinosinusitis with Nasal Polyposis.
Adv Otorhinolaryngol. Basel, Karger, 2016, vol 79, pp 91–102 (DOI: 10.1159/000445137)

Taste Receptors in Upper Airway Immunity

Ryan M. Carey · Robert J. Lee · Noam A. Cohen

Department of Otorhinolaryngology, Perelman School of Medicine, University of Pennsylvania, Ravdin Building, Philadelphia, Pa., USA

Abstract

Taste receptors are well known for their role in communicating information from the tongue to the brain about nutritional value or potential toxicity of ingested substances. More recently, it has been shown that taste receptors are expressed in other locations throughout the body, including the airway, gastrointestinal tract, brain and pancreas. The roles of some 'extraoral' taste receptors are largely unknown, but emerging research suggests that bitter and sweet taste receptors in the airway are capable of sensing bacteria and modulating innate immunity. This chapter focuses on the role of bitter and sweet taste receptors in human airway innate immunity and their clinical relevance to rhinosinusitis. The bitter taste receptor T2R38 expressed in sinonasal cilia detects bitter bacterial quorum-sensing molecules and activates a nitric oxide-dependent innate immune response; moreover, there are polymorphisms in T2R38 that underlie susceptibility to chronic rhinosinusitis (CRS). Bitter and sweet receptors in sinonasal solitary chemosensory cells control secretion of antimicrobial peptides in the upper airway and may have a profound impact on airway infections in patients with CRS and diabetes. Future research on taste receptors in the airway has enormous potential to expand our understanding of host-pathogen immune interactions and provide novel therapeutic targets.

Introduction

The airway constantly encounters inhaled microbial pathogens and the sinonasal cavity serves as the initial line of defense [1–3]. With each breath, there is an interplay between host and pathogen, and in most individuals, mucociliary clearance (MCC) and other components of respiratory epithelial innate immunity are able to prevent infection [4] (fig. 1). When the sinonasal defenses fail, it often results in chronic rhinosinusitis (CRS), a disease characterized by impaired MCC and persistent infection and inflammation [5]. In addition to its tremendous economic burden and poor effects on quality of life [6–10], CRS often requires antibiotics for treatment and currently accounts for approximately 1 in 5 antibiotic prescriptions in adults [11]. Therefore, CRS is likely a major contributor to the ongoing crisis of antibiotic resistance, which makes alternative therapeutic strategies for eradicating infections quite appealing. With a firm understanding of sinonasal immune mechanisms, the endogenous host immune defenses could potentially be stimulated to fight off infection, sparing the usage of antibiotics. Recent studies have demonstrated a connection between sinonasal immunity and bitter

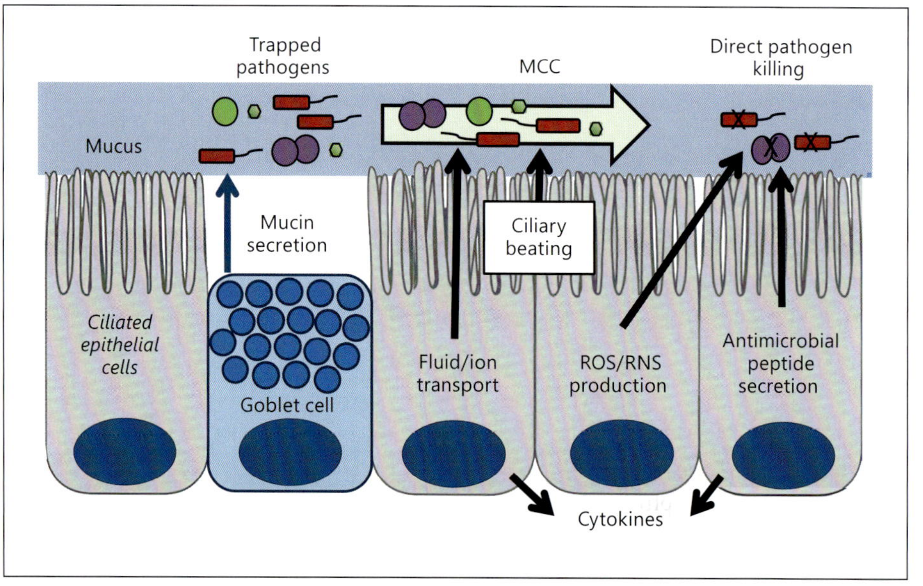

Fig. 1. Mechanisms involved in respiratory epithelial innate immunity. Inhaled pathogens, such as bacteria, virus and fungal spores, become trapped by mucus comprised of sticky mucin macromolecules secreted by respiratory goblet cells [5]. These trapped pathogens are removed from the airway through MCC, the airway's primary physical defense against inhaled microbes and irritants [83]. MCC produced by the beating of motile cilia, requires tight regulation of ion and fluid transport by epithelial cells, which ultimately controls the mucus viscosity [84]. Other components of the respiratory innate immunity rely on direct pathogen killing and inactivation; these modalities include the generation of reactive oxygen and nitrogen species and the production of antimicrobial peptides [2, 46, 83]. With chronic exposure to pathogens, epithelial cells secrete cytokines that activate inflammatory pathways and recruit specific immune cells [83].

and sweet taste receptors, suggesting that these receptors could serve as novel targets for treating respiratory infections and CRS.

Bitter and Sweet Taste Receptors in Immunity

The host immune system has been described by some as the sixth sense because it acts as a sensory system for detecting pathogens [12]. In fact, recent studies have suggested that some bitter and sweet taste receptors are shared by both the immune and taste systems. Bitter and sweet taste receptors, known as T2Rs and T1Rs respectively, are G-protein-coupled receptors that were first identified in the type II taste receptor cells of the tongue [13–15]. The T2Rs detect bitter ingested compounds such as toxic plant alkaloids, and the T1Rs detect sugars such as glucose and sucrose [1, 16]. Taste receptors also exist outside of the tongue in a diverse array of organs including the bladder, urethra, brain, pancreas, testes, GI tract, thyroid and airway [17–20].

One initial hypothesis for extraoral T2R receptors that justified their widespread distribution in the body was that they bind bitter products from pathogenic bacteria or fungi. This theory was supported by early studies of mouse nose contains solitary chemosensory cells (SCCs), which express both T2R bitter and T1R sweet receptors [21–30]. It was determined that these SCCs in the mouse nose respond to the quorum sensing molecules called acyl-homoserine lactones (AHLs), which are secreted by gram-negative bacteria, such as the common airway pathogen *Pseudomonas aeruginosa* [28, 31, 32]. Interestingly, the T2R bitter receptors have a significant number of naturally occurring polymorphisms that underlie individual taste preferences for bitter foods such as green leafy vegetables and beverages such as coffee and beer [33–35]. There is also genetic variation in the T1R sweet receptors that correlates with sweet taste preferences [36–38]. The implications of these genetic variants in the T2Rs and T1Rs could explain differences in immune response and clearance of pathogens. Likewise, it is possible that polymorphisms of these taste receptors at least partially explain the genetic basis of respiratory infections [39–41]. This chapter will review recent studies demonstrating that T2Rs recognize bacterial products, and genetic variation in at least one human T2R correlates with sinonasal infection and CRS. Moreover, the role of T1Rs in regulating sinonasal innate immunity will be discussed.

Bitter Taste Receptors in Ciliated Cells of the Upper Airway

In 2009, researchers demonstrated that bitter taste receptors (T2Rs) were expressed by human bronchial cells and binding of bitter agonists to these T2Rs stimulated a calcium-mediated increase in ciliary beating [42]. They also determined that these T2Rs were localized to the motile cilia lining the epithelium. This finding suggested that motile cilia serve as chemosensory organelles in addition to their previously described role in MCC [5]. The authors hypothesized that T2Rs in bronchial cilia are a way to clear noxious inhaled irritants [42].

It was later discovered that expression of T2Rs extends more proximally in the airway to the sinonasal epithelial cells. One specific isoform, T2R38, is localized to motile cilia of the upper airway [23, 43, 44] (fig. 2). When ciliated epithelial cells were stimulated with known T2R38-specific agonists, such as phenylthiocarbamide (PTC), they exhibited low level calcium responses that activated nitric oxide (NO) synthase (NOS), driving robust intracellular NO production [44]. This signaling pathway depended on 2 important components of the canonical taste signal transduction cascade: phospholipase C isoform β2 (PLCβ2) [1, 16] and the TRPM5 ion channel [45].

Production of NO by airway epithelial cells is an important component of airway defense because NO and its derivatives are damaging to bacterial membranes, enzymes and DNA [46, 47] and thus prevent airway infection [48, 49]. NO also increases ciliary beat frequency through activation of guanylyl cyclase and protein kinase G, which directly phosphorylate ciliary proteins [50]. The NO produced through activation of T2R38 in sinonasal epithelial cells in vitro diffuses into the airway surface liquid (ASL) and is directly bactericidal to *P. aeruginosa*. Furthermore, the NO produced through activation of T2R38 serves as a second messenger to increase ciliary beating and mucocilary clearance [44].

One important piece of evidence in support of the role of T2R38 in airway immunity was the identification of physiologic ligands that activate T2R38. Two major *P. aeruginosa* AHLs, N-butyryl-L-homoserine lactone (C4HSL) and N-3-oxo-dodecanoyl-L-homoserine lactone (C12HSL) [31] were identified as T2R38 agonists [44]. By using purified AHLs and conditioned medium from wild type (wt) *P. aeruginosa* as well as a strain mutated for the enzymes that synthesize AHLs, it was demonstrated that T2R38 detects physiological concentrations of AHLs and activates calcium-dependent NO production. Because many types of gram-negative bacteria secrete AHLs [31], T2R38 likely functions in airway ciliated cells as a sentinel receptor for detecting invading gram-negative bacteria. A diagram of the T2R38 innate immune pathway

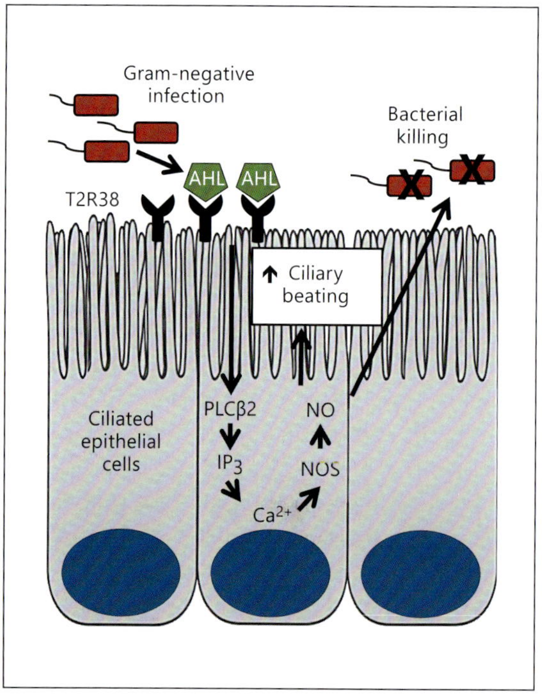

3

Fig. 3. T2R38 bitter taste receptor regulation in human sinonasal epithelial innate immunity. Reading from left to right, gram-negative bacteria secrete AHL molecules to regulate quorum sensing. These AHLs activate T2R38 expressed in human sinonasal cilia [44], activating PLCβ2, which liberates IP3 and causes initiation of a calcium (Ca^{2+}) signal that activates NOS-dependent NO production [43, 44]. NO production has 2 distinct effects (1) it increases ciliary beating and mucociliary transport [43, 44] through activation of the protein kinase G (PKG) pathway [50] and (2) NO diffuses directly into the ASL, where it has direct bactericidal effects [44].

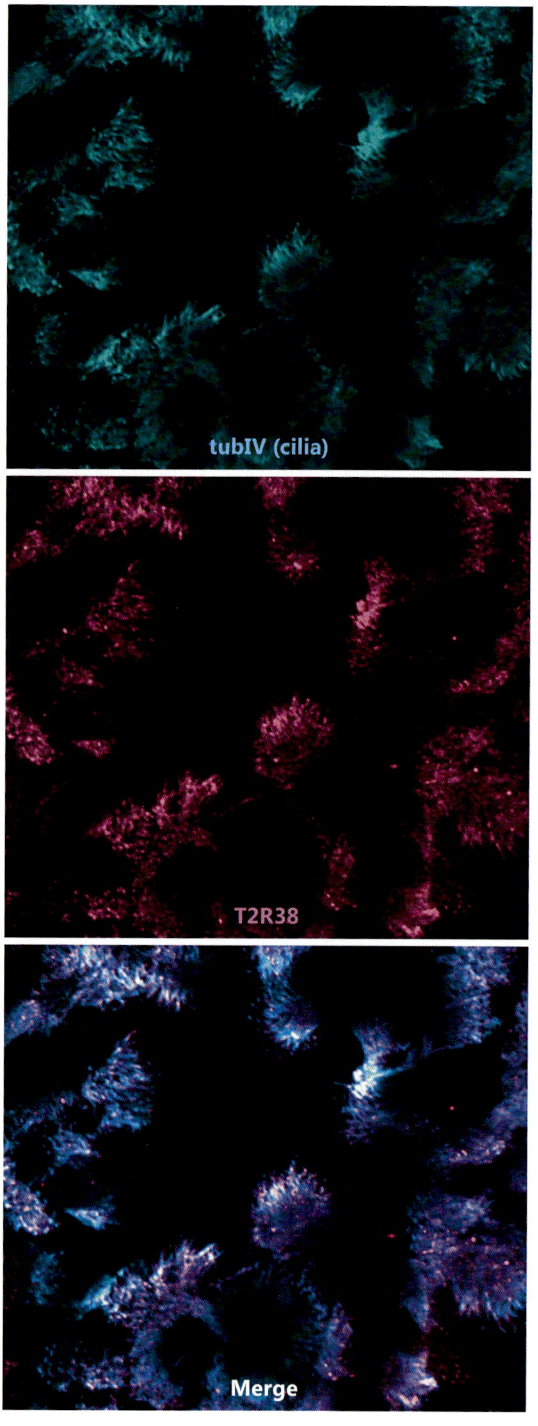

2

Fig. 2. Confocal immunofluorescence micrograph of T2R38 expression in motile cilia from a fixed human sinonasal tissue explant. T2R38 staining and visualization was performed as described in [44], with β-tubulin IV (tubIV) used as a cilia marker. Image by R.J. Lee, Perelman School of Medicine, Philadelphia, Pa., USA.

in sinonasal ciliated epithelial cells is shown in figure 3.

Human T2R38 functionality is dramatically altered by several well-studied polymorphisms in *TAS2R38* [36, 51]. There are 3 polymorphisms that tend to segregate together and are common in Caucasian populations, yielding variants of the protein, one encoding a functional T2R38 and the other a nonfunctional T2R38. The result of these polymorphisms is differences in the amino acids at position 49, 262 and 296 with the functional variant of T2R38 containing proline (P), alanine (A) and valine (V) residues and the nonfunctional variant of T2R38 containing alanine (A), valine (V) and isoleucine (I) at these positions, respectively [51]. The absence of the V at the third position of the AVI variant likely prevents receptor activation [36, 51]. Individuals who are homozygous PAV/PAV (~20% frequency in Caucasians) are considered 'supertasters' and perceive T2R38-specific agonists such as PTC and 6-propyl-2-thiouracil (PROP) as intensely bitter [51]. Conversely, individuals that are homozygous AVI/AVI (~30% frequency in Caucasians) are 'non-tasters' for T2R38-specific agonists. PAV/AVI heterozygotes have varying intermediate levels of taste that correlate with differences of the relative expression levels of the PAV and AVI alleles [36, 50].

The effects of *TAS2R38* polymorphisms were studied by growing primary sinonasal cells from genotyped patients that were PAV/PAV supertasters, AVI/AVI non-tasters or PAV/AVI heterozygotes. The antibacterial NO responses were found to correlate with the *TAS2R38* polymorphism. As compared to cells from AVI/PAV heterozygotes or AVI/AVI non-taster individuals, the PAV/PAV supertaster cells had significantly enhanced NO production, MCC and bacterial killing in response to either PTC or AHLs [44]. This data strongly suggested that *TAS2R38* polymorphisms alter how efficiently sinonasal epithelial cells respond to gram-negative bacteria and prompted further investigation through clinical studies.

Preliminary clinical studies found that PAV/PAV supertasters had a lower frequency of gram-negative sinonasal infection compared to PAV/AVI or AVI/AVI patients with impaired T2R38-dependent responses [44]. *TAS2R38* genotype was compared in patients (N = 56) who had undergone sinonasal surgery for CRS or for non-CRS related concerns (i.e., pituitary pathology) and who had microbiology results of either 'no growth' or normal respiratory flora (e.g., *Staphylococcus epidermis*; n = 35) or positive cultures for gram-negative bacteria (n = 21) or specifically *P. aeruginosa* (n = 14). None of the patients who had gram-negative or *P. aeruginosa* growth had the PAV/PAV genotype. Furthermore, the distribution of AVI/AVI, PAV/AVI and PAV/PAV genotypes was significantly different between control patients and either gram-negative ($p < 0.006$ by χ^2) or *P. aeruginosa* ($p < 0.029$) patients [44]. The control and gram-negative/*P. aeruginosa* patients had no significant differences in the distributions of common polymorphisms of other receptors including TAS2R19, TAS2R30 (also known as TAS2R47) or TAS2R46 with similar minor allele frequencies to TAS2R38.

Additional clinical studies validated the relevance of the preliminary studies of *TAS2R38* genotype in sinonasal disease [52–54]. One retrospective study was performed using *TAS2R38*-genotyped sinonasal tissue samples from 28 patients who had undergone primary functional endoscopic sinus surgery (FESS) [52]. Out of these patients, 46% were AVI/AVI non-tasters, 50% were PAV/AVI heterozygotes and 3.6% were PAV/PAV supertasters. This distribution was significantly different from the approximate expected distributions of 30% AVI/AVI, 50% PAV/AVI and 20% PAV/PAV ($p < 0.043$ by χ^2 analysis), suggesting that PAV/PAV supertasters are less likely to need surgical intervention for CRS [52]. A subsequent prospective study of *TAS2R38* genotype in 70 patients undergoing primary FESS showed that there was a statistically significant difference in the frequency of AVI and PAV alleles compared with the general population [54]. The distribution of diplotypes in the CRS patients were 37% AVI/AVI, 38% PAV/AVI and 8.5% PAV/PAV compared with 29%, 51% and 20%, respectively, in the general population of Philadelphia ($p < 0.0383$ by χ^2 analysis). No significant differences were found in the allele distribution with respect to other known risk factors such as smoking exposure, allergies, asthma, diabetes, nasal polyposis or aspirin sensitivity, indicating that *TAS2R38* is an independent risk factor for CRS requiring FESS [54].

In order to verify that T2R polymorphisms correlate with CRS, 2 Canadian CRS populations were compared with one control population using previously collected pooling-based genome-wide association data that had been screened for single-nucleotide polymorphisms (SNPs) in taste receptors [53]. The *TAS2R38* I296V (*rs10246939*) SNP, thought to underlie the difference in functionality between PAV and AVI variants, was included in this analysis. The I296V SNP frequency differences were ~11 and 15% in the 2 CRS groups compared with the control population, confirming that this SNP is associated with CRS [53]. This study also discovered 3 other missense variants in *TAS2R* genes that were associated with CRS: 2 in *TAS2R49 (rs12226919* and *rs12226920)* and 1 in *TAS2R14 (rs1015443)* [53]. The potential roles of T2R14 or T2R49 in sinonasal immunity remain to be determined.

Additional studies are needed to further explore the role of *TAS2R38* genotype and CRS susceptibility, particularly as it applies to patient outcomes. The existing data have already established the T2R38 pathway as a potential therapeutic target for harnessing the native immune responses to upper respiratory infections. One obstacle is that the large subset of PAV/AVI and AVI/AVI individuals would be less responsive to T2R38 agonists, thus necessitating further exploration of the T2R38-mediated signaling pathway and identification of other T2Rs with similar functions.

Bitter and Sweet Receptors in SCCs of the Upper Airway

In addition to the T2Rs in ciliated epithelial cells, the upper airway also contains SCCs, which express both T2R (bitter) and T1R (sweet) taste receptors [21, 22, 25, 26, 28, 29, 55–57]. SCCs are dedicated chemosensory cells that populate the sinonasal cavity at a frequency of approximately 1 in 100 cells. Mouse nasal SCCs respond to bitter compounds such as denatonium benzoate or bacterial AHLs using similar molecular transduction utilized by oral taste receptor signaling, such as Gα-gustducin, PLCβ2 and TRPM5 [22, 26, 28, 30, 58]. When activated by bitter compounds, mouse nasal SCCs exhibit intracellular calcium responses that cause acetylcholine release [24] which activates trigeminal nociceptors, resulting in breath holding [28] and inflammatory responses [24]. Trigeminal nociceptors can also release various types of neuropeptides into the airway, including vasoactive intestinal peptide and calcitonin gene-related peptide [27, 59]. Therefore, it is possible that in vivo activation of mouse nasal SCC results in local responses such as fluid secretion [56, 60] or increased ciliary beating [61], but this has yet to be experimentally determined.

SCCs were recently identified in humans as well [21, 23, 55]. SCCs expressing T2R47- and T1R2/3 have been identified in primary cell cultures derived from human postsurgical tissues from a variety of sinonasal anatomical regions [23]. Moreover, SCC-like cells in the human vomeronasal duct were observed to express T2R4, T1R1 and T1R2 [55]. It is likely that SCCs are found throughout the human sinonasal cavity, but additional studies of SCC distribution have yet to be completed.

Human SCC physiology has been studied using air-liquid interface (ALI) cell cultures in addition to human sinonasal tissue explants [23]. ALIs are a well-validated cell model that contain a number of cell types including basal, ciliated and goblet cells, [60, 62, 63], and the more recently described SCCs. When human sinonasal ALIs or inferior turbinate explants were stimulated with the bitter agonist denatonium, which activates mouse SCCs [22, 26, 28, 30], an intracellular calcium response originated from discrete cells and initiated a calcium wave that spread to the neighboring cells through gap junctions [23]. Initiation of this calcium signal required known components of taste signaling, including Gα-gustducin, PLCβ2, the inositol 1,4,5-trisphosphate receptor and TRPM5 [23]. Immunofluorescence revealed that the human SCCs co-express the bitter taste receptor T2R47 (also known as T2R30) and the T1R3 sweet receptor subunit. The pharmacological profile of bitter agonists inducing responses in the human SCCs suggest a role for T2R isoforms T2R10, T2R46 and T2R47/T2R30 [23], but not T2R38 as previously shown in mouse SCCs [22, 24, 26, 28, 30]. Human SCCs were not activated by PTC or AHLs, suggesting that human sinonasal T2R38 expression is restricted to ciliated cells. This difference in T2R38 expression represents a species-specific difference between mouse and human.

Surprisingly, the denatonium-induced SCC calcium responses were observed to be blocked in a dose-dependent fashion by apical sugars such as glucose, sucrose [23] and the non-metabolizable sweet agonist sucralose [1, 16, 64]. The inhibition was determined to be dependent on the T1R sweet receptor because the inhibition was removed by application of known antagonists of T1R, lactisole [65] and amiloride [23, 66]. This anatomical and physiological data confirm that human sinonasal SCCs express both bitter and sweet taste receptors, which function in antagonistic roles.

The SCC stimulation had no effect on NO production as seen in T2R38 [23]. Instead, stimulation of the SCC T2Rs activated a robust calcium-dependent secretion of antimicrobial peptides (AMPs), including β-defensins 1 and 2, from the surrounding ciliated epithelial cells [23]. These AMPs were bactericidal to both gram-negative (*P. aeruginosa* and *Klebsiella pneumoniae*) and gram-positive (*Staphylococcus epidermis* and methicillin-resistant *S. aureus*) bacteria [23]. The majority of the AMP secretion with SCC T2R stimulation occurred rapidly within about 5 minutes; this is in contrast to the enhanced AMP production seen over hours in response to stimulation of Toll-like receptor (TLR) [23]. The T2Rs in sinonasal epithelial cells appear to regulate a more rapid release of AMP stores [23], while the TLRs cause upregulation of mRNA for AMPs [67, 68].

Human sinonasal explants exhibited similar AMP secretion as the ALIs, suggesting that in vivo physiology is accurately reflected in human sinonasal ALIs. ALIs derived from bronchial tissue did not exhibit localized SCC-mediated calcium signals or AMP secretion; instead, as previously described, the bronchial responses to bitter agonists were more global, reflecting the activation of ciliated cells rather than SCCs [23, 43]. Taken together, these results suggest that the SCC T2R-mediated AMP secretion is unique to the upper airway. There is a great deal of overlap in SCC signaling between human and mouse ALIs; however, stimulation of mouse nasal SCCs did not result in release of AMPs [23]. As mentioned previously, in vivo stimulation of mouse SCCs was linked to activation of trigeminal nociceptors, which resulted in breath holding [28] and inflammatory responses [24]. It is apparent that the human sinonasal SCCs play a more prominent role in local innate immunity [23], but human SCCs might also activate trigeminal nociceptors and induce neurotransmitter-mediated triggering of gland secretion [69], ciliary beating [61] and inflammation [24]. Future studies of SCCs interaction with neurons will require a different in vitro model because ALIs lack neuronal innervation. Likewise, mouse studies may not be appropriate due to major species-specific differences, and thus, another animal model may be necessary for studying in vivo sinonasal physiology as it relates to SCCs.

One of the more interesting discoveries in human SCC physiology is the inhibition of T2R bitter receptor responses by T1R (sweet receptor) stimulation. As described above, T1R activation by glucose inhibits T2R-activated AMP secretion [23]. This is of particular interest because the glucose concentration normally found in the ASL is approximately 0.5 mM, which appears to be sufficient to activate T1R expressed in the human airway and inhibit SCC-mediated AMP secretion by approximately half [23]. This concentration is 10–100-fold lower than concentrations required to activate T1R-dependent sweet taste [70]. Other extraoral sweet receptors have also been shown to respond to lower sugar concentration such as the T1Rs in pancreatic β-cells [71] and gut endocrine cells [72]. It is likely that the oral T1R sensitivity is tuned to the higher sugar concentrations found in foods, whereas extraoral T1R sensitivities are calibrated to respond to the lower sugar concentrations that are physiologically relevant to the tissues in which they are located. Although the underlying mechanism is unknown, it is possible that the differences in extraoral and oral T1R receptor sugar sensitivity are related to post-translational modifications, alterations in stoichiometry, coupling to alternative signaling pathways or tissue specific accessory subunits. Recent evidence from β-cells suggests that changes in subunit stoichiometry play a role [73]; however, further investigation is required in the airway.

We hypothesize that airway T1R function as 'potentiometers' calibrated to control the magnitude of SCC-T2R-mediated AMP secretion in a physiologic meaningful manner. The T1Rs sense the concentration of glucose in the ASL, which may be an indicator of the onset of infection. More specifically, sinonasal T1Rs would be activated by the normal in vivo ASL glucose concentration (~0.5 mM) of healthy individuals [23]; therefore, the T1R sweet receptors in SCCs would effectively 'desensitize' the SCC T2Rs to the bitter compounds secreted by some bacteria during low-level colonization in healthy individuals. Conversely, during infection, bacteria consume the glucose in the ASL, causing a reduction in the ASL glucose concentration. This would signal the onset of pathogen invasion, relieving the T1R-mediated 'desensitization' and allowing the T2Rs to be activated by bitter compounds secreted by bacteria and trigger an appropriate defense response. The proposed model is presented schematically in figure 4.

This hypothesis, though intriguing and potentially impactful, requires further validation. The model may have particular relevance in CRS and diabetes. Glucose homeostasis in the ASL is controlled by tonic leak through the airway epithelium as well as uptake into airway cells via apical transporters, together maintaining the concentration ~10-fold lower than the serum level [74–76]. This balance can be upset in diabetic patients who have elevated blood glucose levels, increased flux of glucose into the ASL and thus elevated ASL glucose concentrations [74, 77]. CRS patients also have an elevated ASL glucose concentration that is approximately 3- to 4-fold higher than healthy individuals, though not correlated with serum glucose [23]. The elevated ASL glucose concentration seen in CRS is likely due to increased leak from breakdown of the epithelial barrier as a result of chronic infection and inflammation [76]; additionally, pro-inflammatory mediators disrupt tight junctions in human sinonasal cells and increase the paracellular glucose flux in human bronchial cells [78, 79]. The elevated ASL glucose concentration in diabetics may contribute to the observation that diabetics are more prone to airway infections than non-diabetics [76, 80]. A recent retrospective study of CRS patients demonstrated that diabetics had a higher frequency of intraoperative microbiology cultures that included gram-negative bacteria such as *P. aeruginosa* [81]. It has been speculated that low ASL glucose promotes airway sterility by limiting the nutrients available for bacterial consumption [74–76]. In addition to this proposed mechanism, it is possible that the higher ASL glu-

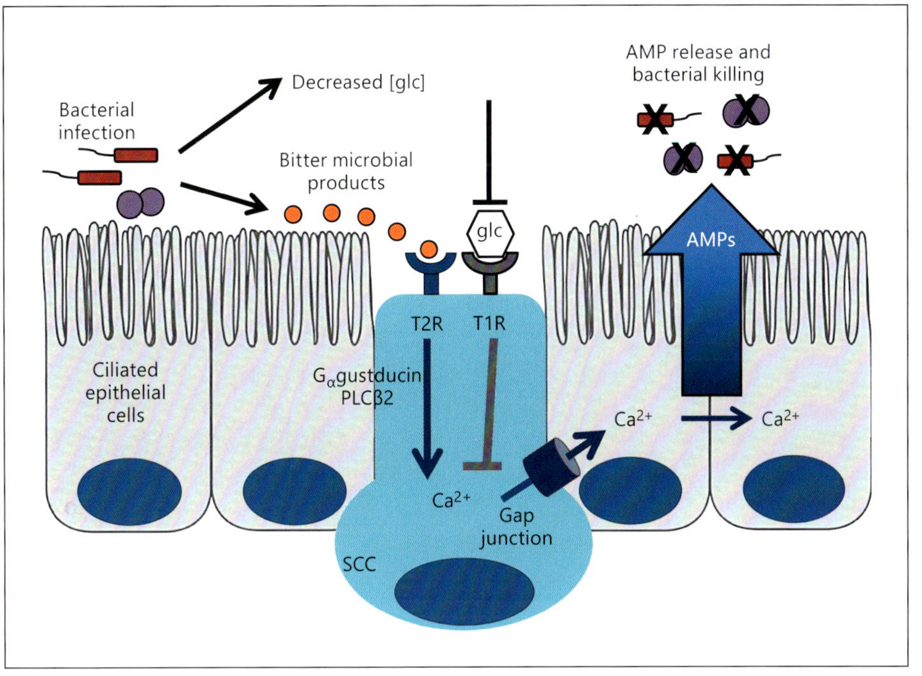

Fig. 4. Human nasal SCCs express taste receptors that regulate airway innate immunity. Reading from left to right, bitter chemicals are secreted by microbes during infection. These bitter molecules activate T2R receptors in SCCs, triggering a calcium (Ca^{2+}) response that propagates to surrounding cells through gap junctions [23]. This calcium signal causes the surrounding epithelial cells to secrete AMPs, which directly kill both gram-positive and gram-negative bacteria. ASL glucose (~0.5 mM in healthy individuals [23]) normally attenuates T2R-mediated signaling through activation of T1R2/3 sweet receptors. During times of infection, bacteria likely consume ASL glucose, thus decreasing the ASL glucose concentration, relieving the T1R2/3-mediated inhibition of T2R signaling and activating AMP secretion [23].

cose in CRS or diabetic patients contributes to disease by repressing T2R-mediated SCCs responses to bitter bacterial molecules through over-activation of T1R sweet receptors. If this were true, topical application of sweet receptor antagonists such as lactisole could be useful therapies for restoring normal sinonasal responses in some patients.

Further studies are necessary to investigate polymorphisms in *TAS1R* genes, which could potentially alter T1R sweet receptor responses to sugars and impact susceptibility to airway infection [36–38]. Increased sugar sensitivity of T1Rs in the airway might lead to increased repression of SCC T2R-mediated AMP secretion. A recent study of Canadian CRS patients and healthy individuals showed allele frequency differences of >10% for 16 different SNPs in *TAS1R* genes [54], highlighting the importance of further investigation.

Conclusions

Emerging data suggest that T2R bitter and T1R sweet taste receptors constitute an integral component of innate immunity in the airway. Multiple taste receptors are expressed in a variety of airway cell types and regulate novel sentinel detection systems in both mice [22, 24, 26, 28, 30, 43] and humans [23, 44]. More recently, T2R38 was determined to be present on the cell membrane of peripheral blood neutrophils, monocytes and lymphocytes and intracellularly in neutrophil vesicles, where it serves as a receptor for C12HSL secreted by *P. aeruginosa* [82]. Additionally, chemosensory cells expressing bitter and umami taste receptors, along with other components of the taste transduction cascade, have been identified in the mammalian urethra; these cells have been shown to respond to stimulation by uropathogenic *Escherichia coli* by triggering release of acetylcholine, which increases bladder detrusor muscle activity in anesthetized rats [18]. Discovery of taste receptors' role in immunity contributes some irony to previous descriptions of the immune system as an additional human 'sense'. Indeed, our immune and taste systems utilize some of the same chemosensory receptors in detecting invading pathogens and perceiving the world. The emerging field of extraoral taste receptors, particularly in the airway, shows promise for expanding our ability to understand and manipulate host-pathogen interactions in human disease.

Conflict of Interest

The authors declare that they have no conflicts of interest.

References

1 Yamamoto K, Ishimaru Y: Oral and extra-oral taste perception. Semin Cell Dev Biol 2013;24:240–246.
2 Parker D, Prince A: Innate immunity in the respiratory epithelium. Am J Respir Cell Mol Biol 2011;45:189–201.
3 Kato A, Schleimer RP: Beyond inflammation: airway epithelial cells are at the interface of innate and adaptive immunity. Curr Opin Immunol 2007;19:711–720.
4 Waterer GW: Airway defense mechanisms. Clin Chest Med 2012;33:199–209.
5 Antunes MB, Gudis DA, Cohen NA: Epithelium, cilia, and mucus: their importance in chronic rhinosinusitis. Immunol Allergy Clin North Am 2009;29:631–643.
6 Blackwell DL, Collins JG, Coles R: Summary health statistics for U.S. adults: national health interview survey 1997. Vital Health Stat 2002;205:1–109.
7 Fokkens WJ, et al: European position paper on rhinosinusitis and nasal polyps 2012. Rhinol Suppl 2012;23:3 p preceding table of contents, 1–298.
8 Gliklich RE, Metson R: The health impact of chronic sinusitis in patients seeking otolaryngologic care. Otolaryngol Head Neck Surg 1995;113:104–109.
9 Khalid AN, Quraishi SA, Kennedy DW: Long-term quality of life measures after functional endoscopic sinus surgery. Am J Rhinol 2004;18:131–136.
10 Ly N, McCaig LF: National hospital ambulatory medical care survey: 2000 outpatient department summary. Adv Data 2002;327:1–27.
11 Bhattacharyya N, Kepnes LJ: Assessment of trends in antimicrobial resistance in chronic rhinosinusitis. Ann Otol Rhinol Laryngol 2008;117:448–452.
12 Bedford FL: The missing sense modality: the immune system. Perception 2011;40:1265–1267.
13 Margolskee RF: The molecular biology of taste transduction. Bioessays 1993;15:645–650.
14 Margolskee RF: Molecular mechanisms of bitter and sweet taste transduction. J Biol Chem 2002;277:1–4.
15 Margolskee RF: Teaching resources. Sensory systems: taste perception. Sci STKE 2005;2005:tr20.
16 Mennella JA, et al: The bad taste of medicines: overview of basic research on bitter taste. Clin Ther 2013;35:1225–1246.
17 Clark AA, et al: TAS2R bitter taste receptors regulate thyroid function. FASEB J 2015;29:164–172.
18 Deckmann K, et al: Bitter triggers acetylcholine release from polymodal urethral chemosensory cells and bladder reflexes. Proc Natl Acad Sci U S A 2014;111:8287–8292.
19 Gu F, et al: Bitter taste receptor mTas2r105 is expressed in small intestinal villus and crypts. Biochem Biophys Res Commun 2015;463:934–941.
20 Wu SV, et al: Expression of bitter taste receptors of the T2R family in the gastrointestinal tract and enteroendocrine STC-1 cells. Proc Natl Acad Sci U S A 2002;99:2392–2397.
21 Barham HP, et al: Solitary chemosensory cells and bitter taste receptor signaling in human sinonasal mucosa. Int Forum Allergy Rhinol 2013;3:450–457.
22 Finger TE, et al: Solitary chemoreceptor cells in the nasal cavity serve as sentinels of respiration. Proc Natl Acad Sci U S A 2003;100:8981–8986.
23 Lee RJ, et al: Bitter and sweet taste receptors regulate human upper respiratory innate immunity. J Clin Invest 2014;124:1393–1405.
24 Saunders CJ, et al: Cholinergic neurotransmission links solitary chemosensory cells to nasal inflammation. Proc Natl Acad Sci U S A 2014;111:6075–6080.

25 Sbarbati A, Osculati F: Solitary chemosensory cells in mammals? Cells Tissues Organs 2003;175:51–55.
26 Tizzano M, et al: Expression of taste receptors in solitary chemosensory cells of rodent airways. BMC Pulm Med 2011; 11:3.
27 Tizzano M, Finger TE: Chemosensors in the nose: guardians of the airways. Physiology (Bethesda) 2013;28:51–60.
28 Tizzano M, et al: Nasal chemosensory cells use bitter taste signaling to detect irritants and bacterial signals. Proc Natl Acad Sci U S A 2010;107:3210–3215.
29 Tizzano M, Merigo F, Sbarbati A: Evidence of solitary chemosensory cells in a large mammal: the diffuse chemosensory system in Bos taurus airways. J Anat 2006;209:333–337.
30 Gulbransen BD, et al: Nasal solitary chemoreceptor cell responses to bitter and trigeminal stimulants in vitro. J Neurophysiol 2008;99:2929–2937.
31 Jimenez PN, et al: The multiple signaling systems regulating virulence in Pseudomonas aeruginosa. Microbiol Mol Biol Rev 2012;76:46–65.
32 Pearson JP, et al: A second N-acylhomoserine lactone signal produced by Pseudomonas aeruginosa. Proc Natl Acad Sci U S A 1995;92:1490–1494.
33 Hayes JE, et al: Allelic variation in TAS2R bitter receptor genes associates with variation in sensations from and ingestive behaviors toward common bitter beverages in adults. Chem Senses 2011;36:311–319.
34 Lanier SA, Hayes JE, Duffy VB: Sweet and bitter tastes of alcoholic beverages mediate alcohol intake in of-age undergraduates. Physiol Behav 2005;83:821–831.
35 Li D, Zhang J: Diet shapes the evolution of the vertebrate bitter taste receptor gene repertoire. Mol Biol Evol 2014;31: 303–309.
36 Bachmanov AA, et al: Genetics of taste receptors. Curr Pharm Des 2014;20: 2669–2683.
37 Fushan AA, et al: Allelic polymorphism within the TAS1R3 promoter is associated with human taste sensitivity to sucrose. Curr Biol 2009;19:1288–1293.
38 Mennella JA, Pepino MY, Reed DR: Genetic and environmental determinants of bitter perception and sweet preferences. Pediatrics 2005;115:e216–e222.
39 Cohen NA, et al: Familial aggregation of sinonasal polyps correlates with severity of disease. Otolaryngol Head Neck Surg 2006;134:601–604.
40 Greisner WA 3rd, Settipane GA: Hereditary factor for nasal polyps. Allergy Asthma Proc 1996;17:283–286.
41 Hamilos DL: Chronic rhinosinusitis patterns of illness. Clin Allergy Immunol 2007;20:1–13.
42 Shah AS, et al: Motile cilia of human airway epithelia are chemosensory. Science 2009;325:1131–1134.
43 Lee RJ, et al: Mouse nasal epithelial innate immune responses to Pseudomonas aeruginosa quorum-sensing molecules require taste signaling components. Innate Immun 2014;20: 606–617.
44 Lee RJ, et al: T2R38 taste receptor polymorphisms underlie susceptibility to upper respiratory infection. J Clin Invest 2012;122:4145–4159.
45 Perez CA, et al: Making sense with TRP channels: store-operated calcium entry and the ion channel Trpm5 in taste receptor cells. Cell Calcium 2003;33:541–549.
46 Fang FC: Perspectives series: host/pathogen interactions. Mechanisms of nitric oxide-related antimicrobial activity. J Clin Invest 1997;99:2818–2825.
47 Marcinkiewicz J: Nitric oxide and antimicrobial activity of reactive oxygen intermediates. Immunopharmacology 1997;37:35–41.
48 Haight JS, et al: Does nasal nitric oxide come from the sinuses? J Otolaryngol 1999;28:197–204.
49 Maniscalco M, Sofia M, Pelaia G: Nitric oxide in upper airways inflammatory diseases. Inflamm Res 2007;56:58–69.
50 Salathe M: Regulation of mammalian ciliary beating. Annu Rev Physiol 2007; 69:401–422.
51 Bufe B, et al: The molecular basis of individual differences in phenylthiocarbamide and propylthiouracil bitterness perception. Curr Biol 2005;15:322–327.
52 Adappa ND, et al: Genetics of the taste receptor T2R38 correlates with chronic rhinosinusitis necessitating surgical intervention. Int Forum Allergy Rhinol 2013;3:184–187.
53 Mfuna Endam L, et al: Genetic variations in taste receptors are associated with chronic rhinosinusitis: a replication study. Int Forum Allergy Rhinol 2014;4:200–206.
54 Adappa ND, et al: The bitter taste receptor T2R38 is an independent risk factor for chronic rhinosinusitis requiring sinus surgery. Int Forum Allergy Rhinol 2014;4:3–7.
55 Braun T, Mack B, Kramer MF: Solitary chemosensory cells in the respiratory and vomeronasal epithelium of the human nose: a pilot study. Rhinology 2011; 49:507–512.
56 Gulbransen B, Silver W, Finger TE: Solitary chemoreceptor cell survival is independent of intact trigeminal innervation. J Comp Neurol 2008;508:62–71.
57 Saunders CJ, Reynolds SD, Finger TE: Chemosensory brush cells of the trachea. A stable population in a dynamic epithelium. Am J Respir Cell Mol Biol 2013;49:190–196.
58 Kotrschal K: Taste(s) and olfaction(s) in fish: a review of specialized sub-systems and central integration. Pflugers Arch 2000;439(3 suppl):R178–R180.
59 Whitear M: Solitary chemoreceptor cells; in Hara TJ (ed): Chemoreception in Fishes. London, Chapman and Hall, 1992, pp 103–125.
60 Lin W, et al: TRPM5-expressing solitary chemosensory cells respond to odorous irritants. J Neurophysiol 2008;99:1451–1460.
61 Lee RJ, et al: Vasoactive intestinal peptide regulates sinonasal mucociliary clearance and synergizes with histamine in stimulating sinonasal fluid secretion. FASEB J 2013;27:5094–5103.
62 Baraniuk JN, Kaliner MA: Neuropeptides and nasal secretion. J Allergy Clin Immunol 1990;86(4 pt 2):620–627.
63 Mosimann BL, et al: Substance P, calcitonin gene-related peptide, and vasoactive intestinal peptide increase in nasal secretions after allergen challenge in atopic patients. J Allergy Clin Immunol 1993;92:95–104.
64 Lee RJ, Foskett JK: cAMP-activated Ca2+ signaling is required for CFTR-mediated serous cell fluid secretion in porcine and human airways. J Clin Invest 2010;120:3137–3148.
65 Lee RJ, Foskett JK: Why mouse airway submucosal gland serous cells do not secrete fluid in response to cAMP stimulation. J Biol Chem 2012;287:38316–38326.

66 Lai Y, et al: Inflammation-mediated upregulation of centrosomal protein 110, a negative modulator of ciliogenesis, in patients with chronic rhinosinusitis. J Allergy Clin Immunol 2011;128:1207–1215.e1.
67 Dimova S, et al: The use of human nasal in vitro cell systems during drug discovery and development. Toxicol In Vitro 2005;19:107–122.
68 Ramanathan M Jr, Lane AP: A comparison of experimental methods in molecular chronic rhinosinusitis research. Am J Rhinol 2007;21:373–377.
69 Hansen A: Olfactory and solitary chemosensory cells: two different chemosensory systems in the nasal cavity of the American alligator, Alligator mississippiensis. BMC Neurosci 2007;8:64.
70 Ooi EH, Wormald PJ, Tan LW: Innate immunity in the paranasal sinuses: a review of nasal host defenses. Am J Rhinol 2008;22:13–19.
71 Ramanathan M Jr, Lane AP: Innate immunity of the sinonasal cavity and its role in chronic rhinosinusitis. Otolaryngol Head Neck Surg 2007;136:348–356.
72 Chiu AG, et al: An animal model for the study of topical medications in sinusitis. Am J Rhinol 2007;21:5–9.
73 Ha KR, et al: A sheep model for the study of biofilms in rhinosinusitis. Am J Rhinol 2007;21:339–345.
74 Kyriazis GA, Soundarapandian MM, Tyrberg B: Sweet taste receptor signaling in beta cells mediates fructose-induced potentiation of glucose-stimulated insulin secretion. Proc Natl Acad Sci U S A 2012;109:E524–E532.
75 Schiffman SS, et al: Selective inhibition of sweetness by the sodium salt of +/–2-(4-methoxyphenoxy)propanoic acid. Chem Senses 1999;24:439–447.
76 Wang JC, et al: Evaluation of domestic and Yucatan swine nasal sinus anatomy as models for future sinonasal research of medications delivered by standard instruments used in functional endoscopic sinus surgery. Int Forum Allergy Rhinol 2013;3:150–156.
77 Jang HJ, et al: Gut-expressed gustducin and taste receptors regulate secretion of glucagon-like peptide-1. Proc Natl Acad Sci U S A 2007;104:15069–15074.
78 Garnett JP, Baker EH, Baines DL: Sweet talk: insights into the nature and importance of glucose transport in lung epithelium. Eur Respir J 2012;40:1269–1276.
79 Kojima I, et al: Sweet taste-sensing receptors expressed in pancreatic β-cells: sweet molecules act as biased agonists. Endocrinol Metab (Seoul) 2014;29:12–19.
80 Kalsi KK, et al: Glucose homeostasis across human airway epithelial cell monolayers: role of diffusion, transport and metabolism. Pflugers Arch 2009; 457:1061–1070.
81 Pezzulo AA, et al: Glucose depletion in the airway surface liquid is essential for sterility of the airways. PLoS One 2011; 6:e16166.
82 Maurer S, et al: Tasting pseudomonas aeruginosa biofilms: human neutrophils express the bitter receptor T2R38 as sensor for the quorum sensing molecule N-(3-oxododecanoyl)-l-homoserine lactone. Front Immunol 2015;6:369.
83 Knowles MR, Boucher RC: Mucus clearance as a primary innate defense mechanism for mammalian airways. J Clin Invest 2002;109:571–577.
84 Gao N, et al: Voltage-gated sodium channels in taste bud cells. BMC Neurosci 2009;10:20.

Noam A. Cohen, MD, PhD
Philadelphia Veterans Affairs Medical Center Surgical Services
3900 Woodland Ave.
Philadelphia, PA 19104 (USA)
E-Mail noam.cohen@uphs.upenn.edu

Advances in Medical and Surgical Therapy

Woodworth BA, Poetker DM, Reh DD (eds): Rhinosinusitis with Nasal Polyposis.
Adv Otorhinolaryngol. Basel, Karger, 2016, vol 79, pp 103–113 (DOI: 10.1159/000445141)

Immunomodulators in the Treatment of Nasal Polyposis

Ashleigh A. Halderman · Andrew P. Lane

Department of Otolaryngology – Head and Neck Surgery, Johns Hopkins University School of Medicine, Baltimore, Md., USA

Abstract

The inflammatory mechanisms that contribute to chronic rhinosinusitis with nasal polyps (CRSwNP) are complex. In the past, medical options for treating CRSwNP have been limited. Emerging classes of immunomodulators such as omalizumab, anti-leukotrienes, anti-IL-4, anti-IL-5, and recognition of the modulating effects of macrolides have shown promising results in the treatment of CRSwNP. Ultimately, large randomized controlled trials are necessary to establish the efficacy of these medications but for now, the area of medical immunomodulators remains an exciting frontier.

Introduction

Chronic rhinosinusitis with nasal polyps (CRSwNP) is a heterogeneous disease process that in Western populations is characterized by T-helper 2 (Th2) cytokine-mediated inflammation, an eosinophilic inflammatory infiltrate, and elevated tissue levels of immunoglobulin E (IgE). The most effective medical treatment for CRSwNP is systemic corticosteroids, but the use of these agents is limited by numerous side effects and the potential for significant and even life-threatening complications. In addition, despite the comparative efficacy of steroids, the improvement experienced by patients is variable in degree and duration. As a result, there has been great interest in developing alternative therapies for CRSwNP. Research advances have elucidated immunologic pathways that contribute to CRSwNP pathogenesis, suggesting potential therapeutic immunomodulatory strategies. In recent years, promising new immunomodulators have been released, and the recognition of effects of other classes of medications, such as macrolide antibiotics, on the immune system has sparked study into their impact on CRSwNP.

Omalizumab

Omalizumab is a monoclonal antibody directed against immunoglobulin E that binds free circulating IgE. By this action, it inhibits IgE binding to high-affinity receptors but also, the decrease in free circulating IgE correlates with a decrease in IgE receptors on cells that initiate and mediate the allergic response, including basophils, dendritic cells and mast cells [1–3]. Omalizumab is given in doses between 75–100 mg in subcutaneous injections every 2 weeks. The dosing is dependent upon IgE levels and weight. In asthmatics, IgE levels are significantly reduced within 24–48 h of the first dose and a significant reduction in symptoms occurs within 1 week [4]. The medication is well tolerated with a good safety profile. A large study showed the incidence of anaphylaxis to be between 0.14–0.2% [5].

Because patients with nasal polyps have local production of mucosal polyclonal IgE and sometimes elevated levels of circulating IgE [6–10], anti-IgE is an intriguing therapeutic option. Currently, FDA approval for anti-IgE therapy is limited to patients with moderate-to-severe or severe allergic asthma that has failed traditional treatment and chronic idiopathic urticaria. As approximately 30% of CRSwNP patients are also asthmatic, clinicians began to observe possible beneficial effects on nasal polyps in asthmatic patients who were on Omalizumab [11]. Thus far, only a few small controlled studies looking at IgE therapy in CRSwNP have been reported (see table 1). Three studies have shown a significant decrease in endoscopic polyp scores in patients on Omalizumab [8, 12, 13]. One study showed significant improvement in the endoscopy score in the anti-IgE group compared to the control group [8]. A second study showed a significant improvement in the nasal endoscopy polyp scores in the anti-IgE group after treatment, but the improvement in the study group was not significantly better than the control group [13]. Because the nasal endoscopy polyp score was significantly worse in the study group compared to the control group prior to starting therapy, the authors cautioned that this may have impacted the comparison between the two groups.

One of the largest randomized double blind placebo controlled studies to date enrolled 24 patients and showed promising results. The primary outcome of this study, total nasal endoscopic polyp score, was significantly reduced in the Omalizumab group compared to placebo [8]. Secondary outcomes included Lund–Mackay scoring of sinus CT scans and a quality of life survey. The Lund–Mackay scores of the study group showed significant improvement following treatment, whereas the control group did not. Symptoms of nasal congestion, anterior rhinorrhea and hyposmia were significantly improved in the anti-IgE group compared to control. Interestingly, asthma quality of life scores significantly improved whereas pulmonary function tests did not.

A similarly sized retrospective chart review by Chandra et al. [14] studied the impact of Omalizumab on both antibiotic and steroid use in patients with both asthma and CRS. They found that Omalizumab therapy was associated with a significant decrease in overall antibiotics use in CRS and that a subset of patients additionally experienced a significant decrease in steroid use. Age, aspirin tolerance and polyp status had no impact upon responsiveness to omalizumab as it related to either antibiotic or steroid use.

Two other smaller studies additionally showed significant improvement in total nasal endoscopic polyp scores following Omalizumab treatment [12, 13]. Despite the evidence for a role of Omalizumab in CRSwNP therapy, numerous questions remain, including whether the benefits are durable, whether the drug impacts the timing or need for revision surgery, and how anti-IgE therapy compares to corticosteroids. Vigorous study in the form of larger randomized double blind placebo controlled studies must be carried out to clarify whether Omalizumab can be considered a treatment option for CRSwNP.

Anti-Leukotrienes

Leukotrienes (LTs) are a family of inflammatory mediators that are implicated as playing a significant role in the pathogenesis of asthma and allergic rhinitis. They are produced by a number

Table 1. Review of evidence for immunomodulator therapy in chronic rhinosinusitis with polyposis

Study	Year	LOE	Study design	Study groups	Clinical endpoint	Conclusions
Anti-IgE						
Gevaert [1]	2013	1B	DBPC RCT	15 patients with CRSwNP given omalizumab, 8 treated with placebo	Total nasal endo-scopic polypscores (TPS)	Significant reduction in TPS after treatment with omalizumab but not placebo: TPS significantly lower in treatment group
Vennera [12]	2011	4	Case series	19 patients with CRSwNP with severe asthma treated with omalizumab	Size of NP	NP size significantly reduced at end of follow-up compared with baseline
Penn [13]	2007	4	Case series	4 patients with CRSwNP after ESS treated with omalizumab and 4 controls	NP score, CT score	NP scores significantly improved in treatment group: CT scores did not significantly improve in either group
Anti-Interleukin 5						
Gevaert [35]	2006	1b	DBPC RCT	Patients with CRSwNP: 8 placebo, 8 treated with 1 mg/kg, 8 treated with 3 mg/kg	NP score	Placebo group-NP score worsened in 3/8 and improved in 1/8, 1 mg/kg group-NP score improved in 5/8, 3 mg/kg group-NP score improved in 4/8
Gevaert [37]	2011	1b	DBPC RCT	Patients with CRSwNP: 10 treated with placebo, 20 with mepolizumab	Total polyp score (TPS)	TPS of treatment group significantly improved over TPS of placebo group
Macrolides						
Varvyan-skaya [43]	2014	2B	RCT	22 patients with CRSwNP treated with Clarithromycin 250 mg QD × 24 weeks, 14 treated with 250 mg QD × 12 weeks, 19 no tx	SNOT-20, VAS, Endoscopy score, LM score	SNOT-20 scores significantly better in both treatment groups over control: VAS no difference: Endoscopy scores significantly better in both treatment groups over control: LM score significantly better in 24 week treatment group over control
Peric [55]	2010	4	Case series	Patients with CRSwNP treated with 500 mg Clarithromycin QD, 22 non-atopic, 18 atopic	Nasal symptom score, Endoscopy score	Significant improvement in symptoms in both group, NP size decreased in 10/22 nonallergic and 9/18 allergic patients
Yamada [44]	2000	4	Case series	20 CRSwNP patients treated with Clarithromycin 400 mg QD × 8–12 weeks	Nasal polyp size, IL-8 levels in nasal lavage	Nasal polyp size decreased in 40% of patients. 60% of patients showed no change in size of polyps, IL-8 levels significantly decreased in responders but not in non-responders

of cells including mast cells, eosinophils, basophils, dendritic cells, monocytes/macrophages and T-lymphocytes through either receptor activation or antibody-antigen interactions [15]. Synthesis of LTs occurs from arachidonic acid by way of the 5-lipoxygenase (5-lo) pathway [16]. Cysteinyl LTs (CysLTs) are released during both the early and late phases of the allergic reactions [16]. They act as pro-inflammatory mediators through two receptors: $CysLT_1$ and $CysLT_2$. Binding to the $CysLT_1$ receptor mediates sustained bronchoconstriction, edema and mucus secretion within the airways whereas the binding to the $CysLT_2$ receptor results in increased inflammation, vascular permeability and fibrosis [17, 18].

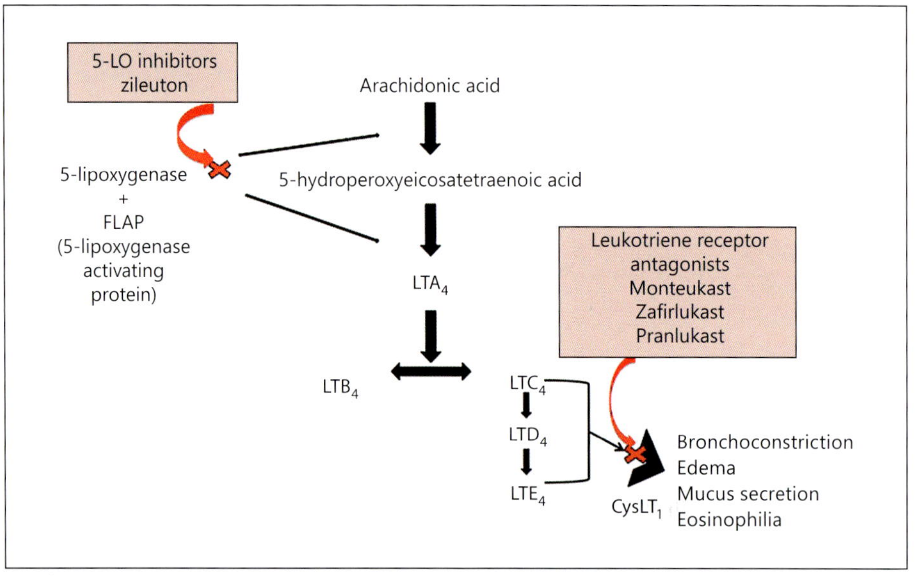

Fig. 1. Arachidonic acid pathway showing location of action of existing anti-leukotriene agents. Arachidonic acid is a precursor from which leukotrienes and prostaglandins are synthesized. The two classes of anti-leukotrienes, 5-LO inhibitors and leukotriene receptor antagonists, act at separate locations within the arachidonic acid pathway to block either the production or activity of leukotrienes.

Pharmacotherapeutic agents targeting LTs, otherwise known as anti-leukotrienes, are classified into two types based on their mechanism of action (fig. 1). LT receptor antagonists bind the LT receptor and block end-organ responses. Montelukast, pranlukast and zafirlukast are included in this group. The second group of medications (including zileuton) inhibit 5-lipoxygenase and therefore biosynthesis of leukotrienes. Generally, both groups of medications are well tolerated. However, in both zileuton and zafirlukast, transaminase elevation and hepatotoxicity have been reported, and therefore patients on these medications should have their liver function monitored. Other side effects of anti-leukotrienes include headache and dyspepsia.

CRSwNP is characterized by increased levels of LTs and their receptors within nasal polyps [19, 20]. The efficacy of anti-leukotrienes in treating diseases often coexistent with CRSwNP, including asthma (exercise and cold induced and both aspirin tolerant and aspirin intolerant) and allergic rhinitis, is well established [21–23]. The 'unified airway' concept suggests that anti-leukotrienes could provide clinical benefit in CRSwNP.

In aspirin-exacerbated respiratory disease (AERD), leukotrienes are theorized to play an integral role in driving the disease process. The evidence for this lies in the findings that levels of leukotrienes, which are elevated in CRSwNP compared to normal controls, are further elevated in patients with AERD [24]. Additionally, the $CysLT_1$ receptor is elevated in the leukocytes and polyp epithelium and stroma in these patients [19, 25]. This data suggests that the subset of patients with CRSwNP who are also aspirin-sensitive may benefit even more from anti-leukotrienes than CRSwNP patients who are aspirin tolerant.

Montelukast has by far been the most extensively studied anti-leukotriene therapeutic in the setting of CRSwNP. Overall, the clinical benefit of montelukast in polyp patients has been fairly minimal. In their meta-analysis and systematic review, Wentzel et al. [26] concluded that leukotriene receptor antagonists were superior to placebo in improving patient symptoms, objective clinical measurements (i.e., nasal endoscopy scores, rhinomanometry and olfactometry) and immune profiles. It did not, however, out-perform the current gold standard of nasal corticosteroids (NCS) in symptom control, and there was some evidence indicating that recurrence rates may be higher with montelukast as monotherapy compared to NCS. Additionally, treatment outcomes did not appear to be affected by asthma status, aspirin tolerance/intolerance and atopy [25].

As mentioned previously, zileuton's mechanism of action is inhibition of 5-lipoxygenase (5-LO), an enzyme that converts arachidonic acid into leukotrienes. Inhibition of this enzyme inhibits the biosynthesis of leukotrienes. Early studies looking at the clinical efficacy of zileuton in the nasal and asthmatic response to allergen and aspirin challenges showed a reduction of acute nasal symptoms following allergen challenge [27, 28]. While these studies were not looking at nasal symptoms in patients with CRS, they were important in establishing nasal response to zileuton. A double-blind placebo-controlled crossover study by Dahlen et al. [29] studied both asthma and nasal symptoms in patients with AERD. Their study supported that AERD patients on zileuton experience an improvement in nasal function in response to the treatment, specifically in hyposmia and rhinorrhea. Both congestion and peak nasal inspiratory flow improved, but did not reach statistical significance in this relatively small study of 40 patients.

To date, no double-blind placebo controlled studies have looked at zileuton in CRSwNP. Two small case series have looked at outcomes in CRSwNP treated with either zafirlukast or zileuton. In each study, the majority of patients were treated with zafirlukast and a small number of patients were treated with zileuton. At the time of these investigations, zileuton was only available in a four times daily dosing schedule, which may have contributed to the low patient numbers. Currently, an extended form of zileuton is available that allows for twice daily dosing. Parnes et al. [30] studied 26 patients treated with zafirlukast and 10 treated with zileuton. Of the patients treated with zileuton, 7 out of 10 saw improvements in their symptom scores. Dentalgia, headache, purulent rhinorrhea, post-nasal drip, nasal congestion, nasal obstruction, olfaction and facial pain and pressure were all significantly improved, although this analysis included all 36 patients together. No objective measures such as endoscopy scores or CT scores were recorded during this study. In an even smaller study, Ulualp et al. [31] evaluated 13 patients on zafirlukast and 2 patients on zileuton. Again, they did not analyze the treatment groups separately. They found significant improvement in major and minor symptoms in 12/15 patients. These 2 studies are too small to draw any conclusions but highlight the fact that larger randomized double-blind placebo-control studies of zileuton in CRSwNP should be considered as limited experience suggests subjective benefits.

Finally, given the different mechanisms of action, it is possible that a combination of a leukotriene receptor antagonist and a 5-lipoxygenase inhibitor may provide more significant benefits than either alone. Di Capite et al. [32] studied this theory in vitro using monteleukast and zileuton. Their work showed that a combination of both medications is more effective than either alone in suppressing activation of mast cells cultured from nasal polyps. Further study is necessary to establish whether these intriguing in-vitro findings have clinical significance.

Anti-IL-5

IL-5 modulates every phase in the life of an eosinophil. It is responsible for maturation of a precursor cell into an eosinophil, activates mature cells in tissue and prolongs the survival of these cells [33]. In 80% of patients with CRSwNP, polyp tissue is characterized by an overabundance of eosinophils [34]. IL-5 synthesis has been shown to be upregulated in polyp tissue, especially in patients with aspirin sensitivity and nonallergic asthma [35].

Anti-IL-5 therapeutics including reslizumab and mepolizumab have been studied in patients with CRSwNP (see table 1). In a small study to establish the safety of a single dose of reslizumab, Gevaert et al. [36] demonstrated that nasal polyp scores decreased significantly in 50% of patients who were treated. When comparing patients who responded to those who did not, they found that responders had significantly higher levels of IL-5 in nasal secretions at baseline than did the nonresponders. This suggested that there may be a subset of CRSwNP patients identified by elevated levels of IL-5 in nasal secretions, who may benefit the most from anti-IL-5 therapies. In addition to the decrease in nasal polyp size in some patients, the authors of this study also reported a significant decrease in serum eosinophil counts, and serum and nasal secretion levels of eosinophil cationic protein (ECP-a marker for eosinophilic inflammation) and the soluble IL-5Rα. Reslizumab was found in this study and others to be associated with rebound eosinophilia after treatment and at times, an exacerbation of symptoms [36, 37]. Overall, the treatment was safe and well tolerated with no major side effects.

A randomized, double-blind, placebo controlled study of mepolizumab in CRSwNP again demonstrated that the nasal polyp scores and CT scores in the treatment group significantly improved compared to the control group [38]. Loss of smell, postnasal drip and congestion improved more in the treatment group compared to the control group, however this change did not reach significance. Perhaps the most impressive symptom improvement in this study was that of hyposmia, which remained improved through 11 months following the last dose whereas the other symptoms normalized within that time frame. A significant decrease in blood eosinophils was seen in the study group compared to the placebo group, however, no significant decrease in nasal IL-5 or IgE was observed. It is important to note that the study size was small and that only 2 doses of mepolizumab were given. It remains possible that longer-term administration of the medication in a larger patient cohort may yield statistically significant results. Contrary to what had been demonstrated in the trial using reslizumab, the study with mepolizumab did not support the previous findings of higher baseline IL-5 levels in nasal secretions in patients who responded to the treatment. Again, mepolizumab was well tolerated with no adverse events due to the medication reported and no rebound eosinophilia was observed after stopping the drug.

Anti-IL-4

Dupilumab is a fully human monoclonal antibody to the alpha subunit of the IL-4 receptor. This subunit is present in both the type I and type II receptors. The type I receptor is activated by IL-4 and is found on lymphocytes and controls Th2 cell differentiation [39]. The type II receptor is activated by both IL-4 and IL-13 and is found on myeloid cells [40]. This makes dupilumab a unique immunomodulatory medication as its one mechanism of action blocks the signaling of two different cytokines. Both IL-4 and IL-13 have been implicated in Th-2 driven inflammation and in the pathophysiology of both asthma and atopy [41, 42]. The medication is given subcutaneously on a weekly basis and is generally well tolerated.

The efficacy of dupilumab for rhinologic symptoms was evaluated by Wenzel et al. [39] in 104 patients with moderate-to-severe asthma and elevated eosinophil levels. At 12 weeks, the study group showed significant improvement in their overall SNOT-22 scores compared to placebo, specifically with the individual symptoms of nasal blockage, cough, post-nasal drip, thick nasal drainage, ear fullness, and need to blow the nose. The Th2 inflammatory biomarkers, thymus and activation-regulated chemokine (TARC), eotaxin-3 and IgE, all significantly decreased in the study group. In addition to the nasal symptoms, this study showed significant improvements in most measures of both lung function and asthma control in the experimental group.

Bachert et al. [43] performed a randomized, double-blind, placebo controlled parallel-group study investigating the effect of dupilumab on nasal polyp burden in patients with CRSwNP. In this study, 60 patients were observed on dupilumab over a 16 week period, during which they also received mometasone furoate nasal spray. The dupilumab-treated group showed a significant improvement in endoscopic polyp score compared to the placebo group. Secondary end points including Lund–Mackay CT score, SNOT-22, and UPSIT scores all significantly improved in the experimental group as well. Individual symptoms that were improved included morning post-nasal drip, nasal congestion, nasal obstruction and anterior rhinorrhea. Asthmatic patients had significant improvements in lung function, the 5-question Asthma Control Questionnaire, UPSIT and SNOT-22 total score. Additionally, Th2 inflammatory biomarkers including total serum IgE, TARC and eotaxin-3 were significantly decreased during the study period. Interestingly, neither this study nor the Wenzel study showed reduction in peripheral eosinophil counts.

In summary, early results of clinical trials with dupilumab suggest efficacy in treating both moderate-to-severe asthma and CRSwNP, at a level at least equivalent to the more well-studied omalizumab and mepolizumab. Future head-to-head or combination studies will be needed to determine the role of dupilumab in the growing arsenal of immunomodulatory monoclonal antibody therapies.

Macrolides

Macrolides are a class of antibiotics, including azithromycin, clarithromycin, and erythromycin, that act as bacterial protein synthesis inhibitors. Along with this antibacterial action, macrolides display anti-inflammatory effects including inhibition of neutrophilic and eosinophilic driven inflammation, downregulation of proinflammatory genes, and improvement of mucociliary clearance [44–46]. For these reasons, long-term macrolide therapy (typically clarithromycin at doses of 200–500 mg twice daily for 2–6 months) has been studied as a therapeutic option in CRSsNP and CRSwNP [44, 45, 47]. Generally, it has been shown that longer courses of macrolide therapy (12 weeks or greater) are more beneficial than shorter courses [44, 48, 49]. A 12 week or greater course of macrolide therapy has been shown to improve SNOT-20 scores, endoscopic scores and saccharine transit time in patients with CRSsNP [46–48]. There appears to be no difference in clinical efficacy between the different types of macrolides, however, erythromycin tends to have a higher incidence of gastrointestinal side effects and may not be tolerated as well [49]. Roxithromycin which is not currently available in the United States has been shown to have greater anti-inflammatory effects than azithromycin or clarithromycin [50].

In vitro studies have demonstrated that macrolides have the ability to inhibit transcriptional activation or reduce DNA-binding activity of nuclear factor kappa B (NF-kB) [46]. NF-kB is a proinflammatory transcription factor whose activity can increase expression of interleukins 2, 6, and 8, tumor necrosis factor alpha and granulocyte-macrophage colony-stimulating factor, among other cytokines and growth factors. Additionally, macrolides have been shown to stabilize the membranes of neutrophils and eosinophils preventing their release of cytoxic mediators via degranulation.

IL-8 is a chemokine produced by nasal gland duct cells and epithelial cells which acts as a neutrophil activating and chemotactic factor [45, 51]. Macrolides have been shown to inhibit lipopolysaccharide-induced IL-8 secretion from nasal epithelial cells which in turn inhibits the chemoattraction and accumulation of neutrophils [52]. They also increase peripheral neutrophil apoptosis [53]. Given the role of IL-8 in neutrophil-driven inflammation, it is not surprising that high levels of IL-8 have been demonstrated in neutrophil-predominant nasal polyps [54]. One study showed that clarithromycin for 8–12 weeks as monotherapy (i.e., without concomitant oral or intranasal steroids) decreased the size of nasal polyps in 40% of patients [45]. No patients experienced an increase in their polyp size while in the study. Further, levels of IL-8 in nasal lavage were found to significantly decrease in those patients whose polyps shrunk while on clarithromycin and did not change in patients who demonstrated no change in polyp size. Interestingly, prior to treatment, those patients whose polyps responded to clarithromycin had significantly higher levels of IL-8 in their nasal lavage than those patients who did not respond and the authors suggest that IL-8 could be a prognostic marker to identify patients who would respond to macrolide therapy.

While targeting IL-8 in patients with neutrophil-predominant nasal polyps may provide some clinical benefit, the majority of polyp patients have high circulating IgE levels and eosinophil-dominated inflammation. While previously postulated that macrolides were not effective in the Th-2-mediated inflammation associated with CRSwNP with and without aspirin sensitivity, more recent studies have suggested that long-term macrolide therapy is effective in atopic patients with NP [55]. A randomized-controlled trial by Varvyanskaya et al. [44] looked at several clinical parameters in patients with nasal polyps treated with 250 mg of clarithromycin a day for 12 and 24 weeks and compared these to a group of controls following ESS. All patients in the study were on nasal steroid sprays. They found that SNOT-20 scores, CT scans and nasal endoscopy scores were all significantly better in the group treated with clarithromycin for 24 weeks compared to the control group at most time points. ECP was measured in the nasal discharge of patients throughout the study and was shown to significantly decrease in both groups who were treated with clarithromycin compared to controls. The group treated for a full 24 weeks showed significantly lower levels of ECP than did the group treated for 12 weeks. In this study, atopic patients were identified with skin prick testing and it was observed that atopic patients had higher visual analog scales than non-atopic patients. Atopy correlated with higher ECP levels that suggest that symptom severity could be related to the amount or intensity of eosinophilic inflammation. Another prospective study supported these findings by showing that clarithromycin therapy was effective in both atopic and non-atopic patients with CRSwNP [56]. Interestingly, other studies have shown that in patients with CRSsNP treated with macrolides, patients with low levels of IgE showed significantly greater clinical benefits in response to the treatment than did patients with CRSsNP and high levels of IgE [47]. These studies are summarized in table 1.

One concern with long-term antibiotic treatment is the possible emergence of bacterial resistance. Several studies investigated macrolide resistance levels in their study populations and did not find any increase in bacterial resistance [44, 47, 49]. In general, across all studies, macrolides were well tolerated with very few instances of intolerance. The most common intolerance and cause for withdrawal from the study for all macrolides was GI upset.

In summary, macrolides appear to favorably modify symptoms of nasal polyposis but their impact on the size and presence of nasal polyps is less impressive. Courses of low-dose therapy 12 weeks or longer appear necessary to impart the greatest clinical benefit. These medications are well tolerated and bacterial resistance after long-term treatment has not been demonstrated. Further clinical studies are necessary to establish the specific therapeutic role macrolides could play in the treatment of CRSwNP.

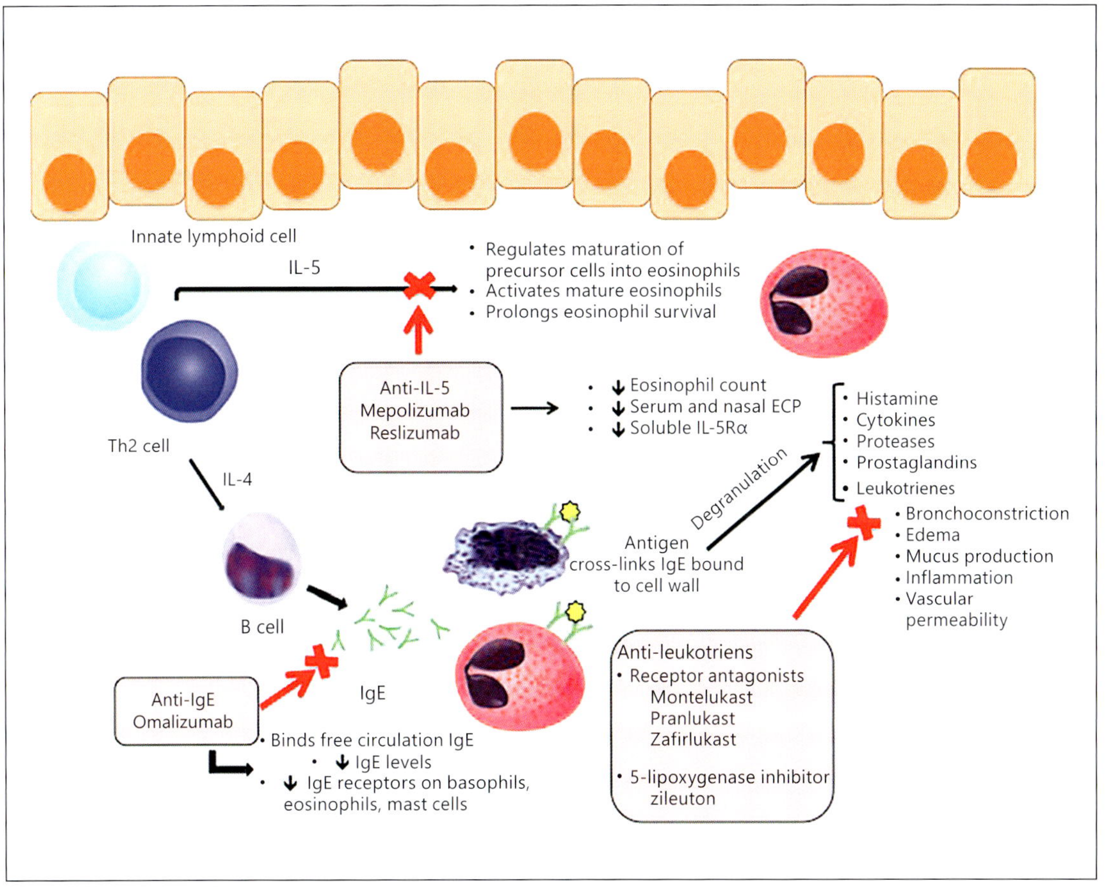

Fig. 2. Complex inflammatory pathways contributing to the pathogenesis of CRSwNP are becoming better understood, offering multiple potential targets for pharmacologic intervention. Immunomodulators, including anti-leukotrienes, anti-IL 5 and anti-IgE, target elements of the CRSwNP inflammatory cascade to suppress and down-regulate.

Conclusion

Inflammatory mechanisms contributing to CRSwNP are complex, presenting multiple potential targets for pharmacologic intervention (fig. 2). Emerging classes of immunomodulators, including anti-leukotrienes, anti-IgE, and anti-IL-5, anti-IL-4, along with evolving anti-inflammatory roles for macrolide antibiotics, have shown promising results in CRSwNP. These agents are being employed to spare systemic steroids in patients with polypoid chronic sinonasal inflammation, and potentially may obviate the need for steroids entirely in some circumstances. However, before immunomodulation can be considered a primary treatment strategy for CRSwNP, large randomized controlled trials are necessary to establish efficacy and to identify biomarkers for guiding choice of therapy. Until that time, immunomodulators will remain an exciting frontier in the medical treatment of this disease.

References

1 Gevaert P, Calus L, Van Zele T, et al: Omalizumab is effective in allergic and nonallergic patients with nasal polyps and asthma. J Allergy Clin Immunol 2013;131:110–116.e1.

2 Incorvaia C, Mauro M, Russello M, Formigoni C, Riario-Sforza GG, Ridolo E: Omalizumab, an anti-immunoglobulin E antibody: state of the art. Drug Des Devel Ther 2014;8:197–207.

3 MacGlashan DW Jr, Bochner BS, Adelman DC, et al: Down-regulation of Fc(epsilon)RI expression on human basophils during in vivo treatment of atopic patients with anti-IgE antibody. J Immunol 1997;158:1438–1445.

4 Milgrom H, Berger W, Nayak A, et al: Treatment of childhood asthma with anti-immunoglobulin E antibody (omalizumab). Pediatrics 2001;108:E36.

5 Corren J, Casale TB, Lanier B, Buhl R, Holgate S, Jimenez P: Safety and tolerability of omalizumab. Clin Exp Allergy 2009;39:788–797.

6 Bachert C, Gevaert P, Holtappels G, Johansson SG, van Cauwenberge P: Total and specific IgE in nasal polyps is related to local eosinophilic inflammation. J Allergy Clin Immunol 2001;107:607–614.

7 Gevaert P, Holtappels G, Johansson SG, Cuvelier C, Cauwenberge P, Bachert C: Organization of secondary lymphoid tissue and local IgE formation to Staphylococcus aureus enterotoxins in nasal polyp tissue. Allergy 2005;60:71–79.

8 Gevaert P, Nouri-Aria KT, Wu H, et al: Local receptor revision and class switching to IgE in chronic rhinosinusitis with nasal polyps. Allergy 2013;68:55–63.

9 Sheahan P, Ahn CN, Harvey RJ, et al: Local IgE production in nonatopic nasal polyposis. J Otolaryngol Head Neck Surg 2010;39:45–51.

10 Zhang N, Holtappels G, Gevaert P, et al: Mucosal tissue polyclonal IgE is functional in response to allergen and SEB. Allergy 2011;66:141–148.

11 Guglielmo M, Gulotta C, Mancini F, Sacchi M, Tarantini F: Recalcitrant nasal polyposis: achievement of total remission following treatment with omalizumab. J Investig Allergol Clin Immunol 2009;19:158–159.

12 Vennera Mdel C, Picado C, Mullol J, Alobid I, Bernal-Sprekelsen M: Efficacy of omalizumab in the treatment of nasal polyps. Thorax 2011;66:824–825.

13 Penn R, Mikula S: The role of anti-IgE immunoglobulin therapy in nasal polyposis: a pilot study. Am J Rhinol 2007;21:428–432.

14 Chandra RK, Clavenna M, Samuelson M, Tanner SB, Turner JH: Impact of omalizumab therapy on medication requirements for chronic rhinosinusitis. Int Forum Allergy Rhinol 2015, Epub ahead of print.

15 Peters-Golden M, Gleason MM, Togias A: Cysteinyl leukotrienes: multi-functional mediators in allergic rhinitis. Clin Exp Allergy 2006;36:689–703.

16 Peters-Golden M, Henderson WR Jr: The role of leukotrienes in allergic rhinitis. Ann Allergy Asthma Immunol 2005;94:609–618; quiz 618–620, 669.

17 Cingi C, Muluk NB, Ipci K, Sahin E: Antileukotrienes in upper airway inflammatory diseases. Curr Allergy Asthma Rep 2015;15:64.

18 Cobanoglu B, Toskala E, Ural A, Cingi C: Role of leukotriene antagonists and antihistamines in the treatment of allergic rhinitis. Curr Allergy Asthma Rep 2013;13:203–208.

19 Chao SS, Graham SM, Brown CL, Kline JN, Hussain I: Cysteinyl leukotriene 1 receptor expression in nasal polyps. Ann Otol Rhinol Laryngol 2006;115:394–397.

20 Baenkler HW, Schafer D, Hosemann W: Eicosanoids from biopsy of normal and polypous nasal mucosa. Rhinology 1996;34:166–170.

21 Cingi C, Ozlugedik S: Effects of montelukast on quality of life in patients with persistent allergic rhinitis. Otolaryngol Head Neck Surg 2010;142:654–658.

22 Cao Y, Wang J, Bunjhoo H, Xie M, Xu Y, Fang H: Comparison of leukotriene receptor antagonists in addition to inhaled corticosteroid and inhaled corticosteroid alone in the treatment of adolescents and adults with bronchial asthma: a meta-analysis. Asian Pac J Allergy Immunol 2012;30:130–138.

23 Park HS: Aspirin-sensitive asthma: recent advances in management. BioDrugs 2000;13:29–33.

24 Swierczynska M, Nizankowska-Mogilnicka E, Zarychta J, Gielicz A, Szczeklik A: Nasal versus bronchial and nasal response to oral aspirin challenge: clinical and biochemical differences between patients with aspirin-induced asthma/rhinitis. J Allergy Clin Immunol 2003;112:995–1001.

25 Corrigan C, Mallett K, Ying S, et al: Expression of the cysteinyl leukotriene receptors cysLT(1) and cysLT(2) in aspirin-sensitive and aspirin-tolerant chronic rhinosinusitis. J Allergy Clin Immunol 2005;115:316–322.

26 Wentzel JL, Soler ZM, DeYoung K, Nguyen SA, Lohia S, Schlosser RJ: Leukotriene antagonists in nasal polyposis: a meta-analysis and systematic review. Am J Rhinol Allergy 2013;27:482–489.

27 Knapp HR: Reduced allergen-induced nasal congestion and leukotriene synthesis with an orally active 5-lipoxygenase inhibitor. N Engl J Med 1990;323:1745–1748.

28 Fischer AR, Rosenberg MA, Lilly CM, et al: Direct evidence for a role of the mast cell in the nasal response to aspirin in aspirin-sensitive asthma. J Allergy Clin Immunol 1994;94(6 pt 1):1046–1056.

29 Dahlen B, Nizankowska E, Szczeklik A, et al: Benefits from adding the 5-lipoxygenase inhibitor zileuton to conventional therapy in aspirin-intolerant asthmatics. Am J Respir Crit Care Med 1998;157(4 pt 1):1187–1194.

30 Parnes SM, Chuma AV: Acute effects of antileukotrienes on sinonasal polyposis and sinusitis. Ear Nose Throat J 2000;79:18–20, 24–25.

31 Ulualp SO, Sterman BM, Toohill RJ: Antileukotriene therapy for the relief of sinus symptoms in aspirin triad disease. Ear Nose Throat J 1999;78:604–606, 608, 613, passim.

32 Di Capite J, Nelson C, Bates G, Parekh AB: Targeting Ca2+ release-activated Ca2+ channel channels and leukotriene receptors provides a novel combination strategy for treating nasal polyposis. J Allergy Clin Immunol 2009;124:1014–1021.e1–e3.

33 Sanderson CJ: Interleukin-5, eosinophils, and disease. Blood 1992;79:3101–3109.

34 Bachert C, Gevaert P, Holtappels G, Cuvelier C, van Cauwenberge P: Nasal polyposis: from cytokines to growth. Am J Rhinol 2000;14:279–290.
35 Bachert C, Wagenmann M, Hauser U, Rudack C: IL-5 synthesis is upregulated in human nasal polyp tissue. J Allergy Clin Immunol 1997;99(6 pt 1):837–842.
36 Gevaert P, Lang-Loidolt D, Lackner A, et al: Nasal IL-5 levels determine the response to anti-IL-5 treatment in patients with nasal polyps. J Allergy Clin Immunol 2006;118:1133–1141.
37 Klion AD, Law MA, Noel P, Kim YJ, Haverty TP, Nutman TB: Safety and efficacy of the monoclonal anti-interleukin-5 antibody SCH55700 in the treatment of patients with hypereosinophilic syndrome. Blood 2004;103:2939–2941.
38 Gevaert P, Van Bruaene N, Cattaert T, et al: Mepolizumab, a humanized anti-IL-5 mAb, as a treatment option for severe nasal polyposis. J Allergy Clin Immunol 2011;128:989–995.e1–e8.
39 Wenzel S, Ford L, Pearlman D, et al: Dupilumab in persistent asthma with elevated eosinophil levels. N Engl J Med 2013;368:2455–2466.
40 Wills-Karp M, Finkelman FD: Untangling the complex web of IL-4- and IL-13-mediated signaling pathways. Sci Signal 2008;1:pe55.
41 Izuhara K, Arima K, Yasunaga S: IL-4 and IL-13: their pathological roles in allergic diseases and their potential in developing new therapies. Curr Drug Targets Inflamm Allergy 2002;1:263–269.
42 Fish SC, Donaldson DD, Goldman SJ, Williams CM, Kasaian MT: IgE generation and mast cell effector function in mice deficient in IL-4 and IL-13. J Immunol 2005;174:7716–7724.
43 Bachert C, Mannent L, Naclerio RM, et al: Effect of subcutaneous dupilumab on nasal polyp burden in patients with chronic sinusitis and nasal polyposis: a randomized clinical trial. JAMA 2016;315:469–479.
44 Varvyanskaya A, Lopatin A: Efficacy of long-term low-dose macrolide therapy in preventing early recurrence of nasal polyps after endoscopic sinus surgery. Int Forum Allergy Rhinol 2014;4:533–541.
45 Yamada T, Fujieda S, Mori S, Yamamoto H, Saito H: Macrolide treatment decreased the size of nasal polyps and IL-8 levels in nasal lavage. Am J Rhinol 2000;14:143–148.
46 Cervin A: The anti-inflammatory effect of erythromycin and its derivatives, with special reference to nasal polyposis and chronic sinusitis. Acta Otolaryngol 2001;121:83–92.
47 Wallwork B, Coman W, Mackay-Sim A, Greiff L, Cervin A: A double-blind, randomized, placebo-controlled trial of macrolide in the treatment of chronic rhinosinusitis. Laryngoscope 2006;116:189–193.
48 Hashiba M, Baba S: Efficacy of long-term administration of clarithromycin in the treatment of intractable chronic sinusitis. Acta Otolaryngol Suppl 1996;525:73–78.
49 Cervin A, Kalm O, Sandkull P, Lindberg S: One-year low-dose erythromycin treatment of persistent chronic sinusitis after sinus surgery: clinical outcome and effects on mucociliary parameters and nasal nitric oxide. Otolaryngol Head Neck Surg 2002;126:481–489.
50 Scaglione F, Rossoni G: Comparative anti-inflammatory effects of roxithromycin, azithromycin and clarithromycin. J Antimicrob Chemother 1998;41(suppl B):47–50.
51 Suzuki H, Takahashi Y, Wataya H, et al: Mechanism of neutrophil recruitment induced by IL-8 in chronic sinusitis. J Allergy Clin Immunol 1996;98:659–670.
52 Suzuki H, Shimomura A, Ikeda K, Furukawa M, Oshima T, Takasaka T: Inhibitory effect of macrolides on interleukin-8 secretion from cultured human nasal epithelial cells. Laryngoscope 1997;107(12 pt 1):1661–1666.
53 Inamura K, Ohta N, Fukase S, Kasajima N, Aoyagi M: The effects of erythromycin on human peripheral neutrophil apoptosis. Rhinology 2000;38:124–129.
54 Allen JS, Eisma R, Leonard G, Lafreniere D, Kreutzer D: Interleukin-8 expression in human nasal polyps. Otolaryngol Head Neck Surg 1997;117:535–541.
55 Videler WJ, van Hee K, Reinartz SM, Georgalas C, van der Meulen FW, Fokkens WJ: Long-term low-dose antibiotics in recalcitrant chronic rhinosinusitis: a retrospective analysis. Rhinology 2012;50:45–55.
56 Peric A, Vojvodic D, Baletic N, Peric A, Miljanovic O: Influence of allergy on the immunomodulatory and clinical effects of long-term low-dose macrolide treatment of nasal polyposis. Biomed Pap Med Fac Univ Palacky Olomouc Czech Repub 2010;154:327–333.

Andrew P. Lane, MD
Department of Otolaryngology, Head and Neck Surgery, Division of Rhinology and Sinus Surgery
Johns Hopkins Outpatient Center, 6th floor, 601 N. Caroline St.
Baltimore, MD 21287-0910 (USA)
E-Mail alane3@jhmi.edu

Advances in Medical and Surgical Therapy

Woodworth BA, Poetker DM, Reh DD (eds): Rhinosinusitis with Nasal Polyposis.
Adv Otorhinolaryngol. Basel, Karger, 2016, vol 79, pp 114–120 (DOI: 10.1159/000445145)

Delivery of Topical Therapies

Kristine A. Smith • Luke Rudmik

Division of Otolaryngology, Head and Neck Surgery, Department of Surgery, University of Calgary, Calgary, Alta., Canada

Abstract

Chronic rhinosinusitis with nasal polyposis (CRSwNP) is an inflammatory disease of the sinonasal passages. Similar to other chronic inflammatory diseases, an essential component of the long-term control is prolonged medical therapy. To minimize the risk of adverse effects and cumulative complications of systemic medications, topical sinonasal therapy has become the primary strategy for prolonged medical therapy. The objective of this review article is to describe the evidence for the most common topical sinonasal delivery techniques. Evidence supports that high-volume irrigations provide the most reliable delivery of medical therapy to the paranasal sinuses. Low-volume nasal sprays and drops provide reliable delivery to the nasal cavity and a degree of penetration into the middle meatus and olfactory cleft; however, they do not reliably penetrate the paranasal sinuses. Sinus surgery and the head down-forward position optimize the delivery of high-volume irrigations into the paranasal sinuses. Additionally, high-volume irrigations assist in overcoming unfavorable nasal anatomy such as septal deviation and turbinate hypertrophy.

Introduction

Chronic rhinosinusitis with nasal polyposis (CRSwNP) is a phenotypic subtype of chronic rhinosinusitis (CRS), an inflammatory disease of the sinonasal passages, which represents approximately 20% of the total CRS population [1, 2]. Similar to other inflammatory conditions, corticosteroid therapy, either topical or systemic, is essential to control the underlying inflammatory process [3, 4]. While systemic corticosteroids can provide excellent control of CRSwNP inflammation and reduce polyp size, the side effects of systemic corticosteroid use preclude long-term use [3, 5]. As such, topical sinonasal delivery methods are the preferred methods of providing prolonged corticosteroid therapy in patients with CRSwNP [2, 6].

Topical delivery of medication to the sinonasal passages is not limited to corticosteroids. There is an evolving interest in administering other types of medical therapy directly to the sinonasal mucosa to avoid potential systemic side effects as

Table 1. Common topical delivery methods

Device	Examples	Estimated time required (min per dose)	Sinonasal delivery sites	Optimal head position	Adverse features
Low-volume*	Nasal drops	3–5	Nasal cavity Olfactory cleft Middle meatus	Lying Head Back	Local irritation Epistaxis Headache
	Nasal spray	0.5–1	Nasal cavity Middle meatus	Lying head low	Head position Intolerance
High-volume**	Neilmed sinus rinse Neti-pot	5–10	Nasal cavity sinus Ethmoid sinus Maxillary sinus Frontal sinus Sphenoid sinus	Head down forward	Eustachian tube dysfunction Local irritation Retained irrigation/leakage Solution preparation

* Less than 50 ml; ** greater than 50 ml.

well as providing higher drug concentrations directly to the diseased sinonasal tissue. In addition to corticosteroids, antibiotics, antihistamines, mucolytics and surfactant-containing solutions have all been used as topical sinonasal therapies [6, 7].

Nasal polyps most commonly originate and recur from the mucosa overlying the ethmoid roof in the middle meatus, but may affect every sinus and even the nasal cavity mucosa of the septum and middle turbinate [3]. The optimal topical sinonasal delivery technique in CRSwNP would enable drugs to penetrate into all the paranasal sinuses as well as the nasal cavity. Current challenges with achieving the optimal delivery of sinonasal medical therapy include gravity pushing medical therapies toward the nasopharynx instead of up into the superiorly located paranasal sinuses, the natural bony lamellae that covers and impairs delivery of drugs directly into the sinus cavities and the potential for anatomic variations to obstruct entrance into the nasal cavity such as septal deviations, inferior turbinate hypertrophy and middle turbinate concha bullosa [6]. With attempts to overcome these inherent topical drug delivery challenges, a variety of delivery methods have been developed and the efficacy of these methods may be affected by a variety of factors. In this paper, the most common delivery methods utilized in clinical practice will be discussed, as well as some of the innovative technology currently being introduced to improve topical delivery of sinonasal medical therapies. The impact of head position, endoscopic sinus surgery (ESS) and nasal anatomy on each delivery method will also be discussed.

Delivery Methods

There is a wide range of methods available that aim to deliver medication to the nasal cavity and paranasal sinuses. The most common methods utilized are high-volume sinonasal irrigations, nasal sprays and nasal drops, which are differentiated primarily by the volume of solution being delivered to the paranasal sinuses. Table 1 outlines the topical delivery methods commonly used in the management of CRSwNP.

High-Volume Sinonasal Irrigations

Technique

Generally, high-volume sinonasal irrigations are defined as a volume of greater than 50 ml, which is directly irrigated through one nostril and expelled through the other [6]. One of the most popularized irrigation methods is the 240 ml squeeze bottle or Neti-Pot. These high-volume irrigation methods may be used to administer saline irrigations but have also become a common method of co-administering additional medications, such as corticosteroids (e.g., budesonide) and various antimicrobials including mupirocin, tobramycin and gentamycin [6, 7]. These medications are added to the saline solution and then irrigated into the nasal cavity in hopes of delivering these therapies directly to the sinonasal mucosa.

Distribution Effectiveness

Several studies have investigated the distribution and penetration of high-volume irrigations into the sinonasal cavities [8–15]. These studies have shown reliable penetration into the paranasal sinuses, with improved penetration after ESS [8, 10–12]. Delivery to the ethmoid sinuses appears to be the most consistent, with decreasing penetration into the maxillary, frontal and sphenoid sinuses, respectively [13]. Complete distribution throughout the nasal cavity is also evident. The larger the volume of the irrigation, the better the distribution throughout the sinonasal cavity, specifically to the lamina papyracea and the olfactory cleft [8]. Overall, less than 5% of high-volume irrigation fluid is retained within the paranasal sinuses [10]. Compared to other delivery methods, high-volume irrigations have superior distribution and penetration into the paranasal sinuses and provide an added benefit of mechanically cleaning the sinonasal cavities and assisting the normal mucociliary clearance to remove potential inflammatory debris [6, 8–15]. Given the improved delivery to the paranasal sinuses, high-volume sinonasal irrigations are the recommended delivery technique when distribution to the paranasal sinuses is the goal of therapy [6].

Adverse Features

Some of the most common adverse events associated with high-volume sinonasal irrigations are Eustachian tube dysfunction (23%), local irritation (1–11%) and headache (7–26%) [16]. Although not an adverse event, the time burden associated with performing sinonasal irrigations can also be a disadvantage for certain patients. On average, sinonasal irrigations are estimated to consume approximately 5–10 min to prepare and administer. Patients may also have to perform rinses multiple times per day, and the time required may reduce compliance.

In 2011, there were 2 suspected deaths from amoebic meningoencephalitis related to contaminated Neti-Pot irrigation with Naegleria fowleri [17]. Until further research elucidates the safety of using tap water, it is preferred that patients use sterile water for irrigation solution. Bacterial contamination of irrigation bottles/pots has been reported in up to 80% of bottles after 2 weeks [18]. Although there is no association between irrigation bottle contamination and sinus infection, most clinicians would agree that it is good practice to regularly disinfect and replace sinonasal irrigation bottles/pots.

Nasal Sprays

Technique

Nasal sprays are a low-volume delivery method where the patient inserts the tip of the medication bottle into the nasal vestibule and aims to the ipsilateral lateral canthus of the eye. The spray mechanism is then activated, most often through a mechanical pump system, to deliver the spray to the nasal cavity. The process consumes approximately 30 seconds.

Distribution Effectiveness

In CRSwNP, corticosteroid nasal sprays have been shown to reduce polyp size and improve nasal obstruction [1, 3, 7, 19]. Studies evaluating the distribution of nasal sprays show excellent penetration into the nasal cavity with limited delivery into the sinus cavities [6]. Recent studies have suggested that greater that 80% of the nasal spray volume penetrates beyond the nasal vestibule into the nasal cavity [20]. With proper technique, the majority of the spray is distributed to the anterior head of the inferior and middle turbinate, with limited distribution to the posterior nasal cavity [21]. However, sprays are unlikely to penetrate into the paranasal sinuses, especially in unoperated sinuses [22]. The middle meatus does receive some distribution; however, it is highly variable and unreliable [6, 23, 24]. Less than 50% of spray volume penetrates into the middle meatus and less than 1% enters the sinuses [22, 24]. As such, nasal sprays are not recommended as the primary method for delivering corticosteroids to the paranasal sinuses [6].

Adverse Features

Nasal sprays are most commonly associated with local irritation and epistaxis, affecting approximately 10% of patients [25]. Headache is also common, affecting 5–25% of patients, depending on the nasal steroid used. While a variety of other wide effects are reported, they tend to be either mild or rare [6, 25]. Nasal sprays are generally well tolerated, easy to administer and consume very little patient time.

Nasal Drops

Technique

Nasal drops are another commonly used low-volume (typically less then 5 ml) delivery technique [6]. In order to administer the medication in such a way that it is retained within the nasal cavity, patients often need to utilize a variety of head positions. The two most efficient head positions for the delivery of nasal drops are the lying head low and lying head back positions. Once in this position, patients administer the drops and are recommended to stay in this position for approximately 3–5 min to prevent immediate drainage into the nasopharynx.

Evidence

The use of drops for the delivery of medication to the nasal cavity and paranasal sinuses is generally limited to corticosteroids. Corticosteroid nasal drops have been shown to reduce polyp side and decrease nasal obstruction with similar efficacy to nasal steroid sprays [24]. Several studies have shown that drops are distributed throughout the nasal cavity, but do not appear to penetrate well into the paranasal sinuses [23, 24, 26, 27]. One advantage of nasal drops is their improved ability to penetrate into the olfactory cleft with certain head positions (e.g., lying head back and lying head low) [6]. CRSwNP patients tend to be more symptomatically affected by olfactory dysfunction; therefore, this delivery method may provide additional benefit in select patients by specifically treating olfactory cleft inflammation and polyposis. In general, however, nasal drops tend to have limited sinus penetration compared to high-volume irrigation methods.

Adverse Features

Similar to nasal sprays, drops are most commonly associated with nasal irritation, epistaxis and poor taste. The time consumed to administer nasal drops is similar to high-volume irrigations since patients are often advised to maintain their head positions for 3–5 min after delivery. Furthermore, the head positions required to provide adequate distribution can be challenging and uncomfortable for certain patients such as those with neck problems [6].

Highlights: Delivery Methods

- High-volume sinonasal irrigation provides the most reliable and comprehensive delivery to the paranasal sinuses, especially after ESS.
- Nasal sprays provide excellent distribution and penetration into the nasal cavity, but have unreliable delivery into the paranasal sinuses.
- Nasal drops may provide improved delivery to the olfactory cleft compared to nasal sprays.

Impact of Sinus Surgery

One of the goals of ESS is to open the paranasal sinuses to facilitate the delivery of topical sinonasal medications. ESS has the greatest impact on the distribution and penetration of medications into the paranasal sinuses, regardless of delivery device [6]. In patients who have not had ESS, distribution to the sinuses is generally inconsistent and limited. Following sinus surgery, distribution improves for all of the paranasal sinuses, especially to the frontal and sphenoid sinuses compared to the ethmoid and maxillary sinuses [6].

The aggressiveness of sinus surgery also influences the distribution of medication. Larger maxillary antrostomy are associated with more effective distribution into the maxillary sinus, while the minimum size for a maxillary antrostomy to improve the delivery of topical medications is approximately 4–5 mm [11, 12, 28]. Endoscopic modified Lothrops and medial maxillectomies may further improve distribution to the frontal and maxillary sinuses, respectively [10, 29–31].

Highlights: Impact of Sinus Surgery

- ESS improves the distribution of topical medications into the paranasal sinuses.
- The minimum size for a maxillary antrostomy required to improve medication delivery is 4–5 mm.
- Modified Lothrop during ESS may improve topical medications into the frontal sinus.

Impact of Head Position

Altering the head position during topical medical therapy may improve delivery into certain paranasal sinuses [8, 32–35]. The head down-forward position improves the delivery to the paranasal sinuses, regardless of device type [6]. Head position has the most effect on sinus distribution in low-volume device [6]. As the volume of the delivery method increases to 200 ml, head position has less impact on the distribution and penetration into the paranasal sinuses [8]. However, low-volume delivery techniques have very little distribution into the sinuses, regardless of head position or a history of ESS [6]. The lying head low and lying head back positions have the greatest distribution to the nasal cavity and olfactory cleft [6].

Highlights: Impact of Head Position

- For high-volume irrigation techniques, the head down-forward position provides the optimal distribution to the paranasal sinuses.
- For low-volume delivery methods, the lying head low and lying head back positions offer the best distribution to the olfactory cleft and nasal cavity.

Impact of Nasal Anatomy

Variants of nasal cavity anatomy, such as septal deviations, narrowed nasal valves and inferior turbinate hypertrophy, have been shown to decrease the distribution of nasal sprays and drops to the nasal cavity. However, high-volume irrigations are able to overcome unfavorable nasal anatomy and penetrate into the paranasal sinuses. The impact of surgery to address these nasal variants has not been studied [6].

Highlights: Impact of Nasal Anatomy

- High-volume irrigations overcome unfavorable nasal anatomy to penetrate the paranasal sinuses.

Summary

To avoid potential adverse effects and cumulative complications of systemic medications, topical sinonasal medications are an essential component during the prolonged management of CRSwNP. A variety of delivery methods exist; however, only high-volume irrigations have reliable delivery to the paranasal sinuses. Low-volume nasal sprays and drops provide reliable delivery to the nasal cavity and a degree of penetration into the middle meatus and olfactory cleft; however, they do not reliably penetrate the paranasal sinuses. Distribution of topical therapies is significantly improved following ESS and the head down-forward position optimizes the delivery of high-volume irrigations to the paranasal sinuses. Additionally, high-volume irrigations overcome unfavorable nasal anatomy to penetrate the paranasal sinuses. Nasal drops and sprays are recommended in patients who cannot tolerate high-volume irrigations.

Funding/Support

There was no funding support for this study.

Conflict of Interest

K.A.S.: None.
L.R.: None.

References

1 Rudmik L, et al: Impact of topical nasal steroid therapy on symptoms of nasal polyposis: a meta-analysis. Laryngoscope 2012;122:1431–1437.
2 Fokkens WJ, et al: EPOS 2012: European position paper on rhinosinusitis and nasal polyps 2012. A summary for otorhinolaryngologists. Rhinology 2012;50: 1–12.
3 Kalish L, et al: Topical steroids for nasal polyps. Cochrane Database Syst Rev 2012;12:CD006549.
4 Rudmik L, Soler ZM: Medical therapies for adult chronic sinusitis: a systematic review. JAMA 2015;314:926–939.
5 Schlosser RJ, Soler ZM: Evidence-based treatment of chronic rhinosinusitis with nasal polyps. Am J Rhinol Allergy 2013; 27:461–466.
6 Thomas WW 3rd, et al: Distribution of topical agents to the paranasal sinuses: an evidence-based review with recommendations. Int Forum Allergy Rhinol 2013;3:691–703.
7 Rudmik L, et al: Topical therapies in the management of chronic rhinosinusitis: an evidence-based review with recommendations. Int Forum Allergy Rhinol 2013;3:281–298.
8 Beule A, et al: Efficacy of different techniques of sinonasal irrigation after modified Lothrop procedure. Am J Rhinol Allergy 2009;23:85–90.
9 Brenner PS, et al: Unexpected consequences of transnasal balloon dilation of the maxillary ostium. Int Forum Allergy Rhinol 2011;1:466–470.
10 Harvey RJ, et al: Fluid residuals and drug exposure in nasal irrigation. Otolaryngol Head Neck Surg 2009;141:757–761.
11 Singhal D, et al: Effect of head position and surgical dissection on sinus irrigant penetration in cadavers. Laryngoscope 2010;120:2528–2531.
12 Grobler A, et al: Pre- and postoperative sinus penetration of nasal irrigation. Laryngoscope 2008;118:2078–2081.
13 Valentine R, et al: A prospective controlled trial of pulsed nasal nebulizer in maximally dissected cadavers. Am J Rhinol 2008;22:390–394.
14 Miller TR, et al: Comparison of topical medication delivery systems after sinus surgery. Laryngoscope 2004;114:201–204.
15 Bleier BS, et al: Temporospatial quantification of fluorescein-labeled sinonasal irrigation delivery. Int Forum Allergy Rhinol 2011;1:361–365.
16 Harvey R, et al: Nasal saline irrigations for the symptoms of chronic rhinosinusitis. Cochrane Database Syst Rev 2007; 18:CD006394.
17 Sowerby LJ, Wright ED: Tap water or 'sterile' water for sinus irrigations: what are our patients using? Int Forum Allergy Rhinol 2012;2:300–302.
18 Psaltis AJ, et al: Contamination of sinus irrigation devices: a review of the evidence and clinical relevance. Am J Rhinol Allergy 2012;26:201–203.
19 Rudmik L, et al: Early postoperative care following endoscopic sinus surgery: an evidence-based review with recommendations. Int Forum Allergy Rhinol 2011; 1:417–430.
20 Shah SA, et al: Regional deposition of mometasone furoate nasal spray suspension in humans. Allergy Asthma Proc 2014, Epub ahead of print.
21 Charlton S, et al: Distribution and clearance of bioadhesive formulations from the olfactory region in man: effect of polymer type and nasal delivery device. Eur J Pharm Sci 2007;30:295–302.
22 Moller W, et al: Pulsating aerosols for drug delivery to the sinuses in healthy volunteers. Otolaryngol Head Neck Surg 2010;142:382–388.

23 Homer JJ, Maughan J, Burniston M: A quantitative analysis of the intranasal delivery of topical nasal drugs to the middle meatus: spray versus drop administration. J Laryngol Otol 2002;116: 10–13.
24 Tsikoudas A, Homer JJ: The delivery of topical nasal sprays and drops to the middle meatus: a semiquantitative analysis. Clin Otolaryngol Allied Sci 2001;26: 294–297.
25 Hamilos D: Chronic rhinosinusitis: management. 2015. http://www.uptodate.com.ezproxy.lib.ucalgary.ca/contents/chronic-rhinosinusitis-management.
26 Cannady SB, et al: Comparison of delivery of topical medications to the paranasal sinuses via 'vertex-to-floor' position and atomizer spray after FESS. Otolaryngol Head Neck Surg 2005;133:735–740.
27 Rudman KL, O'Brien EK, Leopold DA: Radiographic distribution of drops and sprays within the sinonasal cavities. Am J Rhinol Allergy 2011;25:94–97.
28 Saijo R, et al: Particle deposition of therapeutic aerosols in the nose and paranasal sinuses after transnasal sinus surgery: a cast model study. Am J Rhinol 2004;18:1–7.
29 Hwang PH, Woo RJ, Fong KJ: Intranasal deposition of nebulized saline: a radionuclide distribution study. Am J Rhinol 2006;20:255–261.
30 Manes RP, Tong L, Batra PS: Prospective evaluation of aerosol delivery by a powered nasal nebulizer in the cadaver model. Int Forum Allergy Rhinol 2011; 1:366–371.
31 St Martin MB, et al: Deposition of aerosolized particles in the maxillary sinuses before and after endoscopic sinus surgery. Am J Rhinol 2007;21:196–197.
32 Merkus P, et al: Influence of anatomy and head position on intranasal drug deposition. Eur Arch Otorhinolaryngol 2006;263:827–832.
33 Weber R, et al: Videoendoscopic analysis of nasal steroid distribution. Rhinology 1999;37:69–73.
34 Dowley AC, Homer JJ: The effect of inferior turbinate hypertrophy on nasal spray distribution to the middle meatus. Clin Otolaryngol Allied Sci 2001;26: 488–490.
35 Senocak D, Senocak M, Bozan S: Sinonasal distribution of topically applied particles: computerized tomographic detection and the effects of topical decongestion. Otolaryngol Head Neck Surg 2005;133:944–948.

Dr. Luke Rudmik
Division of Otolaryngology, Head and Neck Surgery, Department of Surgery
University of Calgary, Foothills Medical Centre, South Tower Suite 602, 1403 – 29th St. NW
T2N 2T9 Calgary, AB (Canada)
E-Mail lukerudmik@gmail.com

Advances in Medical and Surgical Therapy

Woodworth BA, Poetker DM, Reh DD (eds): Rhinosinusitis with Nasal Polyposis.
Adv Otorhinolaryngol. Basel, Karger, 2016, vol 79, pp 121–130 (DOI: 10.1159/000445148)

Topical Steroids

Gretchen M. Oakley[a, b] · Richard J. Harvey[b, c]

[a]Department of Otolaryngology – Head and Neck Surgery, University of California San Francisco, San Francisco, Calif., USA;
[b]Rhinology and Skull Base Research Group, Applied Medical Research Centre, University of New South Wales, Sydney,
[c]Faculty of Medicine and Health Sciences, Macquarie University, Sydney, Australia

Abstract

Chronic rhinosinusitis with nasal polyps (CRSwNP) is an inflammatory condition with heterogeneous pathophysiology. A cornerstone of the management of this condition is the use of anti-inflammatory agents. Corticosteroids are very effective and the most commonly used, but other drugs with immunodulatory activity such as anti-IL5, doxycycline (Th2), and macrolides (anti-neutrophilic/IL8) have been shown to have efficacy. Although systemic corticosteroids have shown benefit in managing this condition, the frequency of use often required in this condition is associated with significant adverse effects. Topical corticosteroids, particularly when utilized after endoscopic sinus surgery and delivered in a high volume, high pressure manner, provide the desired anti-inflammatory effects with nearly negligible systemic absorption. Studies assessing the long-term use of second generation topical corticosteroids have demonstrated no significant effects on cortisol levels, growth rate, intraocular pressures or lens opacification, or local mucosal atrophy. Patients who often respond most favorably to corticosteroid treatment are those with a Th2-mediated, highly eosinophilic CRSwNP. However, there is a subset of patients who are steroid resistant. In the case of a predominantly neutrophilic CRSwNP, it is important to be aware that patients may respond well to the use of macrolide therapy. Additionally, the use of verapamil has shown promise in increasing steroid responsiveness in a difficult to treat group of patients with steroid resistance. Topical corticosteroids play a key role in the long term management of this complicated inflammatory condition by providing the much needed pharmacologic local control with minimal systemic adverse effects.

Introduction

Chronic rhinosinusitis with nasal polyps (CRSwNP) is an inflammatory disease state of a heterogeneous pathophysiologic process. CRSwNP is a subtype of chronic rhinosinusitis (CRS) with increased disease severity and poorer prognosis than CRS without nasal polyps (CRSsNP). Current concepts in the pathogenesis of CRSwNP focus on the inflammatory processes secondary to dysregulation of local immune

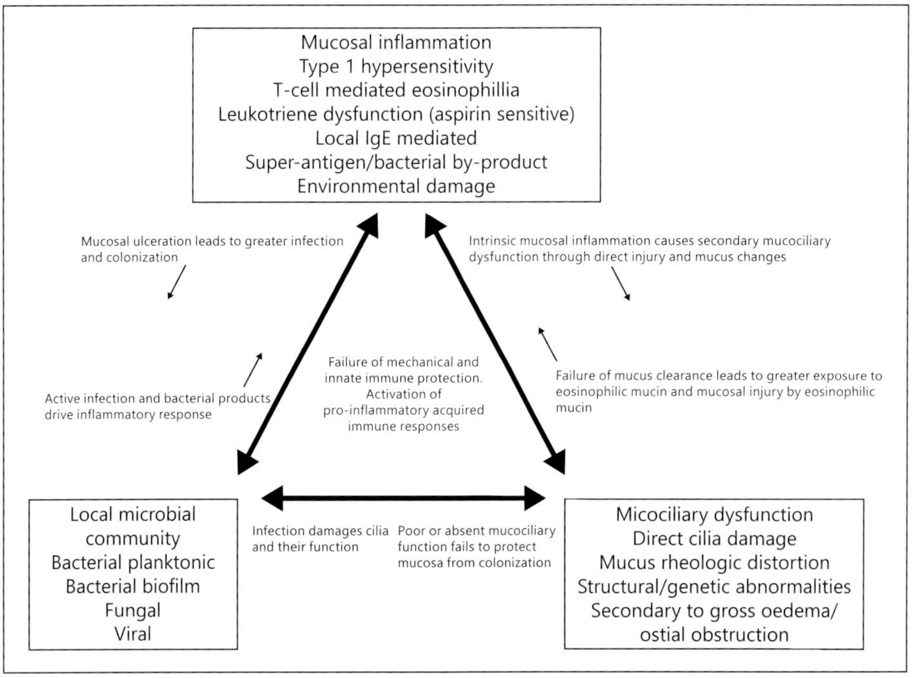

Fig. 1. The pathophysiologic interaction of intrinsic mucosal inflammation, microbial flora and mucociliary dysfunction in CRS. (Courtesy of Division of Rhinology, St. Vincent's Hospital, Sydney; with permission.)

function, impairment of the epithelial barrier, and a sustained inflammatory response to foreign antigens [1] (fig. 1). Although prior research and treatment has focused on common environmental antigens, it is the host response and not simply their presence that is the primary defect. CRSwNP is not a simple disease of osteomeatal complex (OMC) occlusion. Radiographic studies demonstrate that OMC occlusion has no relationship to disease in the dependent sinuses (maxilla, anterior ethmoid and frontal) in CRSwNP [2, 3]. In the case of CRSwNP, patients have diffuse sinus mucosal inflammation which appears unrelated to any local anatomic obstruction. Therefore, surgical interventions or treatment philosophies focused on ventilation or limited OMC correction of the drainage pathways are unlikely to provide significant modification of the underlying chronic inflammatory process or maintain any lasting disease modification.

CRSwNP is characterized by excessive T-helper 2 (Th2) inflammation, eosinophilic infiltration, and decreased regulatory T-cell (Treg) function. Given that CRSwNP is an inflammatory process, corticosteroids have been accepted as a central element in treatment strategies and have proven quite effective. The mechanism of action of corticosteroids combines suppression of gene transcription for proinflammatory products and reduction of airway inflammatory cell infiltration and function [4, 5]. In addition, they affect endothelial cells by inhibiting cell surface molecules, such as cell chemotactic factors and adhesion molecules, as well as inhibiting vascular permeability, and suppressing the production and effects of humoral factors [4]. Although corticosteroids inhibit macrophages, eosinophils, basophils and mast cells, they have much less of an effect on neutrophils [4]. In addition to their influence on cell distribution, corticosteroids also inhibit the initiation and activation of the T-cell cycle and the cytokines secreted by activated T cells [4].

Benefit of Topical Steroids

Although it has been demonstrated that corticosteroids delivered topically have beneficial effects in patients with CRS, the treatment response in studies is very heterogeneous and often poor. How corticosteroids are delivered and whether the sinus cavity has been modified to affect distribution greatly impacts the effectiveness of the drug [6]. The critical issues of delivery device and surgery are addressed elsewhere in this book. A meta-analysis of topical corticosteroid in CRS assessing 40 studies and 3,624 patients has shown that the use of topical corticosteroids after endoscopic sinus surgery was most effective compared to surgery naïve cohorts [7]. When compared to placebo, topical corticosteroids have led to improved overall symptom score, decreased polyp score, reduced polyp size, and prevented polyp recurrence after sinus surgery [7–9]. Notably, these favorable outcomes are greater when the intranasal steroids were delivered with a high volume, high pressure irrigation device and followed endoscopic sinus surgery compared to their counterparts [6, 7, 10]. In a study on high volume irrigation in the postoperative setting that performed subgroup analysis for CRSwNP, the most challenging eosinophilic patients (>10/high power field [HPF]) had as good or better improvement in symptoms, Sino-Nasal Outcome Test 22 (SNOT-22), and endoscopy scores compared to CRSsNP or low tissue eosinophilia (≤10/HPF) [11]. In fact, the use of postoperative intranasal steroids has become recommended practice based on prior evidence-based reviews [12, 13].

The goal of endoscopic sinus surgery is to create a wide open common cavity to enable maximal delivery of topical anti-inflammatory therapy and removal of hypersecretory mucin (fig. 2). There is little basis for surgery as a single modality treatment for CRSwNP and the use of topical steroids in an unoperated sinus cavity often has limited benefit due to their restricted access to the diseased sinus mucosa. There is good evidence to show that topical corticosteroid therapy does not reach the sinus prior to surgery, and the use of simple sprays is ineffective in any state of the sinus [14]. Total sinus distribution of topical irrigation improves significantly to all sinuses after endoscopic sinus surgery [14]. In particular, distribution to the frontal sinuses is almost undetectable pre-operatively and is significantly improved after surgery [14]. Distribution of nasal irrigation is also influenced by the type of delivery device. Delivery via Neti-pot and squeeze bottle techniques is significantly better than the pressurized spray techniques both prior to and after surgery [14].

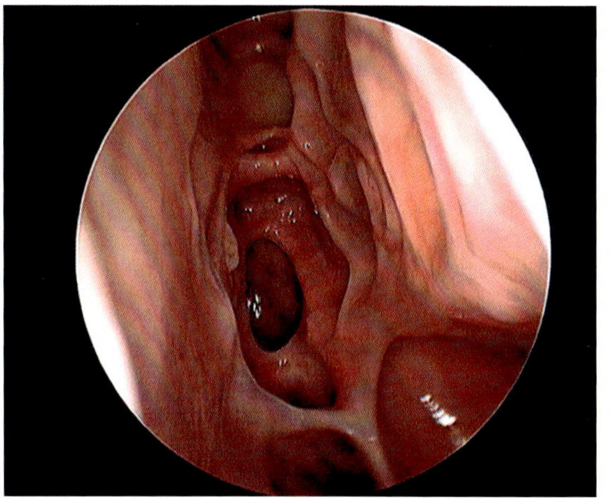

Fig. 2. A wide open sinus cavity following endoscopic sinus surgery. The access for topical corticosteroids to the sinuses in the postsurgical cavity is significantly improved.

Surgery also provides an opportunity to reduce the current inflammatory burden of disease. This concept describes patients with the highest inflammatory load as those having eosinophilic CRS with nasal polyposis and concomitant asthma and/or aspirin intolerance [15]. These patients represent the extreme end of the 'inflammatory spectrum' and experience worse subjective and objective postoperative outcomes, higher recurrence rates and need for revision surgery. It is hypothesized that more radical surgery achieves the goal of eradicating the presence of proinflammatory mediators, such as eosinophils in mucosa, eosinophilic mucin, fungal and staphylococcal antigens, and bacterial load that contribute to the local inflammatory load [15]. Surgical reduction of the inflammatory surface area and consequently the overall inflammatory load may allow subsequent control to be maintained with medical therapies.

Systemic versus Topical Steroids

Use of systemic corticosteroids is a common and effective practice in managing CRSwNP [16]. The effects are mostly limited to the time that the patients are receiving the medication. However, the prolonged use of systemic corticosteroids can be associated with complications involving various organ systems. Many of these effects are either dose and/or duration dependent. The risk–benefit balance will have a great degree of individual variability but there are some guides as to when intermittent systemic delivery needs to be replaced by a wide surgical corridor and the regular delivery of local or topical corticosteroids.

There are 3 concepts to consider when using systemic corticosteroids: maximal dose, cumulative dose, and duration/frequency of treatment course. Serious complications, such as avascular necrosis of the femoral hip, is a rare event and reported in doses over 40 mg and a total cumulative steroid dose of 290–1,000 mg [17]. As a guide, the duration of corticosteroid therapy should be 2–3 weeks in order to suppress the inflammatory process across the life span of the tissue eosinophil. It has been demonstrated that CRSwNP patients receiving more than 3 short courses of systemic corticosteroid treatment per year (more than 21 days per year of treatment, prednisolone 1 mg/kg/day for a 6–10 day course) had reduced bone mineral density [18]. In this study, 10.9 and 43.5% had osteoporosis and osteopenia respectively at the lumbar spine and 48.8% had asymptomatic adrenal insufficiency [18]. Therefore, if more than 2–3 courses of systemic steroid therapy, 2–3 weeks duration each, are required within a 12-month period (with each course of maximal dose <40 mg and maximum cumulative dose of 290–1,000 mg) to control patient symptoms, then consideration for wide endoscopic sinus surgery with the goal of transitioning the patient from systemic therapy to topical corticosteroid therapy is indicated. A history of good response to previous oral corticosteroids can provide important diagnostic information. CRSwNP patients that have proven to be steroid responsive are likely to have greater benefit from postoperative topical corticosteroid therapy [1] (fig. 3).

Safety Concerns with Topicals

Actual Dose Exposure

Topical corticosteroids offer the ability to deliver necessary anti-inflammatory medication to the areas of need with a much lower risk of side effects. While irrigations are used with high volumes and have a larger total drug load, most of the irrigation solution is wasted after contact with the sinus mucosa. Only 5% of the solution will be retained in the sinuses after the squeeze bottle irrigation [19] in the postsurgical setting, which translates to a 50 μg exposure from daily 1 mg budesonide irrigations.

HPA Suppression

Studies assessing the safety profile of topical intranasal corticosteroids have demonstrated that there is no effect on serum, urinary or salivary cortisol levels measured after 6 weeks of twice daily budesonide irrigation use [20, 21]. Similar-

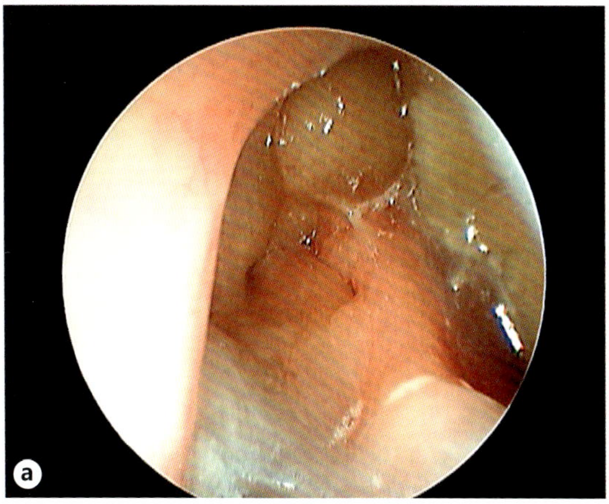

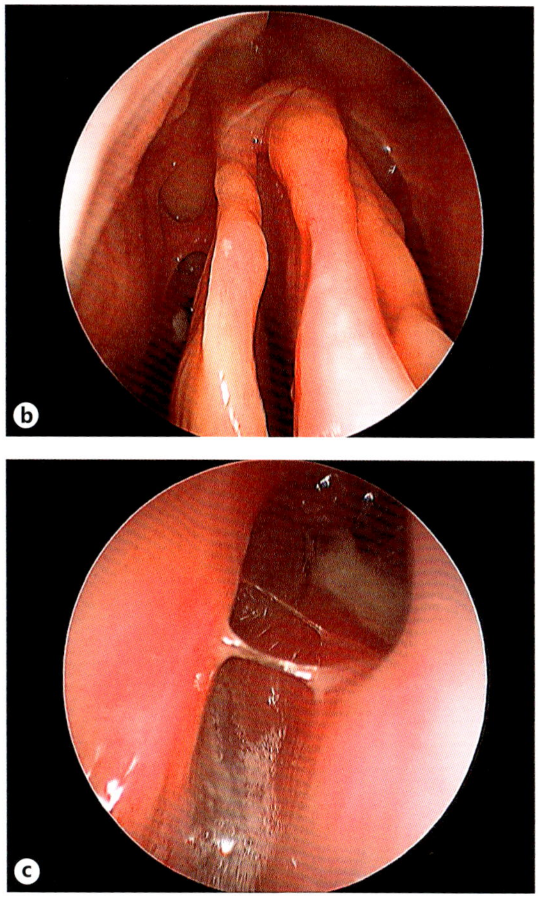

Fig. 3. Endoscopic images of a Lothrop cavity from the right in a steroid sensitive patient who is intermittently compliant with her topical steroid irrigations. **a** 18 months post-endoscopic sinus surgery and Lothrop with poor control of her CRSwNP due to prior noncompliance with her postoperative topical steroid irrigations. **b** Same patient 3 months later with good compliance with steroid irrigations. **c** Same patient an additional 3 months later after again discontinuing her steroid irrigations. The rapid fluctuations in CRSwNP control based on topical steroid use in this patient demonstrates the important role this ongoing medical therapy plays in successful management of this condition.

ly, studies assessing second generation intranasal corticosteroids (mometasone furoate, fluticasone proprionate, fluticasone furoate, ciclesonide) have shown no significant impact on the hypothathalamic-pituitary-adrenal axis [22].

Growth Effects in Children
One study with prepubertal children using twice daily beclomethasone diproprionate for 1 year for perennial allergic rhinitis reported a slowing of growth rate in the steroid group (0.9 cm difference) [23]. However, no effect on height was seen in several prospective studies assessing mometasone, fluticasone proprionate, budesonide, ciclesonide and triamcinolone given at recommended doses for 1 year [24–28].

Ocular Side Effects
A systematic review of randomized controlled trials showed no increase in intraocular pressures, lens opacity, or cataract formation with use of intranasal corticosteroid spray compared to controls [29].

The Myth of Mucosal Atrophy
'Mucosal atrophy' resulting from topical steroid use has been raised as a concern by primary care physicians as these heathcare providers see epidermal atrophy from steroid-based topical skin creams or ointments. However, the respiratory epithelium differs from stratified keratinizing squamous epithelium of the skin, which thins and loses hair/keratin production as a result of the

catabolic effects of corticosteroids. This effect is reversible on skin and not seen in upper or lower respiratory mucosa. A recent systematic review of the literature has shown no evidence of intranasal steroid use causing mucosal atrophy, regardless of type, dose, duration, or indication for use in 11 randomized controlled studies [30].

Minor Effects

Common local side effects of intranasal corticosteroid use include epistaxis, throat irritation, nasal dryness, and burning and stinging sensations, which have proven to be mild, similar to placebo (except for epistaxis), and self-resolving without discontinuation of the medication [31–35]. Rate of epistaxis has been reported to be 5% in intranasal steroid spray users with the side of epistaxis correlating with patient handedness [30], supporting that it is the result of the spray being directed at the septum leading to mucosal dryness, mechanical trauma from the nasal applicator tip against the septum or anterior head of the inferior turbinate, or both. Patient instruction on use of any nasal sprays or irrigations should always be conducted to minimize these issues that could be contributing to epistaxis.

Corticosteroid Potency, Bioavailability and Effectiveness

Beclomethasone diproprionate was introduced as the first steroid to be used in the form of an aerosol, which had the added benefits of high potency with much lower systemic effects. The systemic bioavailability of intranasal corticosteroids is the result of the total of nasal and intestinal absorption and clearance from first pass hepatic metabolism. Although the European position paper on rhinosinusitis and nasal polyps 2012 found that there was no superiority of second generation intranasal corticosteroids (mometasone, fluticasone, ciclesonide) over first generation (budesonide, betamethasone, beclomethasone, triamcinolone and dexamethasone) in terms of final symptom score or polyp reduction [36], the second generation agents are still first choice. One of the main features that separate these groups of corticosteroids is their pharmacokinetic qualities. The second generation corticosteroids have qualities that minimize their systemic bioavailability, thus minimizing their risk of systemic exposure. With each topical application of second generation corticosteroid, 30% of the medication remains in the nose where it binds to glucocorticoid receptors, while the remaining 70% is swallowed and absorbed through the intestinal tract and undergoes a degree of first pass metabolism that varies based on agent: 80–90% for triamcinolone acetonide, 90% for budesonide, and 99% for mometasone furoate nasal spray and fluticasone proprionate [37]. The greater the lipophilicity of the agent, the greater the uptake and retention in targeted mucosa and respiratory tract tissue, the longer the binding time with local glucocorticoid receptors and the less available systemically to cause side effects [22]. The order of lipophilicity begins with mometasone furoate as the highest, followed by fluticasone propionate, beclomethasone dipropionate, budesonide, triamcinolone acetonide and flunisolide as the least lipophilic [24–28]. A meta-analysis by Schafer et al. [38] comparing the efficacy and side effects of 6 different intranasal corticosteroids (therapeutic index) demonstrated that budesonide had the highest efficacy, followed by mometasone furoate and triamcinolone, and that mometasone and triamcinolone had the lowest risk of adverse effects. Figure 4 shows various topical steroid options for management of CRSwNP arranged in order of their respective potencies.

Steroid Resistance

CRSwNP has been shown to be mostly a Th2-mediated inflammatory condition that is characterized by predominantly eosinophilic infiltration and a strong interleukin (IL)-5 cytokine profile. Although a Th1/Th17-mediated, neutrophilic

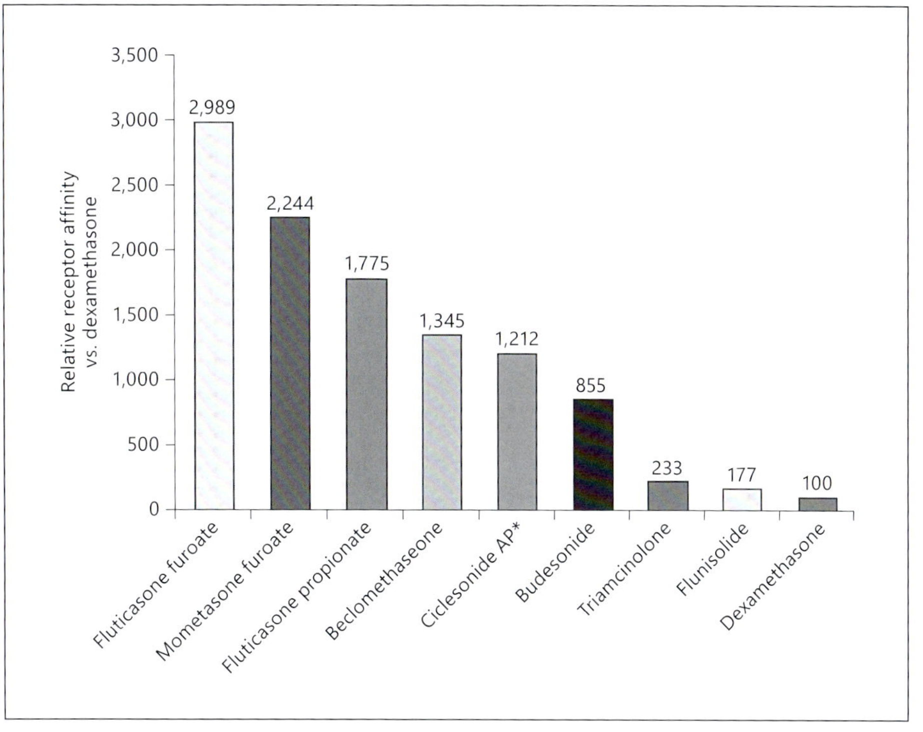

Fig. 4. A representation of topical steroid options arranged in order of potency. (Data from McKenzie [46] and Valotis et al. [47]. Figure reproduced with permission from Derendorf et al. [48].)

rather than eosinophilic CRSwNP has also been demonstrated in a South Chinese population with otherwise similar clinical features to their Caucasian European counterparts [39], studies show that the eosinophilic, Th2/IL-5 process is the more common condition universally for nasal polyposis [40, 41]. An eosinophilic phenotype has been reported in 76% of CRSwNP patients, including a mixed eosinophilic-neutrophilic phenotype in 35.8% [41] (fig. 5). Knowing the predominant inflammatory mediators in a given patient's CRSwNP condition can be beneficial for treatment planning: the greater the eosinophilic component, the better the response to corticosteroids. One study demonstrated a significantly greater reduction in bilateral polyp size, nasal congestion, total nasal symptom scores, and nasal resistance in the eosinophilic group treated with oral corticosteroids than the neutrophilic group [41]. The response to effectively delivered topical corticosteroids should be similar.

The benefit of better categorizing a patient's CRS, and therefore being able to better select the most effective treatment for it, argues for structured histopathology reporting on all CRS patients. For example, patients who do not demonstrate adequate steroid responsiveness, such as those with neutrophilic-dominant CRS, could be started earlier on alternative medical therapies following their endoscopic sinus surgery. Macrolide therapy has been shown to be much more effective in a neutrophilic-dominant CRS rather than an eosinophilic CRS. Their mechanism of action involves blocking proinflammatory cytokines, such as IL-8 and tumor necrosis factor-α, and inhibition of neutrophil migration and adhesion [42]. A randomized, double-blind, placebo-controlled study showed significantly better subjective and objective outcomes in CRS patients treated with 3 months of macrolide therapy compared to controls, particularly in those with low IgE levels [43].

P-glycoprotein is an efflux pump glycoprotein derived from the 'multi-drug resistance' gene that has been shown to be present in nasal mucosa, particularly in CRSwNP [44]. It is theorized that its overexpression may be responsible for the steroid resistance that some patients demonstrate. Verapamil is a calcium channel blocker that functions as a p-glycoprotein inhibitor, which has been shown to increase the intracellular accumulation of steroid in nasal polyps [45]. Verapamil is beginning to be used in CRSwNP patients who prove to be steroid resistant in an effort to downregulate the p-glycoprotein and allow the corticosteroids to be more effective in managing their condition. Research is ongoing in this area.

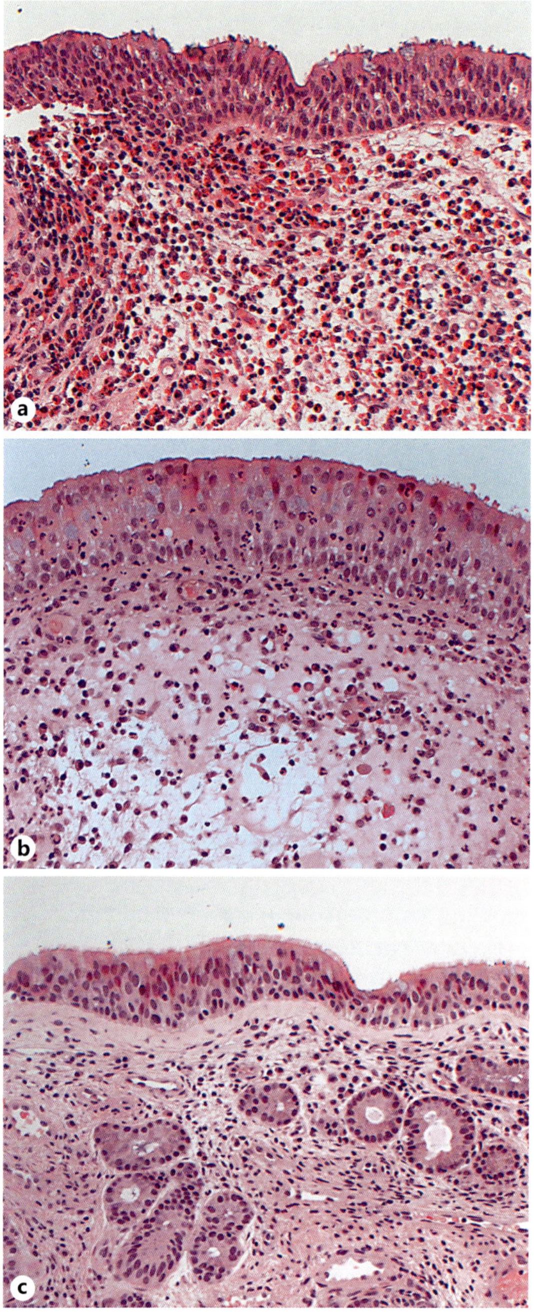

Fig. 5. Histologic appearance of tissue from patients with eosinophilic CRS with >10 eosinophils per HPF (**a**), patients with neutrophilic CRS (**b**) and a normal tissue sample with no CRS (**c**).

Conclusion

CRSwNP is a complicated and heterogeneous condition characterized by a predominantly Th2 and eosinophilia-mediated inflammatory process that can be difficult to treat. Although systemic corticosteroids have shown benefit in managing this condition, the need for regular use and associated adverse effects precludes their use beyond intermittent therapy for most patients. Topical corticosteroids, particularly when utilized after endoscopic sinus surgery and delivered in a high volume, high pressure manner, provide an effective anti-inflammatory regime with nearly negligible systemic effects. They are the cornerstone of the pharmacologic management of corticosteroid-sensitive eosinophilic CRSwNP. Non-eosinophilic endotypes and corticosteroid resistance are areas of unmet clinical need.

References

1 Chin D, Harvey RJ: Nasal polyposis: an inflammatory condition requiring effective anti-inflammatory treatment. Curr Opin Otolaryngol Head Neck Surg 2013; 21:23–30.

2 Leung RM, Kern RC, Conley DB, Tan BK, Chandra RK: Osteomeatal complex obstruction is not associated with adjacent sinus disease in chronic rhinosinusitis with polyps. Am J Rhinol Allergy 2011;25:401–403.

3 Snidvongs K, Chin D, Sacks R, Earls P, Harvey RJ: Eosinophilic rhinosinusitis is not a disease of ostiomeatal occlusion. Laryngoscope 2013;123:1070–1074.

4 Boumpas DT, Chrousos GP, Wilder RL, Cupps TR, Balow JE: Glucocorticoid therapy for immune-mediated diseases: basic and clinical correlates. Ann Intern Med 1993;119:1198–1208.

5 Mullol J, Obando A, Pujols L, Alobid I: Corticosteroid treatment in chronic rhinosinusitis: the possibilities and the limits. Immunol Allergy Clin North Am 2009;29:657–668.

6 Snidvongs K, Kalish L, Sacks R, Sivasubramaniam R, Cope D, Harvey RJ: Sinus surgery and delivery method influence the effectiveness of topical corticosteroids for chronic rhinosinusitis: systematic review and meta-analysis. Am J Rhinol Allergy 2013;27:221–233.

7 Kalish L, Snidvongs K, Sivasubramaniam R, Cope D, Harvey RJ: Topical steroids for nasal polyps. Cochrane Database Syst Rev 2012;12:CD006549.

8 Fandino M, Macdonald KI, Lee J, Witterick IJ: The use of postoperative topical corticosteroids in chronic rhinosinusitis with nasal polyps: a systematic review and meta-analysis. Am J Rhinol Allergy 2013;27:e146–e157.

9 Joe SA, Thambi R, Huang J: A systematic review of the use of intranasal steroids in the treatment of chronic rhinosinusitis. Otolaryngol Head Neck Surg 2008;139:340–347.

10 Thomas WW 3rd, Harvey RJ, Rudmik L, Hwang PH, Schlosser RJ: Distribution of topical agents to the paranasal sinuses: an evidence-based review with recommendations. Int Forum Allergy Rhinol 2013;3:691–703.

11 Snidvongs K, Pratt E, Chin D, Sacks R, Earls P, Harvey RJ: Corticosteroid nasal irrigations after endoscopic sinus surgery in the management of chronic rhinosinusitis. Int Forum Allergy Rhinol 2012;2:415–421.

12 Rudmik L, Hoy M, Schlosser RJ, et al: Topical therapies in the management of chronic rhinosinusitis: an evidence-based review with recommendations. Int Forum Allergy Rhinol 2013;3:281–298.

13 Rudmik L, Soler ZM, Orlandi RR, et al: Early postoperative care following endoscopic sinus surgery: an evidence-based review with recommendations. Int Forum Allergy Rhinol 2011;1:417–430.

14 Harvey RJ, Goddard JC, Wise SK, Schlosser RJ: Effects of endoscopic sinus surgery and delivery device on cadaver sinus irrigation. Otolaryngol Head Neck Surg 2008;139:137–142.

15 Bassiouni A, Naidoo Y, Wormald PJ: When FESS fails: the inflammatory load hypothesis in refractory chronic rhinosinusitis. Laryngoscope 2012;122:460–466.

16 Poetker DM, Jakubowski LA, Lal D, Hwang PH, Wright ED, Smith TL: Oral corticosteroids in the management of adult chronic rhinosinusitis with and without nasal polyps: an evidence-based review with recommendations. Int Forum Allergy Rhinol 2013;3:104–120.

17 Poetker DM, Smith TL: What rhinologists and allergists should know about the medico-legal implications of corticosteroid use: a review of the literature. Int Forum Allergy Rhinol 2012;2:95–103.

18 Bonfils P, Halimi P, Malinvaud D: Adrenal suppression and osteoporosis after treatment of nasal polyposis. Acta Otolaryngol 2006;126:1195–1200.

19 Harvey RJ, Debnath N, Srubiski A, Bleier B, Schlosser RJ: Fluid residuals and drug exposure in nasal irrigation. Otolaryngol Head Neck Surg 2009;141:757–761.

20 Man LX, Farhood Z, Luong A, et al: The effect of intranasal fluticasone propionate irrigations on salivary cortisol, intraocular pressure, and posterior subcapsular cataracts in postsurgical chronic rhinosinusitis patients. Int Forum Allergy Rhinol 2013;3:953–957.

21 Welch KC, Thaler ER, Doghramji LL, Palmer JN, Chiu AG: The effects of serum and urinary cortisol levels of topical intranasal irrigations with budesonide added to saline in patients with recurrent polyposis after endoscopic sinus surgery. Am J Rhinol Allergy 2010;24: 26–28.

22 Sastre J, Mosges R: Local and systemic safety of intranasal corticosteroids. J Investig Allergol Clin Immunol 2012;22: 1–12.

23 Skoner DP, Rachelefsky GS, Meltzer EO, et al: Detection of growth suppression in children during treatment with intranasal beclomethasone dipropionate. Pediatrics 2000;105:E23.

24 Allen DB: Systemic effects of intranasal steroids: an endocrinologist's perspective. J Allergy Clin Immunol 2000;106(4 suppl):S179–S190.

25 Murphy K, Uryniak T, Simpson B, O'Dowd L: Growth velocity in children with perennial allergic rhinitis treated with budesonide aqueous nasal spray. Ann Allergy Asthma Immunol 2006;96: 723–730.

26 Schenkel EJ, Skoner DP, Bronsky EA, et al: Absence of growth retardation in children with perennial allergic rhinitis after one year of treatment with mometasone furoate aqueous nasal spray. Pediatrics 2000;105:E22.

27 Skoner DP, Gentile D, Angelini B, Kane R, Birdsall D, Banerji D: The effects of intranasal triamcinolone acetonide and intranasal fluticasone propionate on short-term bone growth and HPA axis in children with allergic rhinitis. Ann Allergy Asthma Immunol 2003;90:56–62.

28 Skoner DP, Maspero J, Banerji D; Ciclesonide Pediatric Growth Study Group: Assessment of the long-term safety of inhaled ciclesonide on growth in children with asthma. Pediatrics 2008; 121:e1–e14.

29 Ahmadi N, Snidvongs K, Kalish L, et al: Intranasal corticosteroids do not affect intraocular pressure or lens opacity: a systematic review of controlled trials. Rhinology 2015;53:290–302.

30 Verkerk MM, Bhatia D, Rimmer J, Earls P, Sacks R, Harvey RJ: Intranasal steroids and the myth of mucosal atrophy: a systematic review of original histological assessments. Am J Rhinol Allergy 2015;29:3–18.
31 Dijkstra MD, Ebbens FA, Poublon RM, Fokkens WJ: Fluticasone propionate aqueous nasal spray does not influence the recurrence rate of chronic rhinosinusitis and nasal polyps 1 year after functional endoscopic sinus surgery. Clin Exp Allergy 2004;34:1395–1400.
32 Small CB, Hernandez J, Reyes A, et al: Efficacy and safety of mometasone furoate nasal spray in nasal polyposis. J Allergy Clin Immunol 2005;116:1275–1281.
33 Stjärne P, Blomgren K, Cayé-Thomasen P, Salo S, Søderstrøm T: The efficacy and safety of once-daily mometasone furoate nasal spray in nasal polyposis: a randomized, double-blind, placebo-controlled study. Acta Otolaryngol 2006; 126:606–612.
34 Stjärne P, Olsson P, Alenius M: Use of mometasone furoate to prevent polyp relapse after endoscopic sinus surgery. Arch Otolaryngol Head Neck Surg 2009; 135:296–302.
35 Vlckova I, Navrátil P, Kana R, Pavlicek P, Chrbolka P, Djupesland PG: Effective treatment of mild-to-moderate nasal polyposis with fluticasone delivered by a novel device. Rhinology 2009;47:419–426.
36 Fokkens WJ, Lund VJ, Mullol J, et al: EPOS 2012: European position paper on rhinosinusitis and nasal polyps 2012. A summary for otorhinolaryngologists. Rhinology 2012;50:1–12.
37 Lipworth BJ, Jackson CM: Safety of inhaled and intranasal corticosteroids: lessons for the new millennium. Drug Saf 2000;23:11–33.
38 Schafer T, Schnoor M, Wagenmann M, Klimek L, Bachert C: Therapeutic Index (TIX) for intranasal corticosteroids in the treatment of allergic rhinitis. Rhinology 2011;49:272–280.
39 Zhang N, Van Zele T, Perez-Novo C, et al: Different types of T-effector cells orchestrate mucosal inflammation in chronic sinus disease. J Allergy Clin Immunol 2008;122:961–968.
40 Jiang XD, Li GY, Li L, Dong Z, Zhu DD: The characterization of IL-17A expression in patients with chronic rhinosinusitis with nasal polyps. Am J Rhinol Allergy 2011;25:e171–e175.
41 Wen W, Liu W, Zhang L, et al: Increased neutrophilia in nasal polyps reduces the response to oral corticosteroid therapy. J Allergy Clin Immunol 2012;129:1522–1528.e5.
42 Harvey RJ, Wallwork BD, Lund VJ: Anti-inflammatory effects of macrolides: applications in chronic rhinosinusitis. Immunol Allergy Clin North Am 2009; 29:689–703.
43 Wallwork B, Coman W, Mackay-Sim A, Greiff L, Cervin A: A double-blind, randomized, placebo-controlled trial of macrolide in the treatment of chronic rhinosinusitis. Laryngoscope 2006;116: 189–193.
44 Bleier BS: Regional expression of epithelial MDR1/P-glycoprotein in chronic rhinosinusitis with and without nasal polyposis. Int Forum Allergy Rhinol 2012;2:122–125.
45 Kocharyan A, Feldman R, Singleton A, Han X, Bleier BS: P-glycoprotein inhibition promotes prednisone retention in human sinonasal polyp explants. Int Forum Allergy Rhinol 2014;4:734–738.
46 McKenzie AW: Percutaneous absorption of steroids. Arch Dematol 1962;86: 611–614.
47 Valotis A, Högger P: Human receptor kinetics and lung tissue retention of the enhanced-affinity glucocorticoid fluticasone furoate. Respir Res 2007;8:54.
48 Derendorf H, Meltzer EO: Molecular and clinical pharmacology of intranasal corticosteroids: clinical and therapeutic implications. Allergy 2008;63:1292–1300.

Gretchen M. Oakley, MD
Ground Floor, 67 Burton Street
Darlinghurst NSW 2010 (Australia)
E-Mail gmoakley@gmail.com

Advances in Medical and Surgical Therapy

Woodworth BA, Poetker DM, Reh DD (eds): Rhinosinusitis with Nasal Polyposis.
Adv Otorhinolaryngol. Basel, Karger, 2016, vol 79, pp 131–137 (DOI: 10.1159/000445179)

Implantable Devices/Drugs in the Management of Nasal Polyps

Griffin D. Santarelli · Joseph K. Han

Division of Rhinology and Endoscopic Sinus and Skull Base Surgery, Department of Otolaryngology, Head and Neck Surgery, Eastern Virginia Medical School, Norfolk, Va., USA

Abstract

The use of biomaterials, which include nasal packing and sinus stents, has an evolving role in the postoperative management of patients with chronic rhinosinusitis with polyps. Some of these biomaterials include drug-eluting properties. The usage of biomaterials postoperatively is both surgeon and patient specific. The published literature supports the use of these products and demonstrates the ability to limit swelling, lateralization and reduce polyp regrowth postoperatively. However, there are heterogeneity in both available materials and results that the otolaryngologist must factor in to the decision-making algorithm.

Introduction

Chronic rhinosinusitis (CRS) is a prevalent disease process affecting 32 million Americans, representing 16.3% of the population [1]. CRS is a complex disease process with multiple phenotypes and endotypes. The presence of CRS with nasal polyps (CRScNP) or polypoid mucosa has a higher burden of symptoms, revision sinus surgery, higher CT scan scores and greater use of medications [2]. The presence of polyps negatively affects the ability of the otolaryngologist to treat patients and they are characterized by frequent relapses [3]. Key to the high rate of symptom recurrence are the polyps recurring and causing a physical obstruction of the paranasal sinus ostia as well as negative histopathologic changes that include epithelial damage, thickened basement membranes and fibrotic stromal tissue [5].

Currently endoscopic sinus surgery (ESS) is an integral intervention for the patient population that fails maximal medical therapy. The goal of surgery is to optimize sinus ventilation, polyp clearance and patency. However, nasal polyps have a strong tendency to recur after surgery even when aeration is improved [4]. Therefore, current advances have been tailored to improving postoperative aeration and minimizing sinonasal inflammation in hopes of decreasing polypoid regrowth.

This chapter will focus on the most recent advances in implantable drugs and devices used in CRS with and without nasal polyposis.

Biomaterials

Biomaterials are synthetic materials engineered to have an in vivo therapeutic or diagnostic role through interactions with a patient's tissue. Advances in technology have lead to the development of new materials that span a wide spectrum of uses including gene therapy, immunotherapy, implantable devices and surgical materials. The essential requirements of biomaterials are that they are both biofunctional and biocompatible. The spectrum of use dictates the nature and regulations of the materials specifically if they are meant for indefinite implantation versus temporary usage, such as postoperative nasal packing.

Otolaryngology is a field that has embraced technological advances, specifically as it pertains to biomaterials. Uses in Otolaryngology have included cochlear implants, laryngeal stents, microplates for facial trauma and drug-eluting materials after sinus surgery. The use of biomaterials is becoming increasingly prevalent and has led to the American Academy of Otolaryngology-Head and Neck Surgery Society releasing a position statement on the use of biomaterials in September of 2015.

The American Academy of Otolaryngology-Head and Neck Surgery has determined that the use of FDA-approved biomaterials can be utilized in sinonasal procedures to improve patient outcomes and reduce complications. These items, such as implants, stents and packing materials, have functions including, but not limited to, local drug delivery, stenting and hemostasis. FDA-approved biomaterials for rhinologic application are not investigational, and the final decision regarding use of these biomaterials should be determined by the treating physician, factoring in best available scientific evidence, surgeon experience and the clinical situation and individual patient preference.

Nonabsorbale versus Absorbable Spacers

In the CRS patient population, ESS can not only provide symptomatic relief and improve quality of life [6] but can also be associated with poor long-term results in 25% of patients [7]. Poor outcomes are suspected to be secondary to postoperative adhesions, synechiae, polyp recurrence or lateralization of the middle turbinate. In an effort to minimize postoperative complications, middle meatal spacers have been employed following ESS in order to reduce adhesions. Middle meatal spacers can be either absorbable (AS) or nonabsorbable (NAS) and span a wide spectrum of materials, including steroid eluting materials.

Lee and Grewal [9] in a meta-analysis of 8 randomized controlled trials showed that while not statistically significant, a pooled analysis favored a trend toward middle meatal spacers versus no spacers in decreasing the formation of synechiae following ESS. Further subgroup analysis also suggested that nonabsorbable spacers are favored to absorbable spacers. However, in a follow-up systematic review, CRS patients undergoing ESS with placement of a spacer revealed a trend favoring AS compared to NAS in reducing adhesion formation [8].

The difficulty with comparing various spacers, however, is the heterogeneity of materials as well as their mechanism of action. A pooled analysis showed a nonsignificant trend favoring middle meatal spacers for reducing the formation of synechiae (relative risk [RR], 0.40; 95% CI, 0.14–1.12). Also, evaluated in 3 of the 8 studies was the role spacers played in decreasing postoperative sinus infections. There was no statistical significance identified (RR 0.89, 95% CI, 0.52–1.52).

In a meta-analysis by Zhao et al. [8], 6 RCTs revealed a nonsignificant trend favoring AS in reducing adhesion formation compared to NAS (RR, 0.40; 95% CI, 0.15–1.03) but that trend was not apparent if the NAS are left in place for greater than 48 h. Therefore, there's likely a role for longer acting spacers in preventing lateralization and scar formation.

Below is a review of some of the specific materials included in the analysis.

Materials

Merocel/Merogel. Merocel is a nonabsorbable packing made from an open cell foam polymer of hydroxylated polyvinyl acetal. Merocel is a product of Medtronic and created by a chemical reaction resulting in cross-linked polyvinyl alcohol (PVA) with a completely open cell structure. The final PVA sponge material has micropores to limit adhesion and trapping of microparticles/bacteria [10]. It is a biodegradable material that can stent open the ostiomeatal complex and provide hemostatic control by tamponade effect via light pressure.

Merogel, a second Medtronic product, is an absorbable hyaluronic acid nasal dressing. It is a biodegradable woven fleece that may be used 'dry' or 'wet' after ESS. The hyaluronic acid provides a scaffold for healing in the sinonasal cavities through its 'woven fleece' pattern. In a mouse animal model, hyaluronic acid has been shown to promote the deposition of a more dermal-like connective tissue matrix in wound beds, leading to the reduction of scarring complications [11], and also has a bacteriostatic effect and decreases the local inflammatory response [12]. When used in its 'dry' state, Merogel has an absorptive role. In its 'wet' state, the biopolymer gradually transforms into a mucoadhesive gel in approximately 24–48 h [10] and separates mucosal surfaces, slowly dissolving after approximately 2 weeks.

In a study by Franklin and Wright [13], 35 patients with CRScNP undergoing ESS were enrolled to receive either absorbable dressing (Merogel) or nonabsorbable sinus packs (Telfa) in their ethmoid cavities. The absorbable packs were removed 48–72 h and the Merogel was applied in a single sheet endoscopically via the middle meatus. Each patient's ethmoid cavities were randomized to receive either absorbable dressing or the standard nonabsorbable sinus packs, allowing each patient to serve as their own control. Endoscopic evaluation at 2 weeks showed a trend toward improved appearance in the Merogel group. At 1-, 3- and 6-month intervals, there was also a trend toward improved endoscopic appearance with the absorbable packing. Patient symptom scores were included and there was a strong preference in 60% of the patients for the absorbable.

Merogel Packing. Merocel packing was then compared directly to Merogel nasal dressing in a blinded, randomized, controlled trial study at the University of Cincinnati [14]. Thirty-seven patients requiring bilateral FESS for chronic sinusitis were randomized to placement of Merogel within the right or left middle meatus and Merocel on the contralateral side. Patients were evaluated at 2, 4, 6 and 8 weeks postoperatively. A blinded endoscopic follow-up revealed no statistical difference between hyaluronic acid absorbable dressing versus nonabsorbable merogel packing in the prevention of synechiae formation. Secondary analysis also did not show a statistically significant difference in postoperative edema or postoperative infection rates between the 2 groups.

In a follow-up study by Berlucchi et al. [15], Merogel was once again compared to nonabsorbable nasal dressings, including Merocel in a series of 66 patients, with a total of 88 nasal cavity interventions. Follow-up endoscopic evaluation at 2-, 4- and 12-week intervals revealed a lower proportion of nasal adhesions in the MeroGel® group at both 4 ($p = 0.041$) and 12 weeks ($p < 0.001$). Secondary analysis also showed an improved blinded endoscopic appearance in re-epithelialization, presence of granulation tissue and appearance of nasal mucosa of nasal cavities post ESS.

Carboxymethyl Cellulose

Carboxymethyl cellulose (CMC) foam is a biodegradable vegetable-based polysaccharide that actively promotes platelet aggregation upon contact with blood. Sinufoam, as marketed by Smith and Nephew, is a dissolvable CMC viscous fiber. The gel typically dissolves in 1 week and is thought to limit postoperative edema, bleeding and provide a physical barrier, limiting synechiae formation. Similar to hyaluronic acid, CMC has been shown in animal models to promote wound healing through a microfiber cellulose scaffold that promotes dermal fibroblasts propagating and re-epithelialization [16].

Sixty patients were included in a study by Szczygielski et al. [17], with half of the patient population randomized to CMC foam dressing post ESS versus a nonabsorbable packing that was removed in 1 week. Patients were evaluated for middle meatal synechiae formation at 1-, 2-, 4- and 8-week intervals as well as evaluating CMC foam's hemostatic role and patient subjective pain measures. The formation of synechiae, as well as hemostatic control, between the 2 groups was not statistically significant with 4 CMCF patients (6.7%) and 10 in the nonabsorbable packing patients developing synechiae (35.7%; $p = 0.092$). However, subjective pain scores did show a difference favoring the CMC foam packed patient population ($p < 0.0001$). CMC foam therefore can be considered a postoperative adjunct; however, further studies need to be performed to elucidate its true effect on synechiae formation.

Drug-Eluting Sinus Stents

In addition to traditional nasal packing, a subset of biomaterial products with drug-eluting properties have been produced and used more frequently for deployment within the postoperative paranasal sinuses. While the sinus implant prevents synechiae formation by preventing lateralization of the middle turbinate through mechanically medializing the middle turbinate, they also promote local anti-inflammatory treatment by slow release of a corticosteroid that coats the polymer implant. Currently, there is only one FDA-approved drug-eluting implant, the Intersect ENT Propel Stent, but variations of steroid suspensions and coating of traditional packing materials have also been studied in the postoperative setting. The benefit of steroid-eluting biomaterials is 2 fold; it both separates the raw mucosal edges to reduce synechiae and the slow release of corticosteroids decreases mucosal edema and enhances healing while not exposing the patient to the mal-effects of systemic steroid usage [19]. Currently, mometasone furoate is the only topical nasal steroid approved by the FDA for the treatment of nasal polyposis [23].

MicroFlow Spacer

One of the products developed for the slow release of medication is the MicroFlow Spacer by Acclarent Inc. It is an implantable sinus implant designed for release of medication in the ethmoid sinuses as a targeted treatment for sinusitis. Even though this device was FDA approved for saline, it has been used with steroids for an of off-label use. It allows for a delayed release of steroids through the micropores along the catheter sheath.

The device is FDA approved to be implanted for 14 days and is removed in the office. Twenty-three patients, with a total of 40 ethmoid cavities, in a study by Catalano et al. [22] were implanted with triamcinolone acetonide 40 mg/ml infused stents and followed over a period of 6 months. Pre-operative SNOT 20 scores were 2.18 versus a post-operative score of 1.02 ($p < 0.001$) and side-specific Lund–MacKay scores also had a statistically significant improvement from 5.75 to 2.80 ($p < 0.001$). The results of the MicroFlow spacer were promising, but were an off-label use of the patented technology and eventually resulted in legal troubles, limiting the availability of the product [28].

Nasopore

Nasopore is a bioresorbable packing marketed by Stryker to serve as a temporary wound dressing in the sinonasal cavity. Nasopore is a synthetically based polymer that fragments and dissolves in several days with a predictable degradation pattern and prevents synechiae formation and limits epistaxis. Coté and Wright [30] infused nasopore with 2 ml of a 40 mg/ml triamcinolone in an off-label use in a controlled study of patients with CRScNP after ESS. Nineteen patients randomized to the steroid-infused Nasopore packing had statistically significant differences at day 7 and 14 in both the Lund–Kennedy ($p = 0.04$ and $p = 0.03$, respectively) and POSE scores ($p = 0.03$ and $p = 0.001$, respectively) relative to the contralateral nasal cavity packed with nasopore, without steroid impregnation. The positive results on healing were also noted at 3- and 6-month observations (Lund–Kennedy, $p = 0.007$ and $p = 0.02$, respectively; POSE, $p = 0.049$ and $p = 0.01$, respectively).

Propel

Propel is the first and only FDA-approved drug-eluting mometasone furoate sinus implant [21] on the market. In a meta-analysis manuscript, data from 2 prospective, multicenter, randomized, double-blind, controlled clinical trials incorporated to include 143 patients undergoing ESS for CRS and who were treated with 370 μg of the mometasone fuorate embedded sinus implants [25, 26]. Both studies included intra-patient controls and included endoscopic end points graded by clinical investigators and a panel of independent sinus surgeons. The final analysis by the panel supported that the drug-releasing implants reduced postoperative interventions by 35% ($p = 0.0008$), lysis of adhesions by 51%, ($p = 0.0016$) and oral steroid need by 40% ($p = 0.0023$), compared to controls, with a reduction in frank polyposis of 46% ($p < 0.0001$).

Resolve Study Sinus Implant

Recently another study involving a different type of steroid-eluting sinus implant was published, the Resolve Study. In this study, a spring-like implant that conforms to the ethmoid sinuses was implanted after ESS and slowly released steroids over a 3-month period. The Resolve study was a randomized, controlled, blinded study using bioabsorbable steroid-eluting sinus implants for recurrent sinonasal polyposis. This study established that the Resolve implant (1,350 μg of mometasone furoate) has a clinically significant reduction of polyp grade and sinus obstruction [24]. Fifty-three treated patients, compared to 47 sham procedure patients, had a significant reduction in bilateral polyp grade ($p = 0.0269$) and ethmoid sinus obstruction ($p = 0.0001$) at 3 months. In addition, treated patients also experienced a 2-fold improvement in the mean nasal obstruction/congestion score (-1.33 ± 1.47 vs. -0.67 ± 1.45; $p = 0.1365$). There were no serious adverse events and patients were also less likely to be indicated for repeat ESS at the 3-month interval.

Other Studies

A systematic review in 2015 by Rizan and Elhassan [27], included 7 prospective studies where steroid-eluting bioabsorbable intranasal devices were implanted in CRScNP patients after ESS. Patients were followed from 2–6 months in the studies, and there was noted to be a statistically significant difference in adhesion formation, polyp formation, inflammation, Lund–Kennedy scores and perioperative sinus endoscopy scores in patients that underwent device implantation ($p < 0.05$). Three of the studies included the PROPEL spacer, 2 studies used nasopore-infused triamcinolone (80 mg) dressings and a gelfoam and SinuFoam (Dexamethasone 16 mg) infused spacer were included in the final 2 studies.

Complications

Nasal packing and stents are foreign materials and do have the potential to cause complications. The traditionally feared complication with nasal packing has always been toxic shock syndrome

(TSS). A 1986 report of TSS after nasal surgery with packing had an incidence as high as 16.5 per 100,000 and topical or systemic antibiotics did not have a demonstrable protective effect [31]. More recent studies have focused on packing for epistaxis where 149 patients prospectively were enrolled either to antibiotics versus no antibiotics after packing and neither group had any infective complication at follow-up [32]. The microbiome of the nasal cavity does not appear to be affected by packing or prophylactic antibiotics postoperatively. Therefore, while the risk for infectious complications with packing is low, the physician must factor the infectious risk of nasal biomaterials prior to placement and the need for postoperative antibiotics.

In addition to infectious complications, there are publications focusing on sinus biomaterial specific complications such as a retained drug-eluting biomaterial that resulted in recalcitrant CRS [33] and violation of the lamina papyracea of the orbit after placement of an ethmoid drug-eluting biomaterial [34]. There are also concerns that steroid-releasing sinus biomaterials have the potential to affect intraocular pressure or alter the hypothalamic-pituitary axis; however, multiple clinical trials have not resulted in clinically significant changes from baseline of the intraocular pressure or lens opacification and there has been no evidence of systemic steroid exposure or adrenal-pituitary axis suppression.

When packing or stenting material is employed, the onus is on the physician to follow the patient in regular intervals to ensure the packing migrates out, resorbs or is removed appropriately. Regular endoscopy on follow-up visits limits the potential for complications to occur and also allows the postsurgical nasal cavity to be monitored for appropriate healing.

Summary

Nasal packing and stents, including those with drug-eluting properties, have an evolving role in the postoperative management of patients with CRS with polyps. The usage of biomaterials postoperatively is both surgeon and patient specific. There is literature that supports the usage of products to limit swelling, lateralization and reduce polyp regrowth but there is heterogeneity in both available materials and results that the otolaryngologist must factor in to the decision-making algorithm.

References

1 Bachert C, Van Bruaene N, Toskala E, Zhang N, Olze H, Scadding G, et al: Important research questions in allergy and related diseases: 3-chronic rhinosinusitis and nasal polyposis – a GALEN study. Allergy 2009;64:520–533.

2 Banerji A, Piccirillo JF, Thawley SE, Levitt RG, Schechtman KB, Kramper MA, et al: Chronic rhinosinusitis patients with polyps or polypoid mucosa have a greater burden of illness. Am J Rhinol 2007;21:19–26.

3 Fokkens W, Lund V, Mullol J; European Position Paper on Rhinosinusitis and Nasal Polyps Group: European position paper on rhinosinusitis and nasal polyps 2007. Rhinol Suppl 2007;20:1–136.

4 Vento SI, Ertama LO, Hytönen ML, Wolff CH, Malmberg CH: Nasal polyposis: clinical course during 20 years. Ann Allergy Asthma Immunol 2000;85:209–214.

5 Kakoi H, Hiraide F: A histological study of formation and growth of nasal polyps. Acta Otolaryngol 1987;103:137–144.

6 Smith TL, Mendolia-Loffredo S, Loehrl TA, et al: Predictive factors and outcomes in endoscopic sinus surgery for chronic rhinosinusitis. Laryngoscope 2005;115:2199–2205.

7 Ramadan HH: Surgical causes of failure in endoscopic sinus surgery. Laryngoscope 1999;109:27–29.

8 Zhao X, Grewal A, Briel M, Lee JM: A systematic review of nonabsorbable, absorbable, and steroid-impregnated spacers following endoscopic sinus surgery. Int Forum Allergy Rhinol 2013;3:896–904.

9 Lee JM, Grewal A: Middle meatal spacers for the prevention of synechiae following endoscopic sinus surgery: a systematic review and meta-analysis of randomized controlled trials. Int Forum Allergy Rhinol 2012;2:477–486.

10 Merocel Medtronic Product. http://www.merocel.com/.

11 Iocono JA, Ehrlich HP, Keefer KA, Krummel TM: Hyaluronan induces scarless repair in mouse limb organ culture. J Pediatr Surg 1998;33:564–567.
12 Samuels P, Tan AK: Fetal scarless wound healing. J Otolaryngol 1999;28: 296–302.
13 Franklin JH, Wright ED: Randomized, controlled, study of absorbable nasal packing on outcomes of surgical treatment of rhinosinusitis with polyposis. Am J Rhinol 2007;21:214–217.
14 Miller RS, Steward DL, Tami TA, Sillars MJ, Seiden AM, Shete M, Paskowski C, Welge J: The clinical effects of hyaluronic acid ester nasal dressing (Merogel) on intranasal wound healing after functional endoscopic sinus surgery. Otolaryngol Head Neck Surg 2003;128:862–869.
15 Berlucchi M, Castelnuovo P, Vincenzi A, Morra B, Pasquini E: Endoscopic outcomes of resorbable nasal packing after functional endoscopic sinus surgery: a multicenter prospective randomized controlled study. Eur Arch Otorhinolaryngol 2009;266:839–845.
16 Ninan N, Muthiah M, Park I, Kalarikkal N, Elain A, Wong TW, Thomas S, Grohens Y: Wound healing analysis of pectin/carboxymethyl cellulose/microfibrillated cellulose based composite scaffolds. Mater Lett 2014;132:34–37.
17 Szczygielski K, Rapiejko P, Wojdas A, Jurkiewicz D: Use of CMC foam sinus dressing in FESS. Eur Arch Otorhinolaryngol 2010;267:537–540.
18 American Rhinologic Society Position Statement on Biomaterial. https://www.american-rhinologic.org/position_biomaterials (accessed January 24, 2014).
19 Bednarski KA, Kuhn FA: Stents and drug-eluting stents. Otolaryngol Clin North Am 2009;42:857–866.
20 Huang Z, Hwang P, Sun Y, Zhou B: Steroid-eluting sinus stents for improving symptoms in chronic rhinosinusitis patients undergoing functional endoscopic sinus surgery. Cochrane Database Syst Rev 2015;6:CD010436.
21 Propel Implant, Intersect ENT. http://propelopens.com/the-propel-advantage/how-it-works/.
22 Catalano PJ, Thong M, Weiss R, Rimash T: The microflow spacer: a drug-eluting stent for the ethmoid sinus. Indian J Otolaryngol Head Neck Surg 2011;63: 279–284.
23 Small CB, Hernandez J, Reyes A, et al: Efficacy and safety of mometasone furoate nasal spray in nasal polyposis. J Allergy Clin Immunol 2005;116:1275–1281.
24 Han JK, Forwith KD, Smith TL: RESOLVE: a randomized, controlled, blinded study of bioabsorbable steroid-eluting sinus implants for in-office treatment of recurrent sinonasal polyposis. Int Forum Allergy Rhinol 2014;4: 861–870.
25 Murr AH, Smith TL, Hwang PH, et al: Safety and efficacy of a novel bioabsorbable, steroid-eluting sinus stent. Int Forum Allergy Rhinol 2011;1:23–32.
26 Marple BF, Smith TL, Han JK, Gould AR, Jampel HD, Stambaugh JW, Mugglin AS: Advance II: a prospective, randomized study assessing safety and efficacy of bioabsorbable steroid-releasing sinus implants. Otolaryngol Head Neck Surg 2012;146:1004–1011.
27 Rizan C, Elhassan HA: Post-sinus surgery insertion of steroid-eluting bioabsorbable intranasal devices: a systematic review. Laryngoscope 2016;126:86–92.
28 Former Acclarent, Inc. Executives Charged with Securities Fraud and Crimes Related to Sale and Distribution of Medical Devices. https://www.fbi.gov/boston/press-releases/2015/former-acclarent-inc.-executives-charged-with-securities-fraud-and-crimes-related-to-sale-and-distribution-of-medical-devices. U.S. Attorney's Office, 2015.
29 Desrosiers M, Hussain A, Frenkiel S, et al: Intranasal corticosteroid use is associated with lower rates of bacterial recovery in chronic rhinosinusitis. Otolaryngol Head Neck Surg 2007;136: 605–609.
30 Côté DW, Wright ED: Triamcinolone-impregnated nasal dressing following endoscopic sinus surgery: a randomized, double-blind, placebo-controlled study. Laryngoscope 2010;120:1269–1273.
31 Jacobson JA, Kasworm EM: Toxic shock syndrome after nasal surgery. Case reports and analysis of risk factors. Arch Otolaryngol Head Neck Surg 1986;112: 329–332.
32 Pepper C, Lo S, Toma A: Prospective study of the risk of not using prophylactic antibiotics in nasal packing for epistaxis. J Laryngol Otol 2012;126:257–259.
33 Sjogren PP, Parker NP, Boyer HC: Retained drug-eluting stents and recalcitrant chronic rhinosinusitis: a case report. Allergy Rhinol (Providence) 2013; 4:e45–e48.
34 Villari CR, Wojno TJ, Delgaudio JM: Case report of orbital violation with placement of ethmoid drug-eluting stent. Int Forum Allergy Rhinol 2012;2: 89–92.

Joseph K. Han, MD
Division of Rhinology and Endoscopic Sinus and Skull Base Surgery
Department of Otolaryngology, Head and Neck Surgery, Eastern Virginia Medical School
River Pavilion Suite 1100, 600 Gresham Drive
Norfolk, VA 23507 (USA)
E-Mail hanjk@evms.edu

Advances in Medical and Surgical Therapy

Woodworth BA, Poetker DM, Reh DD (eds): Rhinosinusitis with Nasal Polyposis.
Adv Otorhinolaryngol. Basel, Karger, 2016, vol 79, pp 138–147 (DOI: 10.1159/000445151)

Oral Therapeutics for Rhinosinusitis with Nasal Polyposis

Andrew J. Thomas · Jeremiah A. Alt

Division of Head and Neck Surgery, Rhinology-Sinus and Skull Base Surgery Program, Department of Surgery, University of Utah, Salt Lake City, Utah, USA

Abstract

Oral therapeutics for chronic rhinosinusitis with nasal polyps (CRSwNP) include oral corticosteroids (OCS), antibiotics, antifungals and anti-leukotrienes. Of these treatments, the strongest evidence exists to support the use of a short course of OCS for treatment of CRSwNP, and OCS are the most consistently recommended oral therapy in practice guidelines. Antibiotics have demonstrated some utility, which appears more likely related to an anti-inflammatory rather than antimicrobial effect. The non-macrolide antibiotics lack sufficient evidence to support their use, though among this class doxycycline has some limited evidence of benefit in CRSwNP. Greater evidence exists for the use of macrolide antibiotics which have shown reduction of subjective and objective measures of CRSwNP severity. A short course of a macrolide should be considered as an option. Oral antifungals are not recommended in the treatment of CRSwNP given disappointing results and known potential adverse effects, except in allergic fungal rhinosinusitis where they may play a role. Leukotriene antagonists have demonstrated some promise in the treatment of CRSwNP, though studies are limited, but should be considered a potentially useful oral therapeutic. The current level of evidence for these oral therapeutic options for CRSwNP is reviewed in this chapter.

Introduction

Chronic rhinosinusitis (CRS) is a condition of inflammation of the nose and paranasal sinuses with signs and symptoms lasting greater than 12 weeks [1]. When CRS is associated with mucosal polyps, it is specifically classified as CRS with nasal polyps (CRSwNP) [2]. Nasal polyps are hyperplastic growths of the nasal mucosa, which contain primarily type 2 T-helper cell (Th2) inflammatory cells and mediators such as eosinophils and immunoglobulin E (IgE) [3, 4]. Based on this inflammatory profile of polyps, it has historically been suggested that CRSwNP may represent a form of atopic disease. However, no clear link has been established between the presence of nasal polyps and atopic disease; the prevalence of CRSwNP has been shown to be similar between both atopic and non-atopic patients [5], and only 0.5% of atopic patients are reported to have nasal polyps [6]. Though many theories exist, the pathophysiology of CRSwNP remains unclear and likely multifactorial [7, 8].

Treatment guidelines for CRSwNP from the American Academy of Otolaryngology, Head and Neck Surgery (AAO-HNS) recommend topical nasal steroid sprays for long-term treatment of polyps in CRS, with a short course of oral corticosteroids (OCS) if there is no response in 3 months [1]. These guidelines also recommend against chronic antibiotics for CRSwNP but suggest that oral antibiotics of the macrolide class may be useful, particularly because of their anti-inflammatory effects. The European position paper on rhinosinusitis and nasal polyps 2012 (EPOS 2012) similarly supports the use of a short course of OCS, suggests potential utility of short duration macrolide therapy and is unable to conclude about long-term treatment with antibiotics in CRSwNP due to limited data [9]. A 2011 Cochrane review on the use of oral steroids also supports their use for patients with nasal polyposis [10]. This chapter focuses on the current level of evidence for oral therapeutics for the treatment of CRSwNP.

Oral Corticosteroids

Studies evaluating a short course of OCS for CRSwNP have generally demonstrated improvements in both subjective and objective measures of disease severity, and their use is supported by major practice guidelines and systematic reviews [1, 9–11]. OCSs are the only medical therapy that has demonstrated significant improvement in both subjective and objective olfaction scores [12]. Here, we will primarily focus our discussion on the 5 randomized controlled trials (RCTs) evaluating different regimens of OCS for CRSwNP, that have been performed within the last 10 years and provide level 1b evidence to support their use [13–18].

Kroflic et al. [15] performed a RCT of 40 patients with nasal polyposis in 2006, comparing the efficacy of topical furosemide and oral methylprednisolone therapy. Either nebulized furosemide (6.6 mmol/l solution) or oral methylprednisolone (1 mg/kg/day) was given for 7 days prior to sinus surgery, and both groups demonstrated significant improvement in subjective nasal obstruction, olfaction and nasal secretions, as well as polyposis severity by nasal endoscopy. In a double-blind, randomized, placebo-controlled trial (DBRCT) by Hissaria et al. [13], 41 patients with CRSwNP randomized to either oral prednisolone (50 mg/day) or placebo for 14 days. Symptoms reported on the 31-item Rhinosinusitis Outcome Measure as well as objective improvement in polyposis severity (nasal endoscopy and MRI) improved significantly more in the prednisolone group. Overall, this steroid regimen was well tolerated with no serious adverse reactions. Longer term outcomes after 2 weeks were not evaluated.

In a prospective case–control study by Alobid et al. [19], patients with CRSwNP were assigned to a short course of oral prednisone (n = 60) or no treatment (n = 18). After evaluation at 2 weeks, the prednisone group then received long-term intranasal budesonide and was re-evaluated at 12, 24 and 48 weeks. All patients demonstrated reduced quality of life (QOL) scores on the Medical Outcome Study Short Form-36 (SF-36) at initial evaluation. At 2 weeks, the prednisone group demonstrated significant improvement in QOL, scores of nasal symptoms (obstruction and sense of smell) and polyp size score (endoscopy), which was maintained at the 48-week evaluation. This study suggests that long-term treatment with intranasal steroids may maintain the benefits of a short course of oral steroids.

A DBRCT by Kirtsreesakul et al. [14] randomized patients with CRSwNP (n = 109) 3:2 to prednisolone (50 mg) or placebo daily for 14 days. The prednisolone group demonstrated a significantly greater peak expiratory flow index, reduction in nasal polyp size (endoscopy) and improvement in nasal symptoms. However, more severe disease was associated with significantly less improvement in both subjective and objective measures. In another 2011 DBRCT, Van Zele et al. [17] compared the efficacy of oral methylprednisolone to doxycycline in the treatment of CRSwNP. A total of 47 patients were randomized to 20 days of either methylprednisolone taper or doxycycline or placebo. Methylprednisolone resulted in a significant reduction in symptoms of nasal congestion, post-nasal drip (PND) and loss of smell. The OCS group demonstrated significant objective reduction in polyp size (endoscopy) and improved peak nasal inspiratory flow (PNIF), as well as decreased blood eosinophil count, IgE level, eosinophilic cationic protein (ECP; eosinophil degranulation marker) and soluble interleukin (IL)-5R. Despite initial benefit, both symptoms and polyp size returned rapidly after discontinuing OCS. Polyp size was no different from baseline or placebo treatment patients after 12 weeks.

Vaidyanathan et al. [16] further explored the role of combined oral and topical treatment in a 2011 RCT, which randomized 60 patients with CRSwNP to either oral prednisolone (25 mg) or placebo daily for 2 weeks. All patients then received long-term topical fluticasone. Similar to other studies [13], the 2-week course of OCS resulted in significantly reduced hyposmia, reduced nasal symptom score and improved scores on the mini Rhinoconjunctivitis Quality of Life Questionnaire. There was also significant reduction in polyp size (endoscopy), improved PNIF and reduction in serum markers of inflammation and eosinophil activation compared to placebo treatment. The reduction in polyp size and hyposmia after prednisolone treatment remained significant up to 10 weeks. Prednisolone caused transiently suppressed adrenal function and increased bone turnover at 2 weeks, but this returned to normal at 10 weeks. This study demonstrated an initial 2-week course of OCS followed by topical steroids is more effective than topical steroids alone, but the added effect is lost by 28 weeks.

Given the short-term efficacy and minimal adverse effects of a single course of oral steroids, appropriate frequency of repeated OCS courses is an important question to consider. Leung et al. [20] determined the threshold at which the risks of continued medical therapy exceed the risks of performing surgery, focusing on the economic impact. The simulated patient in this model was a CRSwNP patient who experiences the benefits of a short course of OCS without prior adverse events. The risk analysis was performed using direct costs (surgery, medical admissions and medications) and indirect costs (morbidity, mortality and decreased QOL). The threshold number of courses of OCS at which the risks exceeded those of endoscopic sinus surgery (ESS) was 0.21/year (once every 5 years). This threshold was lower for CRSwNP patients with asthma and Samter's triad, at 0.53/year (every 2 years) and 1.81/year (every 6 months), respectively. The society analysis, focusing on the most economical use of resources, demonstrated a higher threshold for surgery: once every 2 years (CRSwNP), 1 year (CRSwNP/asthma) or 5 months (Samter's). For simplicity, responsible resource utilization and bias against surgery, the authors recommend considering endoscopic sinus surgery (ESS) for patients requiring OCS more frequently than once every 2 years for CRSwNP patients, yearly for CRSwNP/asthma or twice per year for patients with Samter's triad.

The 2013 evidence-based review with recommendations (EBRR) on OCS in CRS by Poetker et al. [11] makes a strong recommendation for the use of OCS in the short-term management of CRSwNP. Similarly, the EPOS 2012 European recommendations for treatment of CRSwNP conclude that systemic corticosteroids offer clear though short-lived benefits in the treatment of CRSwNP [9]. The long-term efficacy of an oral steroid taper followed by maintenance with topical nasal steroids appears to be approximately 8–12 weeks [11]. Overall, there is good evidence for the use of oral steroids for short-term management of CRSwNP and the decision of when to progress to ESS after repeated OCS treatments should be individualized, considering patient factors such as presence of asthma and Samter's triad.

Antibiotics

Despite limited evidence, antibiotics are commonly prescribed for the treatment of CRSwNP. While CRSwNP has historically been considered a Th2-driven atopic disease process, more recent research has demonstrated that the distinction between the etiologies of these CRS entities is not clearly defined [21, 22]. Some studies have suggested a microbial role in the pathogenesis of CRSwNP and possible utility of antimicrobials as therapeutics. Theories include the superantigen hypothesis, in which colonizing Staphylococcus aureus secrete super-antigens that then lead to increased IgE and polypoid change [23]. Increased mucosal permeability has been demonstrated in CRS as well as a robust immune response in nasal polyps containing B lymphocytes and immunoglobulins [24, 25]. Bacteria may increase mucosal permeability and susceptibility to environmental triggers of inflammation or cause a greater local immune response due to an already compromised mucosal barrier. This could induce immunoglobulin class-switch and production, activation of eosinophils and formation of polyps [25]. However, there is no clear microbial etiology for CRSwNP and non-macrolide antibiotics have lacked utility.

Non-Macrolide Antibiotics

Van Zele et al. [17] randomized patients with CRSwNP to placebo (n = 19) or doxycycline (n = 14) (200 mg on day 1, then 100 mg daily) for 20 days. Doxycycline resulted in polyp size reduction that persisted up to 12 weeks after dosing, as well as a significant reduction in PND after 2 weeks. However, there was no significant improvement in PNIF or in symptom scores of nasal congestion, rhinorrhea or loss of smell. The mechanism for this benefit (antimicrobial versus anti-inflammatory) is unclear. Based on the results of this study, 3 other RCTs (level 1b evidence), and 2 observational cohort studies (level 4 evidence), the EBRR by Soler et al. [26] recommends considering short-term non-macrolide antibiotics as an option in the treatment of CRS, but with caution that the limited reported benefits may be outweighed by the typical side effects of antibiotics, cost and societal considerations such as the development of antibiotic resistance. For CRSwNP specifically, the evidence for use non-macrolide is even weaker (single level 1b study) and the risks and costs may outweigh any potential benefit. There is currently no evidence for treatment of CRSwNP using non-macrolide antibiotics ≥3 weeks.

Macrolide Antibiotics

Macrolides have anti-inflammatory properties and are effective in treating conditions associated with chronic airway inflammation, such as diffuse panbronchiolitis and cystic fibrosis [27, 28]. Clarithromycin has been shown to decrease the production of pro-inflammatory cytokines (IL-5 and IL-8) in nasal mucosa of patients with CRS [29], and to decrease nuclear factor-kappa B activity [30]. Erythromycin and roxithromycin have also been demonstrated to increase neutrophil apoptosis [28].

A DBRCT by Wallwork et al. [27] in 2006 investigated macrolides as treatment for CRS, but did not separate CRSwNP from CRSsNP. This study found significant improvements in SNOT-20 scores, nasal endoscopy, saccharine transit time, as well as reduced IL-8 levels in lavage fluid, suggesting the utility of this treatment (150 mg roxithromycin daily for 3 months). A DBRCT by Haxel et al. [31] randomized patients to 3 months of low-dose erythromycin treatment (250 mg daily; n = 29) or to placebo (n = 29) starting 2 weeks after ESS for CRS. All patients received topical nasal fluticasone daily. There was no significant difference in ECP in nasal secretions, subjective severity of nasal disease, olfaction, saccharin transit time or in SNOT-20 scores. Significant improvement in endoscopy scores at the end of the medication trial was seen for the erythromycin group, but this was nonsignificant at follow-up 12 weeks later.

A 2014 RCT by Varvyanskaya and Lopatin [32] randomized 66 patients with CRSwNP to no oral medication (controls) or to clarithromycin 250 mg daily for either 12 or 24 weeks. All patients also received topical mometasone furoate. SNOT-20 scores, nasal resistance and nasal endoscopy scores of polyposis were all significantly improved in the macrolide-treated groups compared to controls. Lund–Mackay scores of disease severity on CT improved from pre-op to post-op in all groups, but at 24 weeks there was a significantly greater improvement in the 24-week macrolide group compared to controls. Both macrolide treatment groups had significantly reduced ECP levels at 24 weeks after ESS, whereas levels of ECP in control patients increased up to approximately 3 times baseline at 24 weeks; macrolides may control eosinophilic inflammation and perhaps thereby decrease polyp recurrence.

The above RCTs focused on macrolide treatment following ESS, rather than as primary medical therapy, and only one study specifically focused on CRSwNP patients [32]. The efficacy of macrolide treatment has been demonstrated to be significantly less for patients with polyps, and is improved significantly after polypectomy for patients with multiple polyps [33]. Pre-operative macrolides may also delay polyp recurrence after surgery, as patients treated with clarithromycin 500 mg twice daily for 8 weeks prior to ESS demonstrate significantly less endoscopic evidence of disease recurrence 12 months post-operatively, compared to patients undergoing ESS with no pre-treatment [34]. In prospective cohort studies, patients with CRSwNP treated with clarithromycin for 8 weeks have demonstrated significantly decreased symptoms of nasal obstruction, smell dysfunction, PND and rhinorrhea, as well as reduced polyp size (CT and endoscopy) and decreased levels of IL-8 in nasal fluid [35, 36]. Cohort studies using roxithromycin and erythromycin have also demonstrated subjective and objective benefit, supporting the class effect of the macrolides [37, 38].

Based on the available evidence from a single RCT focused on macrolide treatment in patients with CRSwNP [32] and observational cohort studies, macrolides appear to significantly reduce symptoms as well as objective polyp disease. A majority of the evidence is specifically applicable to the post-ESS setting, rather than as primary medical management. Patients with low IgE levels may obtain more benefit from macrolide therapy than atopic patients [27], and patients with multiple polyps may experience more benefit after undergoing polypectomy [33]. Benefits must be weighed against potential harms. Though there were no significant adverse events reported in the studies evaluated here for CRSwNP, macrolides have been associated with potential risk of arrhythmia, liver function abnormalities, ototoxicity and the potential for development of antibiotic resistance [26, 39]. Particular caution is recommended in patients at risk of cardiac arrhythmia [39]. Adverse effects reported in studies of CRS patients were mild to moderate GI disturbance and rash [26, 40]. The more extensive pulmonary literature on the long-term use of macrolides has described increased risk of bacterial resistance and some increased risk of hearing impairment (RR 1.168; 95% CI 1.030–1.325) [41].

Antifungals

Past attempts to broadly define the underlying pathophysiology of CRS focused on the role of fungus. The 'fungal hypothesis' suggested that eosinophilic inflammation of the sinonasal mucosa resulting from environmental fungi, particularly Alternaria fungi, was responsible for the development of CRS [42–44]. Despite some early enthusiasm for the potential utility of antifungals for

CRS [44], subsequent studies have cast doubt on the utility of antifungal therapy [45, 46]. Fungi have been demonstrated not-only in mucosa of patients with CRS, but in nearly all healthy control patients as well, and treatment of CRS with antifungals has had disappointing results [46, 47].

The use of oral antifungals for CRS is discouraged consistently throughout recent systematic reviews and guidelines, including the most recent AAO-HNS clinical practice guidelines for adult sinusitis, a 2013 EBRR by Soler et al. [26], and the 2012 EPOS guidelines [1, 9]. Harm and cost appears to outweigh potential benefits. There has been some lower level evidence for benefit of oral antifungals (primarily itraconazole and ketoconazole) in the treatment of CRS (primarily AFRS) reported in mostly retrospective case series and using non-validated outcome measures [48]. Thanasumpun and Batra [48] performed a systematic review of 27 of these level 4 (n = 15) and 5 (n = 12) evidence studies, in addition to one single RCT by Kennedy et al. [49] (level 1 evidence), and found significant symptom improvement with oral antifungal therapy and some objective improvement in select studies, with elevated liver enzymes (17–20%) being the most common adverse event reported. Higher level evidence was specifically evaluated in a Cochrane review on the efficacy of oral and topical antifungal agents for the treatment of CRS performed by Sacks et al. [50] in 2011, which identified 6 randomized placebo-controlled trials addressing this question. This meta-analysis identified no significant benefit to antifungal therapy in CRS and a significantly increased incidence of adverse events in the antifungal groups. Only the DBRCT by Kennedy et al. [49] specifically investigated systemic oral antifungal treatment (not topical), and this trial did not distinguish CRSwNP from CRSsNP.

Oral antifungal treatments are discouraged for CRSwNP given the limited data available, negative results described in the meta-analysis and trials above, as well as known potential adverse effects [49–51]. There is, however, likely an exception in the case of allergic fungal sinusitis (AFS). Patients with AFS treated with a month of preoperative itraconazole prior to surgery have significantly improved symptoms (SNOT-20), objective disease severity (CT and endoscopy scores), and fungal load (cultures) compared to patients treated with surgery alone [52]. The potential harms of oral antifungal therapy should be considered carefully, particularly hepatic toxicity with elevated liver function tests reported in 4% of patients, unpleasant side effects including nausea and fatigue, as well as the potential for drug interactions with itraconazole [9]. These recommendations do not apply to invasive fungal sinusitis which is a distinct and dangerous disease process treated with surgical debridement and antifungal therapy.

Leukotriene Antagonists

Leukotrienes (LTs) are inflammatory mediators formed in the breakdown of arachidonic acid by 5-lipoxygenase (5-LO), and are synthesized in a number of inflammatory cell types including eosinophils and mast cells [53]. Leukotriene C4 synthase (LTC4S) activity is specifically required for the production of the cysteinyl leukotrienes (CysLTs) [9]. The CysLTs increase mucous production, cause mucosal edema, release of mast cell cytokines, and promote chemotaxis of neutrophils and eosinophils [54–56]. The CysLTs have been implicated in the pathogenesis of CRSwNP [9]. Increased arachidonic acid metabolism [57, 58] and levels of both CysLTs and CysLT receptors have been demonstrated in the nasal mucosa of patients with CRSwNP [55, 59–61]. Levels of 5-LO, LCT4S, and the CysLTs have been shown to be significantly increased in nasal tissue of patients with CRSwNP relative to CRSsNP and controls [62]. Inhibition of LT activity, either by antagonism of the LT receptor with montelukast, zafirlukast or pranlukast (competitive antagonists of the CysLT1 receptor; LTA), or inhibition of CysLT synthesis with zileuton (selective 5-LO enzyme inhibitor) has therefore been considered as a potential treatment for CRSwNP.

LT antagonists (LTAs) have been used as adjunctive treatments for CRSwNP [55], though their use is not supported by recent practice guidelines. There is no recommendation regarding LTAs in the 2015 AAO-HNS practice guidelines for CRSwNP, and the EPOS 2012 guidelines specifically recommend against the use of LTAs (Grade of recommendation A) [1, 9]. However, 2 recent literature reviews suggest a benefit of LTAs for both symptoms and objective measures of CRSwNP severity [55, 56]. Wentzel et al. [56] identified 2 placebo-controlled RCTs, 3 non-placebo controlled RCTs and 7 case series that evaluated LTA treatment either alone or as adjunct therapy for CRSwNP. Smith and Sautter [55] reviewed 4 of the same trials, as well as an in-vitro study which activated mast cells with CysLT then blocked this activation with a combination of montelukast (LTA) and zileuton (5-LO inhibitor) [56]. Overall, LTAs were found to significantly decrease symptom severity as well as polyposis and inflammatory mediators compared to placebo. Addition of an LTA to topical and oral steroid therapy also demonstrated significant improvement in individual symptoms compared to topical/oral steroid alone, but this benefit was lost soon after discontinuing the LTA [63].

The 2 placebo controlled trials were performed by Schäper et al. in 2011 and Pauli et al. in 2007. Schäper et al. treated CRSwNP patients (n = 24) with 10 mg montelukast daily for 6 weeks and evaluated the same patients with placebo in a crossover design, half randomized to placebo before treatment and half after. This study found a significant improvement with montelukast, from baseline and compared to placebo, for nasal symptoms, objective findings on rhinoscopy, nasal airway flow and olfaction. Montelukast was also associated with significant decreases in inflammatory mediators on nasal lavage and for both peripheral and nasal eosinophils. No adverse effects were noted during the trial [64]. Pauli et al. randomized CRSwNP patients to either 10 mg montelukast daily (n = 20) or placebo (n = 10) for 4 weeks and found a significant improvement in nasal symptoms, practical problems, headaches and non-nasal symptoms with montelukast compared to placebo, though no significant change in nasal ECP or polyp size were identified [65].

An RCT by Vuralkan et al. [66] in 2011 randomized 50 patients with nasal polyposis to post-FESS treatment with either 10 mg montelukast daily (n = 25) or 400 mcg mometasone furoate nasal spray twice daily (n = 25) for 6 months. Both treatment groups demonstrated significant postoperative improvement in SNOT-22 scores and the Lund–Mackay CT score at 6 months, but there was no significant difference between the groups. However, the incidence of polyp recurrence reported in the LTA treatment group (48%) was significantly greater compared to the nasal steroid group (20%). A similar study by Mostafa et al. [67] in 2005 did not identify any difference in recurrence rate between patients with nasal polyps treated post-ESS with either 10 mg montelukast daily (n = 25) or 400 mcg beclomethasone nasal spray daily (n = 20) at 1 year follow-up, though similar and significant improvement in symptom scores were seen throughout the study period in both groups.

Almost all studies have evaluated CysLT receptor antagonists, particularly montelukast, and there is limited data available on the utility of 5-LO inhibitors (zileuton). Two studies used zileuton or zafirlukast as treatment for CRSwNP and found improvements in symptoms and decrease in polyposis reported similar to studies using montelukast [68, 69]. A DBRCT crossover study by Dahlen et al. [70] in 1998 also demonstrated reduction of nasal symptoms such as olfactory dysfunction and rhinorrhea, and increase in PNIF, when zileuton was added to existing medical therapy of inhaled and/or oral steroid in treatment of patients with aspirin-intolerant asthma. The limited research using zileuton in CRSwNP precludes recommendations for its use at this time, though the theoretical utility is an interesting point raised by Smith and Sautter [55]. They suggest that given an observed increase in CysLT2 receptor in the nasal mucosa of patients with CRSwNP, but a lack of antagonist action of montelukast, pranlukast, and zafirlukast at this receptor (all act on CysLT1), inhibition of CysLT synthesis by 5-LO inhibition (zileuton) may be a better strategy. Cell culture experiments suggest the possibility for some combined benefit of CsyLTA and 5-LO inhibitors [55].

Though data on the use of LTAs for CRSwNP is limited, there is evidence from 2 RCTs that demonstrate a significant improvement with montelukast relative to placebo in subjective symptoms, objective findings of disease severity, as well as immunologic evidence of disease. Combination therapy with an LTA and oral or topical steroid demonstrates unclear benefit over single modality treatment. Though no major adverse effects were reported in the literature reviewed here, LTAs have been associated with skin rash, behavior change, tremor or potentially a paradoxical worsening of sinus symptoms and asthma [9, 65]. Specifically, montelukast has shown minimal adverse effects, while zileuton is associated with liver function test abnormalities and potential for hepatotoxicity and zafirlukast is known to decrease warfarin clearance [66, 67]. The benefit of LTA therapy appears to be lost soon after discontinuation [56], but long term treatment appears relatively safe. Overall, LTAs have demonstrated some utility in the treatment of CRSwNP, and additional research is indicated to further define the role of these drugs as well as 5-LO inhibitors as therapeutics for CRSwNP.

Conclusions

While the mainstay of treatment for CRSwNP remains topical nasal steroids, oral therapeutics can be considered as a useful adjunct for patients with an inadequate response to topical therapy. The strongest evidence from multiple RCTs supports the use of a short course of OCS for short-term improvement in both subjective and objective measures of disease severity. There is also evidence suggesting the utility of macrolide antibiotics, which have anti-inflammatory effects, for reducing symptoms and polyp burden. This is reflected in the major practice guidelines for the treatment of CRSwNP, which endorse the use of OCS and suggest potential utility of macrolide class antibiotics. Although the evidence is less robust, LTAs have also demonstrated promise and have a favorable safety profile (particularly montelukast) for potential longer term treatment. Non-macrolide antibiotics and oral antifungals lack evidence of benefit for treatment of CRSwNP. The exception being in AFS where oral antifungals likely have a positive effect by reducing fungal load and the resulting allergic response in the sinuses.

References

1 Rosenfeld RM, Piccirillo JF, Chandrasekhar SS, et al: Clinical practice guideline (update): adult sinusitis. Otolaryngol Head Neck Surg 2015; 152(2 suppl):S1–S39.

2 Lange B, Holst R, Thilsing T, Baelum J, Kjeldsen A: Quality of life and associated factors in persons with chronic rhinosinusitis in the general population: a prospective questionnaire and clinical cross-sectional study. Clin Otolaryngol 2013;38:474–480.

3 Larsen PL, Tos M: Origin of nasal polyps: an endoscopic autopsy study. Laryngoscope 2004;114:710–719.

4 Larsen PL, Tos M: Nasal polyps: epithelium and goblet cell density. Laryngoscope 1989;99:1274–1280.

5 Pearlman AN, Chandra RK, Chang D, et al: Relationships between severity of chronic rhinosinusitis and nasal polyposis, asthma, and atopy. Am J Rhinol Allergy 2009;23:145–148.
6 Caplin I, Haynes JT, Spahn J: Are nasal polyps an allergic phenomenon? Ann Allergy 1971;29:631–634.
7 Hsu J, Peters AT: Pathophysiology of chronic rhinosinusitis with nasal polyp. Am J Rhinol Allergy 2011;25:285–290.
8 Chin D, Harvey RJ: Nasal polyposis: an inflammatory condition requiring effective anti-inflammatory treatment. Curr Opin Otolaryngol Head Neck Surg 2013; 21:23–30.
9 Fokkens WJ, Lund VJ, Mullol J, et al: EPOS 2012: European position paper on rhinosinusitis and nasal polyps 2012. A summary for otorhinolaryngologists. Rhinology 2012;50:1–12.
10 Martinez-Devesa P, Patiar S: Oral steroids for nasal polyps. Cochrane Database Syst Rev 2011;7:CD005232.
11 Poetker DM, Jakubowski LA, Lal D, Hwang PH, Wright ED, Smith TL: Oral corticosteroids in the management of adult chronic rhinosinusitis with and without nasal polyps: an evidence-based review with recommendations. Int Forum Allergy Rhinol 2013;3:104–120.
12 Banglawala SM, Oyer SL, Lohia S, Psaltis AJ, Soler ZM, Schlosser RJ: Olfactory outcomes in chronic rhinosinusitis with nasal polyposis after medical treatments: a systematic review and meta-analysis. Int Forum Allergy Rhinol 2014; 4:986–994.
13 Hissaria P, Smith W, Wormald PJ, et al: Short course of systemic corticosteroids in sinonasal polyposis: a double-blind, randomized, placebo-controlled trial with evaluation of outcome measures. J Allergy Clin Immunol 2006;118:128–133.
14 Kirtsreesakul V, Wongsritrang K, Ruttanaphol S: Clinical efficacy of a short course of systemic steroids in nasal polyposis. Rhinology 2011;49:525–532.
15 Kroflic B, Coer A, Baudoin T, Kalogjera L: Topical furosemide versus oral steroid in preoperative management of nasal polyposis. Eur Arch Otorhinolaryngol 2006;263:767–771.
16 Vaidyanathan S, Barnes M, Williamson P, Hopkinson P, Donnan PT, Lipworth B: Treatment of chronic rhinosinusitis with nasal polyposis with oral steroids followed by topical steroids: a randomized trial. Ann Intern Med 2011;154: 293–302.
17 Van Zele T, Gevaert P, Holtappels G, et al: Oral steroids and doxycycline: two different approaches to treat nasal polyps. J Allergy Clin Immunol 2010;125: 1069–1076.e4.
18 Oxford Centre for Evidence-Based Medicine (CEBM) – Levels of Evidence (March 2009). 2009. http://www.cebm.net/oxford-centre-evidence-based-medicine-levels-evidence-march-2009/ (accessed December 10, 2015).
19 Alobid I, Benitez P, Pujols L, et al: Severe nasal polyposis and its impact on quality of life. The effect of a short course of oral steroids followed by long-term intranasal steroid treatment. Rhinology 2006;44:8–13.
20 Leung RM, Dinnie K, Smith TL: When do the risks of repeated courses of corticosteroids exceed the risks of surgery? Int Forum Allergy Rhinol 2014;4:871–876.
21 Kern RC, Conley DB, Walsh W, et al: Perspectives on the etiology of chronic rhinosinusitis: an immune barrier hypothesis. Am J Rhinol 2008;22:549–559.
22 Tan BK, Schleimer RP, Kern RC: Perspectives on the etiology of chronic rhinosinusitis. Curr Opin Otolaryngol Head Neck Surg 2010;18:21–26.
23 Bachert C, Gevaert P, Holtappels G, Johansson SG, van Cauwenberge P: Total and specific IgE in nasal polyps is related to local eosinophilic inflammation. J Allergy Clin Immunol 2001;107:607–614.
24 Tieu DD, Kern RC, Schleimer RP: Alterations in epithelial barrier function and host defense responses in chronic rhinosinusitis. J Allergy Clin Immunol 2009; 124:37–42.
25 Kato A, Peters A, Suh L, et al: Evidence of a role for B cell-activating factor of the TNF family in the pathogenesis of chronic rhinosinusitis with nasal polyps. J Allergy Clin Immunol 2008;121:1385–1392, 1392.e1–e2.
26 Soler ZM, Oyer SL, Kern RC, et al: Antimicrobials and chronic rhinosinusitis with or without polyposis in adults: an evidenced-based review with recommendations. Int Forum Allergy Rhinol 2013;3:31–47.
27 Wallwork B, Coman W, Mackay-Sim A, Greiff L, Cervin A: A double-blind, randomized, placebo-controlled trial of macrolide in the treatment of chronic rhinosinusitis. Laryngoscope 2006;116: 189–193.
28 Inamura K, Ohta N, Fukase S, Kasajima N, Aoyagi M: The effects of erythromycin on human peripheral neutrophil apoptosis. Rhinology 2000;38:124–129.
29 Wallwork B, Coman W, Feron F, Mackay-Sim A, Cervin A: Clarithromycin and prednisolone inhibit cytokine production in chronic rhinosinusitis. Laryngoscope 2002;112:1827–1830.
30 Miyanohara T, Ushikai M, Matsune S, Ueno K, Katahira S, Kurono Y: Effects of clarithromycin on cultured human nasal epithelial cells and fibroblasts. Laryngoscope 2000;110:126–131.
31 Haxel BR, Clemens M, Karaiskaki N, Dippold U, Kettern L, Mann WJ: Controlled trial for long-term low-dose erythromycin after sinus surgery for chronic rhinosinusitis. Laryngoscope 2015;125:1048–1055.
32 Varvyanskaya A, Lopatin A: Efficacy of long-term low-dose macrolide therapy in preventing early recurrence of nasal polyps after endoscopic sinus surgery. Int Forum Allergy Rhinol 2014;4:533–541.
33 Haruna S, Shimada C, Ozawa M, Fukami S, Moriyama H: A study of poor responders for long-term, low-dose macrolide administration for chronic sinusitis. Rhinology 2009;47:66–71.
34 Peric A, Baletic N, Milojevic M, et al: Effects of preoperative clarithromycin administration in patients with nasal polyposis. West Indian Med J 2014;63: 721–727.
35 Dabirmoghaddam P, Mehdizadeh Seraj J, Bastaninejad S, Meighani A, Mokhtari Z: The efficacy of clarithromycin in patients with severe nasal polyposis. Acta Med Iran 2013;51:359–364.
36 Peric A, Vojvodic D, Baletic N, Peric A, Miljanovic O: Influence of allergy on the immunomodulatory and clinical effects of long-term low-dose macrolide treatment of nasal polyposis. Biomed Pap Med Fac Univ Palacky Olomouc Czech Repub 2010;154:327–333.
37 Katsuta S, Osafune H, Takita R, Sugamata M: [Therapeutic effect of roxithromycin on chronic sinusitis with nasal – polyps clinical, computed tomography, and electron microscopy analysis]. Nihon Jibiinkoka Gakkai Kaiho 2002;105: 1189–1197.
38 Moriyama H, Yanagi K, Ohtori N, Fukami M: Evaluation of endoscopic sinus surgery for chronic sinusitis: post-operative erythromycin therapy. Rhinology 1995;33:166–170.

39 Cervin A, Wallwork B: Efficacy and safety of long-term antibiotics (macrolides) for the treatment of chronic rhinosinusitis. Curr Allergy Asthma Rep 2014;14: 416.
40 Videler WJ, Badia L, Harvey RJ, et al: Lack of efficacy of long-term, low-dose azithromycin in chronic rhinosinusitis: a randomized controlled trial. Allergy 2011;66:1457–1468.
41 Li H, Liu DH, Chen LL, et al: Meta-analysis of the adverse effects of long-term azithromycin use in patients with chronic lung diseases. Antimicrob Agents Chemother 2014;58:511–517.
42 Sasama J, Sherris DA, Shin SH, Kephart GM, Kern EB, Ponikau JU: New paradigm for the roles of fungi and eosinophils in chronic rhinosinusitis. Curr Opin Otolaryngol Head Neck Surg 2005; 13:2–8.
43 Ponikau JU, Sherris DA, Kern EB, et al: The diagnosis and incidence of allergic fungal sinusitis. Mayo Clin Proc 1999; 74:877–884.
44 Ponikau JU, Sherris DA, Kephart GM, Adolphson C, Kita H: The role of ubiquitous airborne fungi in chronic rhinosinusitis. Clin Rev Allergy Immunol 2006; 30:187–194.
45 Ebbens FA, Georgalas C, Fokkens WJ: The mold conundrum in chronic hyperplastic sinusitis. Curr Allergy Asthma Rep 2009;9:114–120.
46 Ebbens FA, Georgalas C, Fokkens WJ: Fungus as the cause of chronic rhinosinusitis: the case remains unproven. Curr Opin Otolaryngol Head Neck Surg 2009; 17:43–49.
47 Lackner A, Stammberger H, Buzina W, et al: Fungi: a normal content of human nasal mucus. Am J Rhinol 2005;19:125–129.
48 Thanasumpun T, Batra PS: Oral antifungal therapy for chronic rhinosinusitis and its subtypes: a systematic review. Int Forum Allergy Rhinol 2011;1:382–389.
49 Kennedy DW, Kuhn FA, Hamilos DL, et al: Treatment of chronic rhinosinusitis with high-dose oral terbinafine: a double blind, placebo-controlled study. Laryngoscope 2005;115:1793–1799.
50 Sacks PL, Harvey RJ, Rimmer J, Gallagher RM, Sacks R: Topical and systemic antifungal therapy for the symptomatic treatment of chronic rhinosinusitis. Cochrane Database Syst Rev 2011;8: CD008263.
51 Khalil Y, Tharwat A, Abdou AG, et al: The role of antifungal therapy in the prevention of recurrent allergic fungal rhinosinusitis after functional endoscopic sinus surgery: a randomized, controlled study. Ear Nose Throat J 2011;90:E1–E7.
52 Patro SK, Verma RK, Panda NK, Chakrabarti A, Singh P: Efficacy of preoperative itraconazole in allergic fungal rhinosinusitis. Am J Rhinol Allergy 2015;29:299–304.
53 Parnes SM: Targeting cysteinyl leukotrienes in patients with rhinitis, sinusitis and paranasal polyps. Am J Respir Med 2002;1:403–408.
54 Holgate ST, Peters-Golden M, Panettieri RA, Henderson WR Jr: Roles of cysteinyl leukotrienes in airway inflammation, smooth muscle function, and remodeling. J Allergy Clin Immunol 2003;111(1 suppl):S18–S34; discussion S34–S36.
55 Smith TL, Sautter NB: Is montelukast indicated for treatment of chronic rhinosinusitis with polyposis? Laryngoscope 2014;124:1735–1736.
56 Wentzel JL, Soler ZM, DeYoung K, Nguyen SA, Lohia S, Schlosser RJ: Leukotriene antagonists in nasal polyposis: a meta-analysis and systematic review. Am J Rhinol Allergy 2013;27:482–489.
57 Ogino S, Irifune M, Harada T, Kikumori H, Matsunaga T: Arachidonic acid metabolites in human nasal polyps. Acta Otolaryngol Suppl 1993;501:85–87.
58 Jung TT, Juhn SK, Hwang D, Stewart R: Prostaglandins, leukotrienes, and other arachidonic acid metabolites in nasal polyps and nasal mucosa. Laryngoscope 1987;97:184–189.
59 Jang YJ, Rhee CK, Oh CH, Ryoo HG, Kim HG, Ha M: Arachidonic acid metabolites in antrochoanal polyp and nasal polyp associated with chronic paranasal sinusitis. Acta Otolaryngol 2000;120:531–534.
60 Baenkler HW, Schafer D, Hosemann W: Eicosanoids from biopsy of normal and polypous nasal mucosa. Rhinology 1996; 34:166–170.
61 Chao SS, Graham SM, Brown CL, Kline JN, Hussain I: Cysteinyl leukotriene 1 receptor expression in nasal polyps. Ann Otol Rhinol Laryngol 2006;115:394–397.
62 Perez-Novo CA, Watelet JB, Claeys C, Van Cauwenberge P, Bachert C: Prostaglandin, leukotriene, and lipoxin balance in chronic rhinosinusitis with and without nasal polyposis. J Allergy Clin Immunol 2005;115:1189–1196.
63 Meltzer EO, Hamilos DL, Hadley JA, et al: Rhinosinusitis: establishing definitions for clinical research and patient care. J Allergy Clin Immunol 2004;114(6 suppl):155–212.
64 Schaper C, Noga O, Koch B, Ewert R, Felix SB, Glaser S, Kunkel G, Gustavus B: Anti-inflammatory properties of montelukast, a leukotriene receptor antagonist in patients with asthma and nasal polyposis. J Investig Allergol Clin Immunol 2011;21:51–58.
65 Pauli C, Fintelmann R, Klemens C, Hilgert E, Jund F, Rasp G, Hagedorn H, Kramer MF: [Polyposis nasi – improvement in quality of life by the influence of leukotrien receptor antagonists]. Laryngorhinootologie 2007;86:282–286.
66 Vuralkan E, Saka C, Akin I, Hucumenoglu S, Unal BU, Kuran G, Ocal B: Comparison of montelukast and mometasone furoate in the prevention of recurrent nasal polyps. Ther Adv Respir Dis 2012;6:5–10.
67 Mostafa BE, Abdel Hay H, Mohammed HE, Yamani M: Role of leukotriene inhibitors in the postoperative management of nasal polyps. ORL J Otorhinolaryngol Relat Spec 2005;67:148–153.
68 Parnes SM, Chuma AV: Acute effects of antileukotrienes on sinonasal polyposis and sinusitis. Ear Nose Throat J 2000;79: 18–20, 24–25.
69 Fruth K, Pogorzelski B, Schmidtmann I, et al: Low-dose aspirin desensitization in individuals with aspirin-exacerbated respiratory disease. Allergy 2013;68: 659–665.
70 Dahlen B, Nizankowska E, Szczeklik A, et al: Benefits from adding the 5-lipoxygenase inhibitor zileuton to conventional therapy in aspirin-intolerant asthmatics. Am J Respir Crit Care Med 1998; 157(4 pt 1):1187–1194.

Jeremiah A. Alt, MD, PhD
Division of Head and Neck Surgery, Rhinology-Sinus and Skull Base Surgery Program
Department of Surgery, University of Utah, 30 N 1900 E Rm 3C120
Salt Lake City, UT 84132-2101 (USA)
E-Mail Jeremiah.Alt@hsc.utah.edu

Woodworth BA, Poetker DM, Reh DD (eds): Rhinosinusitis with Nasal Polyposis.
Adv Otorhinolaryngol. Basel, Karger, 2016, vol 79, pp 148–157 (DOI: 10.1159/000445153)

Advances in Surgery: Extended Procedures for Sinonasal Polyp Disease

Jessica E. Southwood · Todd A. Loehrl · David M. Poetker

Division of Rhinology and Sinus Surgery, Department of Surgery, Zablocki VA Medical Center, Milwaukee, Wis., USA

Abstract

In the standard functional endoscopic sinus surgery (FESS) procedure, the amount of dissection is often determined by the extent of disease with the goal to preserve as much normal mucosa as possible while restoring ventilation and reestablishing mucociliary clearance. A subset of patients with chronic rhinosinusitis with nasal polyposis (CRSwNP), however, may continue to have persistent mucosal inflammatory and aggressive polyp regrowth despite standard FESS and maximal pharmacology therapy, leading to recurrent and recalcitrant disease. Advanced endoscopic surgery techniques such as the modified endoscopic medial maxillectomy, endoscopic modified Lothrop procedure, otherwise known as a Draf 3 frontal sinusotomy, and nasalisation or radical ethmoidectomy are extensive surgical procedures to maximize disease clearance while providing sizeable drainage pathways for effective postoperative surveillance and topical delivery of medications. Studies have shown a decreased risk of revision surgery as well as a longer time interval for revision surgery in patients with refractory CRSwNP who have undergone extensive sinus surgery for polyps.

Introduction

Sinonasal polyp disease has a prevalence estimated at 0.2–4% in worldwide studies with a peak incidence in the fifth decade of life [1, 2]. Nasal polyps are often associated with chronic rhinosinusitis, categorized in the broad phenotype of chronic rhinosinusitis with nasal polyposis (CRSwNP), a chronic disease with a prolonged clinical course. Curative treatment is difficult to achieve in CRSwNP and management is primarily aimed at reducing symptom severity. The mechanism by which surgery improves symptom control in CRSwNP is incompletely understood. The lack of high-quality evidence focusing on CRSwNP as well as the heterogeneity of the disease itself leads to significant practice variation in planning the extent of surgery [3, 4]. Furthermore, the rate of postoperative polyp recurrence has been reported to be as high as 60% [5, 6]. Widespread mucosal inflammation with diffuse polyposis, or more severe inflammatory disease like that associated with cystic fibrosis (CF), may be better treated with more extensive surgery to increase access for delivery of topical therapies in the postoperative period [7]. The following chapter focuses on extensive endoscopic surgical techniques for treating recalcitrant CRSwNP.

Middle Turbinate Resection

Controversy exists as to the decision to resect the middle turbinate due to the described risks of atrophic rhinitis, cerebrospinal fluid leak, anosmia, loss of surgical landmarks, postoperative epistaxis and iatrogenic frontal sinusitis [8–10]. Those who advocate resection discuss improvement in intraoperative and postoperative visualization, decreased synechiae, improved patency of sinus ostia allowing for improved ventilation and enhanced delivery of topical medications [11, 12]. It is theorized that the mucosa of the middle turbinates itself may act as a conduit for potential polyp formation and the removal of this surface area of mucosa may help to control polyp regrowth [11, 13]. Marchioni et al. [14] performed a prospective study in a homogeneous case series of patients that underwent surgery exclusively for severe nasal polyposis, comparing the results of those whose middle turbinate was resected and those whose middle turbinate was preserved. There was a statistically significant difference in proportion and time to relapse between the patients who underwent turbinate resection and those with turbinate preservation. Three of 22 patients in the turbinate resection group had recurrence of polyposis on nasal endoscopy versus 17 of 34 patients in the preservation group. The patients who underwent surgery with middle turbinate preservation were 4 times more likely to develop recurrent disease than the patients who underwent middle turbinate resection (hazard ratio 4.06 with 95% CI 1.19–19.89) over the 36 month follow-up period. Wu et al. [11] found the beneficial effect of middle turbinate resection to significantly delay the time until revision surgery for patient with polyps up to 8 years following initial surgery.

Soler et al. [13] performed a multi-institutional observational study which demonstrated no difference in quality-of-life status after bilateral middle turbinate (BMT) resection versus turbinate preservation. Endoscopic exam, olfactory function using the Smell Identification Test and three quality-of-life instruments (Rhinosinusitis Disability Index, Chronic Sinusitis Survey and Medical Outcomes Study Short Form-36 Health Survey), were used to evaluate outcomes. There were 47 patients representing the BMT resection group and 195 patients representing the BMT preservation group with an average follow-up of 17.4 months for all subjects. The decision to resect or preserve the middle turbinate was based on the surgeon's judgment, taking into account the disease process as evidence by symptoms, CT imaging and intraoperative findings. The technique of middle turbinate resection was described as removal of the anteroinferior two-thirds of the middle turbinate using through-cutting instruments, leaving the superior sagittally oriented portion as a landmark and a small posterior stump in the area of the sphenopalatine foramen. Patients undergoing BMT resection were statistically more likely to have comorbidities associated with inflammatory processes and increased disease burden with higher incidence of nasal polyposis (BMT resection 55.3% vs. BMT preservation 37.4%, $p = 0.025$), and prior sinus surgery (BMT resection 85% vs. BMT preservation 61.5% $p = 0.002$) as well as asthma and aspirin intolerance. Patients undergoing BMT resection also tended to undergo more extensive sinus surgery with a higher rate of concurrent total ethmoidectomy, sphenoidotomy and frontal sinusotomy than those with BMT preservation. There were greater improvements in endoscopy and Smell Identification Test scores following BMT resection compared to turbinate preservation after controlling for confounding factors. Soler et al. [13] conclude that the decision to preserve or resect the middle turbinate can be left to the discretion of the surgeon with little or no negative consequences after sinus surgery.

Keys to the middle turbinate resection include taking the turbinate superiorly at the anterior attachment and performing a frontal sinusotomy (Draf 2A or B) to prevent lateralization of the middle turbinate remnant and obstruction of the frontal recess. Additionally, take great care to visualize the tips of the endoscopic scissors to avoid penetrating the skull base. Finally, consider electrosurgical cautery of the posterior stump to avoid post-operative hemorrhage.

Modified Endoscopic Medial Maxillectomy

Standard maxillary antrostomy is greater than 90% effective in managing chronic maxillary sinusitis [15], allowing for improved aeration and drainage of the maxillary sinus as well as increased delivery of topical medications. Despite the high efficiency rates of this procedure, some patients with CRSwNP fail standard maxillary antrostomy for reasons still incompletely understood. Some theories suggest failure is related to the underlying pathophysiology of dysfunctional mucociliary transport as well as obstructed ostia with polyp regrowth as well as chronic inflammatory mucosal disease [16]. The modified endoscopic medial maxillectomy (MEMM) surgical technique is an accepted approach to benign sinonasal tumor resection such as inverted papillomas and juvenile nasopharyngeal angiofibromas [17, 18], however its role in recalcitrant inflammatory disease specifically polypoid disease is less well defined. MEMM has been shown to increase the total sinus irrigation delivery in topical distribution studies in comparison to standard maxillary antrostomy [19]. The increased access to the maxillary sinus after MEMM permits large-volume, positive-pressure application of topical medications and affords increased mechanical removal of mucus to an area otherwise limited by access. Inflammatory maxillary disease is improved likely as a result of increased delivery of intranasal irrigation and improved access and drainage of the inferior and dependent portions of the maxillary sinus [20, 21]. Unlike gravity-aided drainage pathways of the frontal and ethmoid sinuses, mucociliary clearance must work against gravity in the maxillary sinus. The MEMM allows more proficient gravity dependent drainage of the maxillary sinuses postoperatively.

MEMM involves resection of the medial wall of the maxillary sinus and a subtotal inferior turbinectomy [21]. Some authors advocate for preservation of the anterior one-third of the inferior turbinate to prevent atrophic rhinitis and that a posterior stump of the inferior turbinate is maintained to allow cauterization of the branches of the sphenopalatine artery [20]. The mucosa of the lateral nasal wall of the inferior meatus is elevated in a subperiosteal plane with the base of the flap on the floor of the nose. After the medial maxillary wall is resected, the appropriate boundaries of the MEMM are the floor of the nose inferiorly, the posterior wall of the maxillary sinus posteriorly (with care to avoid the descending palatine nerve), and the lacrimal duct anteriorly. After completion of the MEMM, wide access to the maxillary sinus is achieved and polyps are removed without stripping the mucosa. Finally, the previously raised mucosal flap is laid across the exposed bone of the inferior maxilla into the maxillary sinus (fig. 1).

Konstantinidis and Constantinidis [22] reviewed the indications for a medial maxillectomy and suggest various modifications of the procedure such as preserving the anterior aspect of the medial maxillary wall, which can be performed depending of the pathology and extent of disease. For more anterior access of the maxillary sinus, the medial maxillary wall may be removed, however this is not without the risk of nasolacrimal duct injury. Cho and Hwang [23] describe the endoscopic maxillary mega-antrostomy which involves extending the antrostomy through the

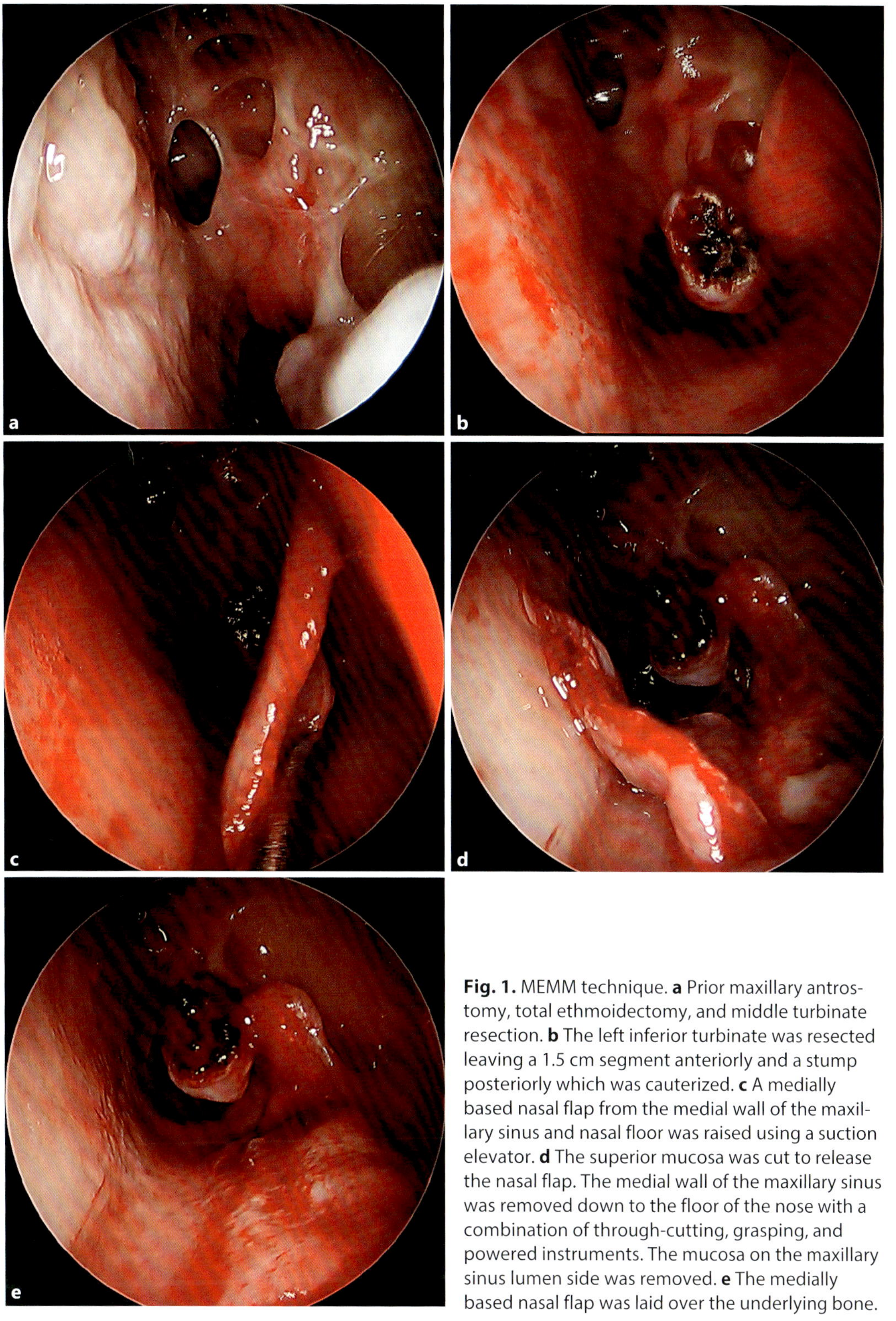

Fig. 1. MEMM technique. **a** Prior maxillary antrostomy, total ethmoidectomy, and middle turbinate resection. **b** The left inferior turbinate was resected leaving a 1.5 cm segment anteriorly and a stump posteriorly which was cauterized. **c** A medially based nasal flap from the medial wall of the maxillary sinus and nasal floor was raised using a suction elevator. **d** The superior mucosa was cut to release the nasal flap. The medial wall of the maxillary sinus was removed down to the floor of the nose with a combination of through-cutting, grasping, and powered instruments. The mucosa on the maxillary sinus lumen side was removed. **e** The medially based nasal flap was laid over the underlying bone.

posterior half of the inferior turbinate down to the floor of the nose in recalcitrant maxillary sinusitis. In their series, 74% of patients reported complete resolution of symptoms with no patients requiring revision during the 11-month follow-up.

In addition to greater topical drug delivery for treatment of inflammatory paranasal sinus disease and affording improved dependent drainage postoperatively, resection of the medial maxillary wall allows for intraoperative access to the inferior and dependent portions of the maxillary sinus, an otherwise difficult area to clear polypoid mucosa. MEMM has been shown to improve the surgical success rate for persistent inflammatory sinus disease of the maxillary sinus [20, 21]. The canine puncture technique described by Sathananthar et al. [24] is also an effective method for removal of maxillary sinus polyps and inflammatory disease in the inferior aspect of the maxillary sinus. However, the MEMM procedure has the continued advantages of improving access to the maxillary sinus in the postoperative setting and improving gravity dependent drainage.

Woodworth et al. reported a success rate of MEMM in 18 out of 19 patients who had failed prior sinus surgery with an average follow-up of 19.5 months [21]. The majority of patients (14) had previously undergone Caldwell-Luc procedures at outside institutions and were predisposed to abnormal mucociliary clearance. The only complication was one nasolacrimal duct injury. Another study demonstrated resolution of recalcitrant maxillary sinusitis in 37 out of 46 patients (80%) who failed on average 3.4 prior surgeries before undergoing MEMM [20]. The average time to recurrence of maxillary sinusitis was 11.7 months for the remaining 20% of patients, however no patients in the series required revision surgery within the 37 month follow-up period [20].

MEMM has been studied in certain subgroups of patients with CRSwNP known to have refractory disease such as cystic fibrosis (CF) and allergic fungal rhinosinusitis (AFRS). CF patients represent a cohort of patients with disturbed mucociliary clearance who may continue to display problematic sinus disease after multiple previous functional endoscopic sinus surgery (FESS) even with patent maxillary antrostomy [25]. The severity of polypoid disease in patients with CF may predict the future likelihood of requiring revision FESS. The normal mucociliary clearance pathway works against gravity and is impaired in CF patients leading to the accumulation of mucopurulence in the largest of the sinus cavities despite previous adequate maxillary antrostomy. The maximum beneficial treatment and goals of the patients that require intervention are to provide a permanent accessible means for medicinal and mechanical removal of inspissated mucus and polyps. Virgin et al. [25] prospectively evaluated 22 CF patients after undergoing MEMM who had previously failed multiple FESS (mean of 4.9 prior sinus operations). Aggressive sinus surgery combined with medical therapy improved not only symptom and endoscopic scores, but also significantly reduced the frequency of pulmonary exacerbations requiring hospitalization (2.0 ± 1.4 vs. 3.2 ± 2.4, respectively; $p < 0.05$). Review of investigations regarding the use of MEMM in patients with CF and chronic rhinosinusitis show low complication rates for this procedure [26].

AFRS patients represent another cohort of CRSwNP patients who may potentially benefit from more extensive sinus surgery. Although medical therapy such as systemic and topical steroids and immunotherapy seem to be beneficial in disease management, endoscopic sinus surgery is the mainstay of treatment in the setting of persistent obstruction with nasal polyposis and accumulation of allergic fungal mucin. The goals of surgery include extirpation of allergic mucin and fungal debris, permanent ventilation of drainage pathways while maintaining intact mucosa, and postoperative access for monitoring of previously diseased areas [27]. Thulasidas and Vaidyanathan performed MEMM in 37 maxillary sinuses of 24 patients with recalcitrant maxillary sinusitis, four of which had a diagnosis of AFRS [27]. The average time for follow-up in the AFRS patients was 19 months. All patients in the series including those with AFRS had disease control without evidence of recurrence.

Draf 3 Frontal Sinusotomy

The endoscopic modified Lothrop procedure (EMLP), otherwise known as a Draf 3 frontal sinusotomy or frontal drillout, is a salvage procedure for failed frontal sinusotomy or Draf 2b. Frontal ostium size has previously been reported as a risk factor for failure of the Draf 2b procedure. The smaller the ostia, the greater the risk of adhesion formation or risk of polyp recurrence leading to complete occlusion of the frontal sinus ostium. The smaller ostium is also less likely to act as a conduit for saline irrigations or other topical therapies.

The surgical borders of the endoscopic Lothrop cavity are well characterized. Laterally the boundaries are the orbital plates of the frontal bone and the periosteum of the skin overlying the frontal process of the maxilla. The first olfactory fasicle of the olfactory bulb marks the posterior border. The anterior table of the frontal sinus demarcates the anterior limit of dissection. Traditionally angled endoscopes are used to identify one frontal recess which is then followed by bony removal (fig. 2). In severe inflammatory disease however, identifying the frontal recess may prove challenging. Chin et al. describe an 'outside-in' EMLP technique in which dissection of the frontal recess is initially avoided until bone removal below the frontal sinus floor to the periosteum of the skin permits wide access [28]. The frontal recess is actually dissected last and the development of the Lothrop cavity occurs en route with early limits of dissection defined during surgery (table 1). One advantage of this technique is the avoidance of inflamed mucosa in the frontal recess early in the procedure to minimize bleeding as well as to improve visualization of the ethmoid roof in relationship to the posterior frontal table or anterior skull base. The authors state that the risk of injury to the skull base is avoided during this anterior to posterior ap-

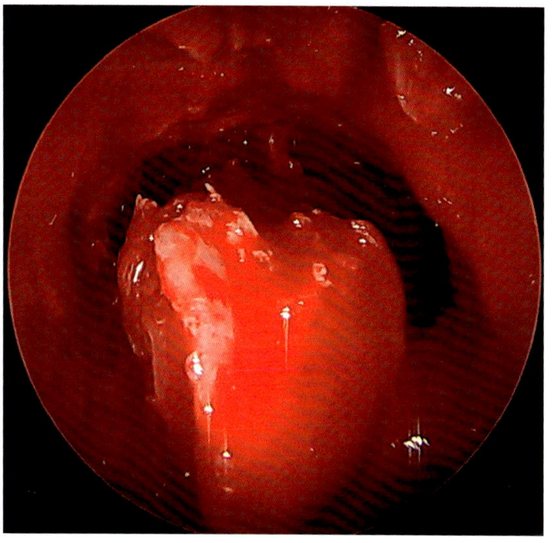

Fig. 2. Completed Draf 3.

Table 1. Surgical steps for the outside-in modified endoscopic lothrop procedure modified from Chin et al. [28]

Surgical step	Description
1	Clear mucosa over frontal process using the medial orbital wall as the lateral border
2	Create a septal window
3	Clear mucosal lining of the nasal cavity underneath the floor of the frontal sinus
4	Drill the remaining superior bony septum
5	Develop the periosteal plane on each side
6	Remove bone between the lateral borders
7	Dissect bone anterior to the frontal recess
8	Complete the cavity by removing bone between the cavity and the true frontal recess (using a 2-mm Kerrison rongeur)

proach by identification of the first olfactory fascicle and the posterior edge of the septal window anterior to the cribriform. Stereotactic image guidance, while helpful in confirming surgical landmarks, is not significantly helpful in identifying the periosteum during this method. Chin et al. [28] describe 15 out of 30 patients that had a diagnosis of CRSwNP, all with at least one prior sinus surgery, 11 underwent the outside-in EMLP technique and 3 underwent the standard Lothrop procedure. Other patients in their study had various pathology including chronic rhinosinusitis without nasal polyposis as well as benign and malignant sinonasal tumors. In the CRSwNP patients, the frontal recess was either occupied by polyps or scarred off. Patients with CRSwNP undergoing the outside-in EMLP had on average a shorter procedure time than the standard Lothrop for all surgical patients (34.6 ± 11.56 vs. 69.6 ± 64.5 min). The procedure time was not explicitly stated for the three CRSwNP patients who underwent the standard Lothrop procedure. The mean operative time included the time point from the commencement of drilling to connection to the frontal recess. Other operative components such as creation of the anterior septal window and removal of mucosa over the frontal recess were not included. There were no complications other than one patient with transient skin edema and no major complications.

Naidoo et al. [29] reviewed the long-term outcomes of the Draf 3 or frontal drill-out over a 10-year time period. AFRS and recurrent Staphylococcus aureus infections were stated as potential risk factors for failure of the EMLP. In this study 229 patients underwent EMLP with a success rate of 95% (217 of 229). Patients had undergone on average 3.8 standard ESS procedures prior to the EMLP. Over half of the patients (135 of 229) had a diagnosis of CRSwNP. Patients underwent an EMLP only after standard FESS had failed and had evidence of recurrent polypoid disease with persistence of symptoms despite maximal medical therapy. Patients with CF were excluded from this patient cohort. Only 12 patients developed disease recurrence and persistence of symptoms requiring revision EMLP. The average length of follow-up was 45 months. All patients noted an improvement in overall postoperative symptom score which included nasal obstruction, facial pain, anosmia, anterior rhinorrhea and post nasal drip. No patient complained of worsening in their symptoms following surgery. Of the 12 patients requiring revision surgery, half (6 of 12) developed recurrent polyposis occluding the frontal neo-ostium. Allergic fungal sinusitis with recurrence of fungal debris and polyposis was noted to be a significant risk of failure in the EMLP revision group, occurring in 7 of 12 patients. The underlying immunologic dysfunction in AFRS patients leads to recurrent polyposis which may occlude the frontal sinus and inhibit ventilation and adequate delivery of topical steroid therapy. Other factors such as persistent colonization of the sinuses which is influenced by antibiotic sensitivity, environmental and immune factors, may lead to scar tissue or osteogenesis and narrowing of the frontal neo-ostium.

One technique, aimed at improving outcomes includes the use of mucosal grafts to cover the exposed bone at the anterior border of the dissection (fig. 3). Illing et al. [30] describe their technique of using either mucosa harvested from a turbinate or from the planned septectomy site to cover the exposed bone. They recently reported a 100% clinical success rate in patients at least 12 months out from the technique.

The Draf 3 procedure has been shown to decrease the risk of revision sinus surgery in CRSwNP, especially in asthma and aspirin intolerant patients. In a study by Bassiouni and Wormald [31], the group of patients undergoing the Draf 3 procedure had undergone previous complete sphenoethmoidectomies and had medically resistant frontal sinus polyps. In addition to the Draf 3 procedure, these patients underwent a revision sphenoethmoidectomy and partial removal of the middle turbinate. The middle turbinate was always

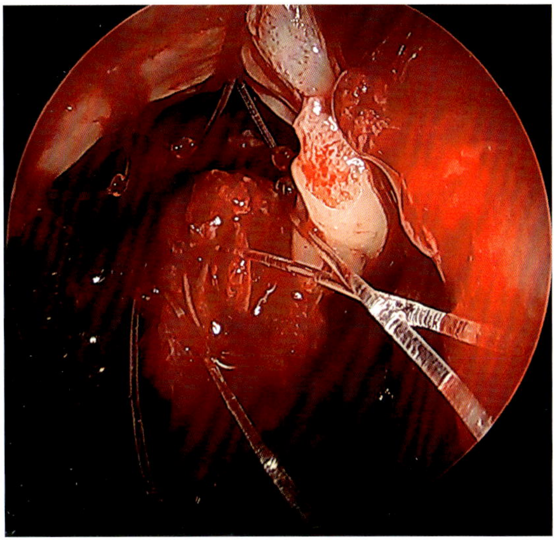

Fig. 3. Completed Draf 3 with a mucosal graft covering the anterior exposed bone. A Propel® drug eluding stent is used to hold the graft in place.

partially removed in the Draf 3 procedure; however, it was never removed in the standard ESS group. The overall revision rate reported in this retrospective cohort study in 338 consecutive operations was 18% (follow-up duration >12 months, median of 29 months), with a 37% revision rate in the FESS group versus 7% in the Draf 3 group ($p < 0.001$). Survival analysis showed that the Draf 3 significantly reduced the risk of revision surgery (hazard ratio = 0.258, $p = 0.0026$).

Nasalisation or Radical Ethmoidectomy

Nasalisation (or nasalization) is described as a radical ethmoidectomy whereby all the bony lamellae and mucosa of the ethmoid is removed in addition to a large maxillary antrostomy, sphenoidotomy, frontal ostium exposure and resection of the middle turbinate [6]. The mucosa on the walls of the large sinuses and around the frontal ostia is preserved. Septal deviation may also be addressed at the time of sinus surgery if thought to impede delivery of topical steroid sprays.

Radical ethmoidectomy is advocated by some authors in the presence of very extensive polyps in the paranasal cavities to decrease the likelihood of early recurrence and functional failure [6, 32, 33]. The goal of nasalisation surgery is to transform the ethmoid labyrinth into an open corridor that can be reached by topical steroids [33]. The essential elements to nasalisation are (1) a large antrostomy and sphenoidotomy, (2) resection of the middle turbinate, (3) removal of as much of the ethmoid partitions and mucosa as safely as possible and (4) procession of the dissection anteriorly towards the frontal ostium [33].

Jankowski et al. [6] compared the improvement of symptoms associated with radical ethmoidectomy or nasalisation to functional standard ethmoidectomy in patients with severe sinonasal polyposis 5 years after the respective surgery. The criteria for comparison were the recurrence rate of nasal polyps using visual assessment on nasal endoscopy and CT imaging, and functional symptom results from patients free of revision surgery who responded to a questionnaire using visual analogue scales. The questionnaire included symptoms of nasal obstruction, rhinorrhea, post-nasal drip, anosmia and the severity of each with 0 = disabling or severely persistent symptoms and 10 = normal or complete absence of symptoms. The overall nasal functional benefit was scored 8.41 ± 0.40 after nasalisation and 5.69 ± 0.83 after ethmoidectomy $p = 0.002$ in patients who did not require revision surgery. The total recurrence rate was 22.7% in the nasalisation group and 58.3% in the ethmoidectomy group ($\chi^2 = 10.41$, $p < 0.01$). The nasalisation group underwent significantly less revision procedures compared to the ethmoidectomy group (4 revision procedures in 3 of 33 patients of the nasalisation group vs. 14 revision procedures in 7 of 25 patients of the ethmoidectomy group, $\chi^2 = 10.3$, $p < 0.01$). Results of this study must be considered with the clear limitation that no validated outcome measures were used.

Bonfils discussed the functional results of 194 patients with nasal polyps after complete sphenoethmoidectomy and inferior resection of the middle turbinate [32]. Clinical symptoms and steroid use were monitored before and after surgery using an actuarial analysis via the Kaplan–Meier life table method 3- and 5-years post-operatively. The 5-year nasal obstruction control rate was 65.8%, the severe posterior rhinorrhea control rate was 82.9% and the anosmia control rate was 65.8%. Patients considered to have secondary polyposis disease such as granulomatosis with polyangiitis, formerly known as Wegener's granulomatosis, Churg–Strauss syndrome or CF were excluded from this study. There were 55 patients who had undergone a previous sinonasal surgery including simple polypectomy (n = 16, 8.2%), Caldwell–Luc (n = 5, 2.6%), middle meatus antrostomy (n = 6, 3.1%), partial ethmoidectomy (n = 25, 12.9%) or septoplasty (n = 3, 1.5%). Only 8 patients (4.1% study population) developed recurrent nasal polyposis requiring additional surgery with a mean delay between the two procedures of 74 ± 13 months. The number of short courses of oral steroids decreased significantly from 4.31 ± 0.23 courses preoperatively to less than one per year in the seven years following nasalisation surgery.

Conclusion

The goals of polyp management in CRSwNP are to improve the airway and facilitate delivery of medications. Aggressive disease calls for aggressive surgery in order to remove obstructive polyps, create an open cavity for topical medication delivery and mechanical debridement, as well as postoperative monitoring of polyp reoccurrence. Advanced endoscopic sinus surgery such as middle turbinate resection, MEMM, Draf 3 and nasalisation may not be appropriate for the majority of CRSwNP patients; however, those with recalcitrant disease who have failed prior FESS and those with underlying mucociliary dysfunction have shown improvement in disease control with these techniques.

References

1 Lange B, Holst R, Thilsing T, Baelum J, Kjeldsen A: Quality of life and associated factors in persons with chronic rhinosinusitis in the general population: a prospective questionnaire and clinical cross-sectional study. Clin Otolaryngol 2013;38:474–480.

2 Johansson L, Akerlund A, Holmberg K, Melén I, Bende M: Prevalence of nasal polyps in adults: the skövde population-based study. Ann Otol Rhinol Laryngol 2003;112:625–629.

3 Hopkins C, Browne JP, Slack R, et al: The national comparative audit of surgery for nasal polyposis and chronic rhinosinusitis. Clin Otolaryngol 2006; 31:390–398.

4 Sharma R, Lakhani R, Rimmer J, Hopkins C: Surgical interventions for chronic rhinosinusitis with nasal polyps. Cochrane Database Syst Rev 2014; 11:CD006990.

5 Wynn R, Har-El G: Recurrence rates after endoscopic sinus surgery for massive sinus polyposis. Laryngoscope 2004; 114:811–813.

6 Jankowski R, Pigret D, Decroocq F, Blum A, Gillet P: Comparison of radical (nasalisation) and functional ethmoidectomy in patients with severe sinonasal polyposis. A retrospective study. Rev Laryngol Otol Rhinol (Bord) 2006;127: 131–140.

7 Chin D, Harvey RJ: Nasal polyposis: an inflammatory condition requiring effective anti-inflammatory treatment. Curr Opin Otolaryngol Head Neck Surg 2013; 21:23–30.

8 Kennedy DW: Middle turbinate resection: evaluating the issues – should we resect normal middle turbinates? Arch Otolaryngol Head Neck Surg 1998;124: 107.

9 Nurse LA, Duncavage JA: Surgery of the inferior and middle turbinates. Otolaryngol Clin North Am 2009;42:295–309, ix.

10 Vleming M, Middelweerd RJ, de Vries N: Complications of endoscopic sinus surgery. Arch Otolaryngol Head Neck Surg 1992;118:617–623.

11 Wu AW, Ting JY, Platt MP, Tierney HT, Metson R: Factors affecting time to revision sinus surgery for nasal polyps: a 25-year experience. Laryngoscope 2014; 124:29–33.

12 Toffel PH: Secure endoscopic sinus surgery with partial middle turbinate modification: a 16-year long-term outcome report and literature review. Curr Opin Otolaryngol Head Neck Surg 2003;11: 13–18.

13 Soler ZM, Hwang PH, Mace J, Smith TL: Outcomes after middle turbinate resection: revisiting a controversial topic. Laryngoscope 2010;120:832–837.

14 Marchioni D, Alicandri-Ciufelli M, Mattioli F, et al: Middle turbinate preservation versus middle turbinate resection in endoscopic surgical treatment of nasal polyposis. Acta Otolaryngol 2008; 128:1019–1026.

15 Kennedy DW, Zinreich SJ, Shaalan H, Kuhn F, Naclerio R, Loch E: Endoscopic middle meatal antrostomy: theory, technique, and patency. Laryngoscope 1987; 97(8 pt 3 suppl 43):1–9.

16 Richtsmeier WJ: Top 10 reasons for endoscopic maxillary sinus surgery failure. Laryngoscope 2001;111(11 pt 1):1952–1956.
17 Fyrmpas G, Konstantinidis I, Constantinidis J: Endoscopic treatment of juvenile nasopharyngeal angiofibromas: our experience and review of the literature. Eur Arch Otorhinolaryngol 2012;269: 523–529.
18 Carta F, Verillaud B, Herman P: Role of endoscopic approach in the management of inverted papilloma. Curr Opin Otolaryngol Head Neck Surg 2011;19: 21–24.
19 Harvey RJ, Goddard JC, Wise SK, Schlosser RJ: Effects of endoscopic sinus surgery and delivery device on cadaver sinus irrigation. Otolaryngol Head Neck Surg 2008;139:137–142.
20 Wang EW, Gullung JL, Schlosser RJ: Modified endoscopic medial maxillectomy for recalcitrant chronic maxillary sinusitis. Int Forum Allergy Rhinol 2011;1:493–497.
21 Woodworth BA, Parker RO, Schlosser RJ: Modified endoscopic medial maxillectomy for chronic maxillary sinusitis. Int Forum Allergy Rhinol 2006;20:317–319.
22 Konstantinidis I, Constantinidis J: Medial maxillectomy in recalcitrant sinusitis: when, why and how? Curr Opin Otolaryngol Head Neck Surg 2014;22: 68–74.
23 Cho DY, Hwang PH: Results of endoscopic maxillary mega-antrostomy in recalcitrant maxillary sinusitis. Am J Rhinol 2008;22:658–662.
24 Sathananthar S, Nagaonkar S, Paleri V, Le T, Robinson S, Wormald PJ: Canine fossa puncture and clearance of the maxillary sinus for the severely diseased maxillary sinus. Laryngoscope 2005;115: 1026–1029.
25 Virgin FW, Rowe SM, Wade MB, et al: Extensive surgical and comprehensive postoperative medical management for cystic fibrosis chronic rhinosinusitis. Am J Rhinol Allergy 2012;26:70–75.
26 Chaaban MR, Kejner A, Rowe SM, Woodworth BA: Cystic fibrosis chronic rhinosinusitis: a comprehensive review. Am J Rhinol Allergy 2013;27:387–395.
27 Thulasidas P, Vaidyanathan V: Role of modified endoscopic medial maxillectomy in persistent chronic maxillary sinusitis. Int Arch Otorhinolaryngol 2014;18:159–164.
28 Chin D, Snidvongs K, Kalish L, Sacks R, Harvey RJ: The outside-in approach to the modified endoscopic lothrop procedure. Laryngoscope 2012;122:1661–1669.
29 Naidoo Y, Bassiouni A, Keen M, Wormald PJ: Long-term outcomes for the endoscopic modified lothrop/draf III procedure: a 10-year review. Laryngoscope 2014;124:43–49.
30 Illing EA, Cho DY, Riley KO, Woodworth BA: Draf III mucosal graft technique: long-term result. Int Forum Allergy Rhinol 2016;6:514–517.
31 Bassiouni A, Wormald PJ: Role of frontal sinus surgery in nasal polyp recurrence. Laryngoscope 2013;123:36–41.
32 Bonfils P: Evaluation of the combined medical and surgical treatment in nasal polyposis. I: functional results. Acta Otolaryngol 2007;127:436–446.
33 Jankowski R, Bodino C: Evolution of symptoms associated to nasal polyposis following oral steroid treatment and nasalization of the ethmoid – radical ethmoidectomy is functional surgery for NPS. Rhinology 2003;41:211–219.

David M. Poetker, MD, MA
Division of Rhinology and Sinus Surgery
Department of Otolaryngology and Communication Sciences
Medical College of Wisconsin
9200 West Wisconsin Avenue
Milwaukee, WI 53226 (USA)
E-Mail dpoetker@mcw.edu

Woodworth BA, Poetker DM, Reh DD (eds): Rhinosinusitis with Nasal Polyposis.
Adv Otorhinolaryngol. Basel, Karger, 2016, vol 79, pp 158–167 (DOI: 10.1159/000445155)

Outcomes in Medical and Surgical Treatment of Nasal Polyps

Aria Jafari • Adam S. DeConde

Department of Surgery, Division of Otolaryngology – Head and Neck Surgery, University of California San Diego, San Diego, Calif., USA

Abstract

Chronic rhinosinusitis with nasal polyps is a heterogeneous disease with a variety of medical and surgical options available to the patient and provider. Consensus statements and recent trends in outcomes research advocate that treatment be driven by patient-reported outcome measures. To this end, there has been increasing sophistication and nuance in both the outcome instruments themselves, as well as the method in which they are collected and interpreted. This is reflected in concepts such as the minimally clinically important difference and domain stratification, which have helped clinicians understand patient motivations and response to treatment. Medical management with topical and possibly systemic corticosteroids is considered the initial treatment strategy of choice, with endoscopic sinus surgery (ESS) reserved for patients who fail to improve. While there is strong evidence for surgical intervention over continued medical therapy in recalcitrant patients, a variety of additional targeted medical treatments and refinements to the nature and extent of ESS have been proposed to further maximize outcomes. Here, with the understanding that limitations continue to exist in our ability to fully answer many treatment-related questions, we present the current cumulative evidence for a patient-centered and outcomes-focused approach to manage this uniquely challenging disease.

Introduction

Chronic rhinosinusitis with nasal polyposis (CRSwNP) is a heterogeneous disease defined by the phenotype of chronic sinus inflammation with polyp formation. Navigation of treatment strategies for this condition is challenging for

Table 1. Key criteria of quality for clinical research instruments

Criteria	Definition
Reliability	stability of data administered at different times to the same group (test-retest reliability) or ability to produce similar results using different items from the same instrument (internal consistency) or equivalence of different observers producing the same assessment using the same instrument (inter-rater reliability)
Validity	extent to which an instrument measures what it intends
Responsiveness	ability of a measure to detect change over time

Table 2. Selected disease-specific quality of life measurement in sinonasal disease

Instrument	Year	Questions, n	Reliability	Validity	Responsiveness	Ease of use
RSOM-31	1995	31	++	++	++	+
RSDI	1997	30	+++	++	++	++
SNOT-20	1998	20	+++	++	+++	++
SNOT-22	2000	22	+++	+++	+++	+++

RSOM-31 = Rhinosinusitis outcome measure; RSDI = rhinosinusitis disability index; SNOT-20 = sinonasal outcome test-20; SNOT-22 = sinonasal outcome test-22; + = not strongly demonstrated; ++ = strongly demonstrated; +++ = very strongly demonstrated.

both patients and providers as a variety of medical and surgical options are available. While there is debate concerning the specific interventions, there is clear consensus that optimization of patient reported outcome measures (PROMs) is the primary goal of treatment [1, 2].

Since the introduction of PROMs for chronic rhinosinusitis (CRS) in the 1990s, their collection and analysis has become increasingly sophisticated. These refinements have been a boon to our understanding of how symptoms and quality of life (QOL) are influenced by specific interventions, but require an informed clinician to interpret the data. To this end, this chapter seeks to summarize the latest outcomes research on management of CRSwNP, inclusive of all etiologies of nasal polyps contributing to sinonasal symptomatology, in a way that is memorable for clinicians and easily translatable to patient care.

Primary Outcome Instruments

The ideal PROM instrument captures all impacts of CRS on a patient's QOL, achieves good reliability, internal consistency, validity and correlates with overall health with minimal survey burden [3] (table 1). Over the past 20 years, a variety of measures have been investigated and refined and most correlate closely [4] (table 2). The most recent iteration is the Sinonasal Outcome Test-22 (SNOT-22) and it has been longitudinally validated, translated internationally, and found to correlate with anchor questions of overall change after interventions [5]. Furthermore, pre-operative (baseline) SNOT-22 scores have been advocated as a useful clinical tool in predicting which patients will achieve symptom improvements following surgery [6]. A limitation of the SNOT-22 is that it does not capture medication use or disease duration. The Chronic Sinusitis Survey (CSS) is a 6-item test and an important complementary tool that incorporates this additional data [4]. The complexity of rhinologic disease may ultimately necessitate the integration of multiple PROM instruments to best capture the true impact on QOL [4, 7].

The Minimal Clinically Important Difference
Longitudinal comparisons of baseline and interval PROM scores have served as the basis for evaluating interventions for CRSwNP. The minimal clinically important difference (MCID) is the smallest difference in score perceived as beneficial by a patient [8]. This concept links PROM score change with practical patient benefit, thereby increasing the clinical interpretability and allowing researchers to use this numerical threshold in describing frequencies of achieving clinically meaningful treatment success. Hopkins et al. [5] integrated this intuitive approach into the SNOT-22 instrument and found the MCID to be 9.

Domain Stratification and Utility Scores
Aggregate reporting of PROM scores is useful in large cohorts of patients, but may be oversimplified for a patient or clinician seeking the potential impact of a given intervention on symptoms. Factor analysis of the SNOT-22 has revealed 5 correlated but discrete measured health domains in CRS [9]. Reporting of domains allows for a refined understanding of how interventions impact each domain, and how symptoms influence treatment selection. For instance, DeConde et al. [10] found that patients electing surgery over continued medical therapy have comparable sinonasal symptomatology but carry greater burdens of psychological and sleep symptomatology. Utility scores, or a quantification of value for a patient's health state, also correlate most strongly with these domains [11]. Thus, domain stratification and utility valuation are important symptom-based methods of enhancing clinical precision in determining which patients will benefit from which interventions.

Secondary Outcome Instruments
A variety of secondary outcome measures, or outcomes that do not directly address QOL, have been described to provide additional information to the treating practitioner. These include nasal breathing, radiographic (Lund–Mackay) [12], endoscopic (Lund–Kennedy) [13] and olfactory scores [14]. The secondary outcome measures provide important information that guides treatment for the practitioner as well as validates treatment outcomes in research. Although secondary outcome measures do not correlate perfectly with PROMs, endoscopy accounts for 33% of the variance seen in PROMs [DeConde, in press].

Medical Outcomes

CRSwNP can have a significant impact on QOL due to nasal obstruction, congestion, discharge and loss of sense of smell [15]. The goals of treatment are to improve QOL, as reported in PROMs, eliminate or reduce the size and number of polyps, restore nasal airflow and improve olfaction [16]. Medical treatment is the initial strategy in these patients, with surgery considered for recalcitrant patients.

Topical Corticosteroids
Corticosteroids disrupt the inflammatory pathway at many levels and are implicated in the infiltration and activation of eosinophils and chemotactic cytokines [17]. In 2012, a Cochrane Review based on 40 studies and 3,624 patients showed that topical corticosteroids consistently demonstrate significant benefit in PROMs, polyp size

Table 3. Summary of outcomes in medical treatment of nasal polyps

	Highest LOE	Outcomes					Recommendation
		PROMs	polyp size/ endoscopy score	nasal airflow	olfaction	CT	
Topical corticosteroids	Ia	+++	+++	+++	ND	*	A
Oral corticosteroids	Ia	+++	+++	+++	++	++	A
Leukotriene antagonists	II	++	++	*	+	*	B
Aspirin desensitization	II	+	*	*	+	+	C
Antibiotics	Ib	ND	+	ND	ND	*	C
Antimycotics	Ib	+/–	+/–	ND	*	*	C
Immune-modulators	II	+	+	ND	*	+	D

LOE = Level of evidence; ND = significance not clearly demonstrated; * = determination unable to be made due to limited evidence; + = improvements demonstrated in few studies, none with high level of evidence; ++ = improvements demonstrated in several studies with moderate level of evidence, or few studies with high level of evidence; +++ = improvements demonstrated in several studies, most or all with high level of evidence; – = worsening demonstrated in few studies, none with high level of evidence.

and nasal airflow. However, no significant improvement in sense of smell was shown [16]. In general, topical nasal corticosteroids are well tolerated, with limited systemic absorption and adverse events limited to nasal irritation and epistaxis. Level 1 evidence supports usage of topical corticosteroids for CRSwNP and should be a part of first-line therapy [1] (table 3).

Oral Corticosteroids

Systemic corticosteroids are used in cases of symptomatic CRSwNP that have failed nasal topical treatment, but there is heterogeneity concerning the specific indication, dosage and duration. In 2010, a Cochrane Review showed improvement in PROMs, polyp size, nasal airflow, as well as sense of smell, which was not demonstrated in topical corticosteroid treatment. Furthermore, when compared to topical corticosteroids alone, the use of oral corticosteroids preceding topical treatment showed more durable improvements in polyp size and sense of smell [18]. Despite the benefit, using systemic corticosteroids must be weighed against the adverse effects, which include gastrointestinal complications, growth suppression, diabetes mellitus, hypertension, psychiatric effects, osteopenia, osteoporosis and avascular necrosis [19]. In a non-randomized study where patients were treated with repeated 7–10 day courses of 1 mg/kg/day on average about 7 times per year 5 years, significant (>40%) rates of osteopenia and osteoporosis and adrenal insufficiency (48.4%) on laboratory testing were observed [20]. Another RCT evaluating the use of 50 mg daily of prednisone for 2 weeks showed that about half of the adverse events were psychiatric (insomnia and mood disturbance) with insomnia as significantly more common in the treatment group [21]. Level 1 evidence supports short-course of systemic corticosteroids with dosage between 30 and 50 mg with or without taper for up to 2 weeks followed by topical corticosteroid treatment (table 3).

Leukotriene Antagonists

Leukotrienes (LT) are produced by eosinophils and bind to receptors triggering inflammation. LTs and their receptors are seen at increased levels in nasal polyps and can therefore serve as therapeutic targets. Two RCTs have been performed studying treatment of LT antagonists (montelukast) in patients with CRSwNP. Collectively, these studies showed improvement of PROMs, polyp size, nasal airflow and immunologic parameters when compared to placebo [22, 23]. However, in a non-placebo controlled RCT, there was no overall difference in these parameters between the LT group and nasal corticosteroids [24]. The greatest benefit of LT antagonists over nasal corticosteroids was headache, facial pain, sneezing, nasal pruritus, post-nasal drip and smell disturbance [25, 26]. LT antagonists can be considered as adjunctive treatment in patients with predominantly allergic-type nasal symptoms.

Aspirin Desensitization

Aspirin exacerbated respiratory disease (AERD) is a condition characterized by nasal polyps, asthma and aspirin (ASA) intolerance [27]. Patients with this condition have been shown to have higher polyp burden and rates of recurrence [28]. To improve outcomes, adjuncts to corticosteroid and LT antagonist treatment, such as ASA desensitization, have been studied. In general, this treatment involves the administration of increasing doses of ASA under clinical supervision until a maintenance dose can be taken. RCTs comparing ASA desensitization therapy to placebo are lacking, due to the inability to adequately blind patients to treatment. As such, literature is limited to cohort and case–control studies. In a long-term review of 65 patients who underwent ASA desensitization, Stevenson et al. [29] demonstrated significant reductions in sinonasal symptoms, olfactory dysfunction, use of systemic corticosteroids and number of endoscopic sinus surgery (ESS) procedures. In a more recent study of post-ESS patients, significant improvement in PROMs, endoscopic scores with desensitization treatment was shown [30]. Based on these limited (level II) data, ASA desensitization may be helpful in the treatment of CRSwNP in AERD especially after ESS (table 3).

Antibiotics

This treatment has been thought to benefit patients through both antimicrobial and potentially intrinsic anti-inflammatory effects. In a RCT, Van Zele et al. [31] showed improvement in polyp size only and reduced levels of inflammatory markers after a 20-day course of doxycycline compared to placebo. However, another RCT evaluating long-term macrolide treatment in patients with CRS (52% with nasal polyps) failed to show improvement in PROMs, polyp size, nasal airflow or sense of smell [32]. There is additional data demonstrating potential benefit in PROMs and endoscopic scores in long-term (3 months) macrolide antibiotic treatment in patients with low IgE (<200 μg/l), but this study excluded patients with nasal polyps [33]. Overall, there is data to support the use of oral doxycycline in CRSwNP and potentially long-term oral macrolides in patients with low IgE levels.

Antimycotics

Targeting fungi with antifungal therapy holds the possibility of decreasing sinonasal inflammation based on the hypothesis that ubiquitous airborne fungi trigger the pathogenesis of CRSwNP [34]. Unfortunately, the literature shows mixed results, and risk of systemic side effects. For systemic therapy, a double-blind placebo controlled RCT evaluating the use of terbinafine in 53 patients over 6 weeks demonstrated no improvement in PROMs, CT scores [35]. In a subsequent retrospective case-series study of patients with allergic fungal sinusitis (AFS) treated with at least 3 months of itraconazole, Chan et al. [36] found that most patients demonstrated no change in endoscopic scores and little or no change in PROMs, in addition, 19% had elevated liver function tests requiring one patient to stop therapy. A recent RCT demonstrated that patients given itraconazole pre-operatively for 4 weeks prior to surgery experienced significant improvements in SNOT-20 with itraconazole therapy alone (31.28 ± 13.79 to 15.72 ± 9.34, $p = <0.001$). Unfortunately, at the 2-month postoperative time point, there were no clinically significant differences between the 2 groups. This study does keep the question open as to what role itraconazole plays 'maximizing' medical therapy prior to proceeding to ESS for AFS. Two of the 27 patients that received itraconazole essentially had complete resolution of symptomatic disease and cancelled surgery [37].

Topical treatment has also been investigated as a safer alternative given theoretically decreased systemic absorption [35, 38]. However, in a RCT of 60 patients with CRS, 8-weeks of topical amphotericin B treatment demonstrated worsening of PROMs (non-validated instruments) in the treatment group and no difference in endoscopy scores [39]. Use of both systemic and topical antimycotics is not supported by the literature and may be harmful to patients [2].

Immune Modulators

Inflammatory mediators IL-5 and IgE have been shown to be present at high levels in polyp homogenates, nasal secretions and blood serum in patients with nasal polyps [40]. Recently, antibodies-mediated therapies directed at these targets have been studied. A RCT by Gevaert et al. [41] showed that PROMs (non-validated instruments), polyp size and nasal airflow failed to improve with anti-IL-5 therapy compared to controls; however, patients with elevated nasal IL-5 levels (>40 pg/ml) were more likely to have reduction in polyp size. These findings have been confirmed in another small RCT with 24 patients that demonstrated improvement in PROMs, polyp size and radiographic (CT scores) [42]. Level II evidence does indicate benefit for the use of immune modulators for patients, but larger studies will be required to clarify their role in treatment of CRSwNP (table 3).

The outcomes for medical treatment in nasal polyps, including level of evidence and recommendations, is summarized in table 3.

Surgical Outcomes

When medical management fails to adequately control symptoms, surgical intervention should be considered in patients with CRSwNP [1]. The growth in the quality of data supporting surgical intervention for CRS has evolved dramatically over the past 20 years. Early studies from single-institutions found relatively high rates of improvement (73–98.4%) but lacked standardized and validated outcome measures [43, 44]. Use of validated outcome measures in multi-institutional cohorts demonstrated that patients do achieve an MCID after ESS approximately 75% of the time [45, 46]. Analysis of the data found that presence of polyps either made no difference [46] or were predictive of greater improvement in QOL [44]. When compared to patients electing continued medical therapy, patients electing surgery patients with CRS are more likely to achieve an MCID on the RSDI physical subscale (OR 3.36, 95% CI 1.15–9.87; $p = 0.027$) and CSS symptom subscale (OR 2.65, 95% CI 1.06–6.66; $p = 0.038$) [47]. In evaluation of medical versus surgical therapy in a North American cohort of patients with CRSwNP, surgical patients are more likely to improve cardinal symptoms [48].

It is important to note that a handful of RCT's have not found a difference between patients receiving medical or surgical management [49–52]. The fundamental shortcoming of these studies lies in the fact that patients had not failed preliminary medical therapy as is standard of care in the US. This data reaffirms that all patients should undergo a trial of failed medical therapy prior to surgical therapy.

Extent of Sinus Surgery

Although data support the use of surgery with continued medical therapy in medically recalcitrant CRSwNP, there remains room for improvement in this intervention. Long-term data reflects the potentially relentless nature of this disease with the mean time to revision surgery approximately 5 years [53]. Further analysis revealed that resection of the middle turbinates' prolonged the meantime to revision surgery by 6 months. The question remains as to what is the ideal surgical extent for patients undergoing ESS for CRSwNP.

The least invasive method of addressing mechanical obstruction is simple polypectomy and offers an in-office alternative to ESS for patients that cannot tolerate or would like to avoid general anesthesia. A recent analysis by Rudmik et al. [54] demonstrates cost-effectiveness of simple polypectomy in the office for a select group of patients with isolated symptoms of nasal obstruction. This method involves the removal of polyps alone, without disruption of the mucosa or bone from nearby ostia or sinuses. The concern with this procedure does not address the underlying source of inflammation, as demonstrated by a 75% recurrence rate on endoscopy in an 8-year follow-up study [55].

ESS in addition to polypectomy both removes the nasal polyposis and marsupializes the sinus cavity with the sinonasal cavity. Browne et al. [56] compared outcomes of patients undergoing polypectomy alone to polypectomy and additional surgery. Additional surgery was defined as surgery to at least one of following regions: middle meatus/uncinate process, anterior or posterior ethmoid, sphenoid or frontal sinuses. While the authors found that there were no significant improvements in PROMs, slight improvement in recurrence rates were observed in the additional surgery group. However, the limit of the additional surgery group was the ethmoid sinus in 85% of patients, suggesting that the true effects of more extensive surgery, including frontal or sphenoid surgery, may not have been captured by this study. A multi-institutional observational study demonstrated a trend of improvement in postoperative PROMs including olfactory measures in complete surgery (defined by bilateral maxillary antrostomies, bilateral total ethmoidectomies, bilateral sphenoidotomies and bilateral frontal sinusotomies (Draf IIa, IIb, or III)) as compared to a targeted approach in CRS [57].

The role of middle turbinate resection has also been investigated as a possible important surgical target in CRSwNP. In a 2006 study by Jankowski et al. [58], ESS with removal of the middle turbinate was compared to endoscopic ethmoidectomy and improvements in PROMs, CT score and polyp recurrence were noted in the group with more extensive surgery. Additional evidence for resection of the middle turbinate in addition to standard ESS has been demonstrated by a retrospective cohort study where patients with CRSwNP who underwent this procedure had a delay in time to revision surgery [53]. Concerns about the clinical detriment of middle turbinate resection can be assuaged by multicenter data showing no diminished QOL is associated with middle turbinate resection [59].

Finally, extended sinusotomies, particularly in the frontal sinus, may play an important role in long-term control of CRSwNP. The frontal recess is a common site of early failure in CRSwNP due to the inherent anatomic bottleneck created by the orbits, frontal beak and septum. In a retrospective review of 339 patients, Naidoo et al. [60] found that patients with nasal polyps were among the highest risk groups for endoscopic failure of standard frontal sinusotomy. Even after complete sphenoethmoidectomies, maxillary antrostomies and Draf 2a frontal sinusotomies, there is a 19.8% endoscopic recurrence rate of polyps at 6 months [61]. However, in the same retrospective review, the revision rate after ESS with Draf 2a was 37% compared to 7% for patients that underwent Draf 3s ($p < 0.001$) [61]. These data suggest that while ESS and current medical therapies may be inadequate at controlling mucosal inflammation in one-fifth of patients, extended sinusotomies, particularly the Draf III, may be an important adjunct in a subset of patients with CRSwNP.

Conclusion

Improvement in QOL is the primary end point that all clinicians seek to optimize in patients with CRSwNP. Balancing a variety of medical and surgical interventions with a patchwork quilt of evidence requires an educated clinician and an informed patient. Consensus statements emphasize patient education and PROMs as evidence for treatment success, accentuating the shift toward patient-centered results in research and clinical care [1, 2]. Specific attention to patient's disease within a greater context is especially important in CRSwNP, as it is a benign condition with a high rate of recurrence that can be detrimental to QOL.

Medical therapies remain the first-line therapy in CRSwNP, and surgery remains an important option for recalcitrant cases. Topical corticosteroids are a well-established initial treatment of choice, with systemic treatment as an important adjunct. In medically recalcitrant cases, surgery is the most effective way to improve QOL. Controversy remains as to what is the appropriate extent of surgery in terms of efficacy and cost effectiveness. In order to answer the question of the appropriate surgical extent, randomized study designs, with long-term follow-up (5-years) would preferably be undertaken. Unfortunately, definitive study designs can be cost prohibitive, leaving clinicians and patients gleaning ideal interventions through synthesis of diverse studies and data.

Conflict of Interest

Adam S. DeConde is a consultant for IntersectENT, Inc. (Menlo Park, Calif., USA) which is not affiliated with this work.

References

1 Fokkens WJ, Lund VJ, Mullol J, et al: EPOS 2012: European position paper on rhinosinusitis and nasal polyps 2012. A summary for otorhinolaryngologists. Rhinology 2012;50:1–12.
2 Rosenfeld RM, Piccirillo JF, Chandrasekhar SS, et al: Clinical practice guideline (update): adult sinusitis executive summary. Otolaryngol Head Neck Surg 2015;152:598–609.
3 Kimberlin CL, Winterstein AG: Validity and reliability of measurement instruments used in research. Am J Health Syst Pharm 2008;65:2276–2284.
4 Quintanilla-Dieck L, Litvack JR, Mace JC, Smith TL: Comparison of disease-specific quality-of-life instruments in the assessment of chronic rhinosinusitis. Int Forum Allergy Rhinol 2012;2:437–443.
5 Hopkins C, Gillett S, Slack R, Lund VJ, Browne JP: Psychometric validity of the 22-item sinonasal outcome test. Clin Otolaryngol 2009;34:447–454.
6 Rudmik L, Soler ZM, Mace JC, DeConde AS, Schlosser RJ, Smith TL: Using preoperative SNOT-22 score to inform patient decision for Endoscopic sinus surgery. Laryngoscope 2015;125:1517–1522.
7 Morley AD, Sharp HR: A review of sinonasal outcome scoring systems – which is best? Clin Otolaryngol 2006;31:103–109.
8 Jaeschke R, Singer J, Guyatt GH: Measurement of health status. Ascertaining the minimal clinically important difference. Control Clin Trials 1989;10:407–415.
9 DeConde AS, Bodner TE, Mace JC, Smith TL: Response shift in quality of life after endoscopic sinus surgery for chronic rhinosinusitis. JAMA Otolaryngol Head Neck Surg 2014;140:712–719.
10 DeConde AS, Mace JC, Bodner T, et al: SNOT-22 quality of life domains differentially predict treatment modality selection in chronic rhinosinusitis. Int Forum Allergy Rhinol 2014;4:972–979.
11 Remenschneider AK, D'Amico L, Gray ST, Holbrook EH, Gliklich RE, Metson R: The EQ-5D: a new tool for studying clinical outcomes in chronic rhinosinusitis. Laryngoscope 2015;125:7–15.
12 Lund VJ, Mackay IS: Staging in rhinosinusitus. Rhinology 1993;31:183–184.
13 Lund VJ, Kennedy DW: Staging for rhinosinusitis. Otolaryngol Head Neck Surg 1997;117(3 pt 2):S35–S40.
14 Doty RL, Shaman P, Kimmelman CP, Dann MS: University of Pennsylvania smell identification test: a rapid quantitative olfactory function test for the clinic. Laryngoscope 1984;94(2 pt 1):176–178.
15 Bachert C: Evidence-based management of nasal polyposis by intranasal corticosteroids: from the cause to the clinic. Int Arch Allergy Immunol 2011;155:309–321.
16 Kalish L, Snidvongs K, et al: Topical steroids for nasal polyps. Cochrane Database Syst Rev 2012;12:CD006549.
17 Badia L, Lund V: Topical corticosteroids in nasal polyposis. Drugs 2001;61:573–578.

18 Vaidyanathan S, Barnes M, Williamson P, Hopkinson P, Donnan PT, Lipworth B: Combined oral and intranasal corticosteroid therapy for nasal polyps. Ann Intern Med 2011;155:277–278.
19 Martinez-Devesa P, Patiar S (ed): Oral Steroids for Nasal Polyps. Chichester, John Wiley & Sons, Ltd., 1996.
20 Bonfils P, Halimi P, Malinvaud D: Adrenal suppression and osteoporosis after treatment of nasal polyposis. Acta Otolaryngol 2006;126:1195–1200.
21 Hissaria P, Smith W, Wormald PJ, et al: Short course of systemic corticosteroids in sinonasal polyposis: a double-blind, randomized, placebo-controlled trial with evaluation of outcome measures. J Allergy Clin Immunol 2006;118:128–133.
22 Schäper C, Noga O, Koch B, et al: Anti-inflammatory properties of montelukast, a leukotriene receptor antagonist in patients with asthma and nasal polyposis. J Investig Allergol Clin Immunol 2011;21:51–58.
23 Pauli C, Fintelmann R, Klemens C, et al: [Polyposis nasi – improvement in quality of life by the influence of leukotrien receptor antagonists]. Laryngorhinootologie 2007;86:282–286.
24 Vuralkan E, Saka C, Akin I, et al: Comparison of montelukast and mometasone furoate in the prevention of recurrent nasal polyps. Ther Adv Respir Dis 2012;6:5–10.
25 Mostafa BE, Abdel Hay H, Mohammed HE, Yamani M: Role of leukotriene inhibitors in the postoperative management of nasal polyps. ORL J Otorhinolaryngol Relat Spec 2005;67:148–153.
26 Stewart RA, Ram B, Hamilton G, Weiner J, Kane KJ: Montelukast as an adjunct to oral and inhaled steroid therapy in chronic nasal polyposis. Otolaryngol Head Neck Surg 2008;139:682–687.
27 Samter M, Beers RF Jr: Intolerance to aspirin. Clinical studies and consideration of its pathogenesis. Ann Intern Med 1968;68:975–983.
28 Amar YG, Frenkiel S, Sobol SE: Outcome analysis of endoscopic sinus surgery for chronic sinusitis in patients having Samter's triad. J Otolaryngol 2000;29:7–12.
29 Stevenson DD, Hankammer MA, Mathison DA, Christiansen SC, Simon RA: Aspirin desensitization treatment of aspirin-sensitive patients with rhinosinusitis-asthma: long-term outcomes. J Allergy Clin Immunol 1996;98:751–758.
30 Cho KS, Soudry E, Psaltis AJ, et al: Long-term sinonasal outcomes of aspirin desensitization in aspirin exacerbated respiratory disease. Otolaryngol Head Neck Surg 2014;151:575–581.
31 Van Zele T, Gevaert P, Holtappels G, et al: Oral steroids and doxycycline: two different approaches to treat nasal polyps. J Allergy Clin Immunol 2010;125:1069–1076.e4.
32 Videler WJ, BADIA L, Harvey RJ, et al: Lack of efficacy of long-term, low-dose azithromycin in chronic rhinosinusitis: a randomized controlled trial. Allergy 2011;66:1457–1468.
33 Wallwork B, Coman W, Mackay-Sim A, Greiff L, Cervin A: A double-blind, randomized, placebo-controlled trial of macrolide in the treatment of chronic rhinosinusitis. Laryngoscope 2006;116:189–193.
34 Ponikau JU, Sherris DA, Kephart GM, Adolphson C, Kita H: The role of ubiquitous airborne fungi in chronic rhinosinusitis. Curr Allergy Asthma Rep 2005;5:472–476.
35 Kennedy DW, Kuhn FA, Hamilos DL, et al: Treatment of chronic rhinosinusitis with high-dose oral terbinafine: a double blind, placebo-controlled study. Laryngoscope 2005;115:1793–1799.
36 Chan KO, Genoway KA, Javer AR: Effectiveness of itraconazole in the management of refractory allergic fungal rhinosinusitis. J Otolaryngol Head Neck Surg 2008;37:870–874.
37 Patro SK, Verma RK, Panda NK, Chakrabarti A, Singh P: Efficacy of preoperative itraconazole in allergic fungal rhinosinusitis. Am J Rhinol Allergy 2015;29:299–304.
38 Rupa V, Jacob M, Mathews MS, Seshadri MS: A prospective, randomised, placebo-controlled trial of postoperative oral steroid in allergic fungal sinusitis. Eur Arch Otorhinolaryngol 2010;267:233–238.
39 Weschta M, Rimek D, Formanek M, Polzehl D, Podbielski A, Riechelmann H: Topical antifungal treatment of chronic rhinosinusitis with nasal polyps: a randomized, double-blind clinical trial. J Allergy Clin Immunol 2004;113:1122–1128.
40 Alobid I, Mullol J: Role of medical therapy in the management of nasal polyps. Curr Allergy Asthma Rep 2012;12:144–153.
41 Gevaert P, Lang-Loidolt D, Lackner A, et al: Nasal IL-5 levels determine the response to anti-IL-5 treatment in patients with nasal polyps. J Allergy Clin Immunol 2006;118:1133–1141.
42 Gevaert P, Van Bruaene N, Cattaert T, et al: Mepolizumab, a humanized anti-IL-5 mAb, as a treatment option for severe nasal polyposis. J Allergy Clin Immunol 2011;128:989–995.e1–e8.
43 Kennedy DW, Senior BA: Endoscopic sinus surgery. A review. Otolaryngol Clin North Am 1997;30:313–330.
44 Terris MH, Davidson TM: Review of published results for endoscopic sinus surgery. Ear Nose Throat J 1994;73:574–580.
45 Smith TL, Mendolia-Loffredo S, Loehrl TA, Sparapani R, Laud PW, Nattinger AB: Predictive factors and outcomes in endoscopic sinus surgery for chronic rhinosinusitis. Laryngoscope 2005;115:2199–2205.
46 Smith TL, Litvack JR, Hwang PH, et al: Determinants of outcomes of sinus surgery: a multi-institutional prospective cohort study. Otolaryngol Head Neck Surg 2010;142:55–63.
47 Smith TL, Kern RC, Palmer JN, et al: Medical therapy vs surgery for chronic rhinosinusitis: a prospective, multi-institutional study. Int Forum Allergy Rhinol 2011;1:235–241.
48 DeConde AS, Mace JC, Alt JA, Soler ZM, Orlandi RR, Smith TL: Investigation of change in cardinal symptoms of chronic rhinosinusitis after surgical or ongoing medical management. Int Forum Allergy Rhinol 2015;5:36–45.
49 Alobid I, Benitez P, Bernal-Sprekelsen M, et al: Nasal polyposis and its impact on quality of life: comparison between the effects of medical and surgical treatments. Allergy 2005;60:452–458.
50 Lildholdt T, Fogstrup J, Gammelgaard N, Kortholm B, Ulsoe C: Surgical versus medical treatment of nasal polyps. Acta Otolaryngol 1988;105:140–143.
51 Lildholdt T, Rundcrantz H, Bende M, Larsen K: Glucocorticoid treatment for nasal polyps. The use of topical budesonide powder, intramuscular betamethasone, and surgical treatment. Arch Otolaryngol Head Neck Surg 1997;123:595–600.
52 Ragab SM, Lund VJ, Scadding G: Evaluation of the medical and surgical treatment of chronic rhinosinusitis: a prospective, randomised, controlled trial. Laryngoscope 2004;114:923–930.

53 Wu AW, Ting JY, Platt MP, Tierney HT, Metson R: Factors affecting time to revision sinus surgery for nasal polyps: a 25-year experience. Laryngoscope 2014; 124:29–33.
54 Rudmik L, Smith KA, Kilty S: Endoscopic polypectomy in the clinic: a pilot cost-effectiveness analysis. Clin Otolaryngol 2015;41:110–117.
55 Larsen K, Tos M: A long-term follow-up study of nasal polyp patients after simple polypectomies. Eur Arch Otorhinolaryngol 1997;254(suppl 1):S85–S88.
56 Browne JP, Hopkins C, Slack R, et al: Health-related quality of life after polypectomy with and without additional surgery. Laryngoscope 2006;116:297–302.
57 DeConde AS, Suh JD, Mace JC, Alt JA, Smith TL: Outcomes of complete vs targeted approaches to endoscopic sinus surgery. Int Forum Allergy Rhinol 2015; 5:691–700.
58 Jankowski R, Pigret D, Decroocq F, Blum A, Gillet P: Comparison of radical (nasalisation) and functional ethmoidectomy in patients with severe sinonasal polyposis. A retrospective study. Rev Laryngol Otol Rhinol (Bord) 2006;127: 131–140.
59 Soler ZM, Hwang PH, Mace J, Smith TL: Outcomes after middle turbinate resection: revisiting a controversial topic. Laryngoscope 2010;120:832–837.
60 Naidoo Y, Bassiouni A, Keen M, Wormald PJ: Risk factors and outcomes for primary, revision, and modified Lothrop (Draf III) frontal sinus surgery. Int Forum Allergy Rhinol 2013;3:412–417.
61 Bassiouni A, Wormald PJ: Role of frontal sinus surgery in nasal polyp recurrence. Laryngoscope 2013;123:36–41.

Adam S. DeConde, MD
Department of Surgery/Division of Otolaryngology, Head and Neck Surgery
University of California, 200 W. Arbor Drive, #8895
San Diego, CA 92103 (USA)
E-Mail adeconde@ucsd.edu

Author Index

Subject Index